Hot Topics in Lung Infections

Editors

RACHAEL A. LEE
HELEN W. BOUCHER

INFECTIOUS DISEASE CLINICS OF NORTH AMERICA

www.id.theclinics.com

Consulting Editor
HELEN W. BOUCHER

March 2024 • Volume 38 • Number 1

ELSEVIER

1600 John F. Kennedy Boulevard • Suite 1800 • Philadelphia, Pennsylvania, 19103-2899.
http://www.theclinics.com

INFECTIOUS DISEASE CLINICS OF NORTH AMERICA Volume 38, Number 1
March 2024 ISSN 0891–5520, ISBN-13: 978-0-443-29380-1

Editor: Kerry Holland
Developmental Editor: Varun Gopal

Infectious Disease Clinics of North America (ISSN 0891–5520) is published in March, June, September, and December by Elsevier Inc., 360 Park Avenue South, New York, NY 10010-1710. Periodicals postage paid at New York, NY and additional mailing offices. Subscription prices are $379.00 per year for US individuals, $100.00 per year for US students, $432.00 per year for Canadian individuals, $472.00 per year for international individuals, $100.00 per year for Canadian students, and $200.00 per year for international students. For institutional access pricing please contact Customer Service via the contact information below. To receive student rate, orders must be accompanied by name of affiliated institution, date of term, and the *signature* of program/residency coordinator on institution letterhead. Orders will be billed at individual rate until proof of status is received. Foreign air speed delivery is included in all *Clinics* subscription prices. All prices are subject to change without notice. **POSTMASTER**: Send address changes to *Infectious Disease Clinics of North America,* Elsevier Health Sciences Division, Subcription Customer Service, 3251 Riverport Lane, Maryland Heights, MO 63043. **Customer Service: 1-800-654-2452 (US). From outside the US and Canada, call 1-314-447-8871. Fax: 1-314-447-8029. E-mail: JournalsCustomerService-usa@ elsevier.com (print support) or JournalsOnlineSupport-usa@elsevier.com (online support).**

Infectious Disease Clinics of North America is also published in Spanish by Editorial Inter-Médica, Junin 917, 1er A 1113, Buenos Aires, Argentina.

Reprints. For copies of 100 or more, of articles in this publication, please contact the Commercial Reprints Department, Elsevier Inc., 360 Park Avenue South, New York, New York 10010-1710. Tel. 212-633-3874, Fax: 212-633-3820, E-mail: reprints@elsevier.com.

Infectious Disease Clinics of North America is covered in *MEDLINE/PubMed (Index Medicus), Current Contents/ Clinical Medicine, Science Citation Alert, SCISEARCH,* and *Research Alert.*

Contributors

CONSULTING EDITOR

HELEN W. BOUCHER, MD, FACP, FIDSA
Dean and Professor of Medicine, Tufts University School of Medicine, Chief Academic
Officer, Tufts Medicine, Boston, Massachusetts, USA

EDITORS

RACHAEL A. LEE, MD, MSPH, FIDSA
Chief Healthcare Epidemiologist, Associate Professor, Department of Medicine, Division
of Infectious Diseases, University of Alabama at Birmingham, Birmingham, Alabama

HELEN W. BOUCHER, MD, FACP, FIDSA
Dean and Professor of Medicine, Tufts University School of Medicine, Chief Academic
Officer, Tufts Medicine, Boston, Massachusetts, USA

AUTHORS

MOHAMMED ALSAEED, MD
Clinical Fellow, Division of Infectious Diseases, Multi-Organ Transplant Program,
Department of Medicine, University of Toronto, University Health Network, Toronto,
Ontario, Canada; Senior Registrar, Division of Infectious Diseases, Department of
Medicine, Prince Sultan Military Medical City, Riyadh, Saudi Arabia

ROBERT A. BALK, MD
Professor of Medicine, Division of Pulmonary, Critical Care, and Sleep Medicine, Rush
University Medical Center, Rush Medical College, Chicago, Illinois, USA

CHRISTOPHER D. BERTINI, Jr, MD
Department of Internal Medicine, UTHealth Houston McGovern Medical School, Houston,
Texas, USA

RODRIGO CAVALLAZZI, MD
Division of Pulmonary, Critical Care, and Sleep Disorders, University of Louisville,
Louisville, Kentucky, USA

JARED D. CHRISTENSEN, MD, MBA
Associate Professor, Department of Radiology, Duke University Medical Center, Durham,
North Carolina, USA

JENNIFER FEBBO, MD
Assistant Professor, University of New Mexico, Albuquerque, New Mexico, USA

CRISTINA VAZQUEZ GUILLAMET, MD
Associate Professor, Division of Infectious Diseases, Washington University School of
Medicine, St. Louis, Missouri, USA

SHAHID HUSAIN, MD, MS, FECMM, FRCP
Professor of Medicine, Staff Physician, Director of Transplant Infectious Disease, Division of Infectious Diseases, Multi-Organ Transplant Program, University Health Network, University of Toronto, Toronto, Ontario, Canada

LAUREN A. IGNERI, PharmD, BCPS, BCCCP
Clinical Pharmacy Specialist, Critical Care, Department of Pharmacy, Cooper University Healthcare, Camden, New Jersey

ANDRE C. KALIL, MD, MPH
Professor of Medicine, Department of Internal Medicine, Division of Infectious Diseases, University of Nebraska Medical Center, Omaha, Nebraska, USA

LOREN KETAI, MD
Professor Emeritus, Department of Radiology, University of New Mexico, Albuquerque, New Mexico, USA

FAREED KHAWAJA, MD
Department of Infectious Diseases, Infection Control, and Employee Health, Assistant Professor, The University of Texas MD Anderson Cancer Center, Houston, Texas, USA

JONATHAN L. KOFF, MD
Director, Adult Cystic Fibrosis Program, Yale University Center for Phage Biology and Therapy, Associate Professor, Department of Internal Medicine, Section of Pulmonary, Critical Care and Sleep Medicine, Yale School of Medicine, New Haven, Connecticut, USA

MARIN H. KOLLEF, MD
Professor, Division of Pulmonary and Critical Care Medicine, Washington University School of Medicine, St. Louis, MO, USA

GABRIELA MAGDA, MD
Assistant Professor of Medicine, Columbia University Lung Transplant Program, Division of Pulmonary, Allergy, and Critical Care Medicine, Columbia University Irving Medical Center, Columbia University Vagelos College of Physicians and Surgeons, New York, New York, USA

MARK L. METERSKY, MD
Professor of Medicine, Division of Pulmonary, Critical Care and Sleep Medicine, University of Connecticut School of Medicine, UConn Health, Farmington, Connecticut, USA

BRYAN O'SULLIVAN-MURPHY, MD, PhD
Medical Instructor, Department of Radiology, Duke University Medical Center, Durham, North Carolina, USA

THOMAS S. MURRAY, MD, PhD
Associate Professor, Department of Pediatrics, Section of Infectious Diseases and Global Health, Yale School of Medicine, New Haven, Connecticut, USA

H. PAGE MCADAMS, MD
Professor, Department of Radiology, Duke University Medical Center, Durham, North Carolina, USA

CHIAGOZIE I. PICKENS, MD
Department of Medicine, Pulmonary and Critical Care Division, Northwestern University Feinberg School of Medicine, Chicago, Illinois, USA

RACHEL RAFEQ, PharmD
PGY2 Residency Program Director, Clinical Pharmacy Specialist, Emergency Medicine, Department of Pharmacy, Cooper University Healthcare, Camden, New Jersey

JULIO A. RAMIREZ, MD
Norton Infectious Diseases Institute, Norton Healthcare, Louisville, Kentucky, USA

JONATHAN REVELS, DO
Assistant Professor, University of New Mexico, Albuquerque, New Mexico, USA

AJAY SHESHADRI, MD, MS
Department of Pulmonary Medicine, Associate Professor, The University of Texas MD Anderson Cancer Center, Houston, Texas, USA

GAIL STANLEY, MD
Clinical Fellow, Department of Internal Medicine, Section of Pulmonary, Critical Care and Sleep Medicine, Yale School of Medicine, Adult Cystic Fibrosis Program, Yale University Center for Phage Biology and Therapy, New Haven, Connecticut, USA

SARAH SUNGURLU, DO
Assistant Professor of Medicine, Division of Pulmonary, Critical Care, and Sleep Medicine, Rush University Medical Center, Rush Medical College, Chicago, Illinois, USA

LACEY WASHINGTON, MD
Associate Professor, Department of Radiology, Duke University Medical Center, Durham, North Carolina, USA

RICHARD G. WUNDERINK, MD
Department of Medicine, Pulmonary and Critical Care Division, Northwestern University Feinberg School of Medicine, Chicago, Illinois, USA

Contents

> Pneumonia is a lower respiratory tract infection caused by the inability to
> clear pathogens from the lower airway and alveoli. Cytokines and local in-
> flammatory markers are released, causing further damage to the lungs
> through the accumulation of white blood cells and fluid congestion, leading
> to pus in the parenchyma. The Infectious Diseases Society of America de-
> fines pneumonia as the presence of new lung infiltrate with other clinical
> evidence supporting infection, including new fever, purulent sputum, leu-
> kocytosis, and decline in oxygenation. Importantly, lower respiratory infec-
> tions remain the most deadly communicable disease. Pneumonia is
> subdivided into three categories: (1) community acquired, (2) hospital ac-
> quired, and (3) ventilator associated. Therapy for each differs based on the
> severity of the disease and the presence of risk factors for methicillin-re-
> sistant *Staphylococcus aureus* or *Pseudomonas aeruginosa*.

> The chest radiograph is the most common imaging examination performed
> in most radiology departments, and one of the more common indications
> for these studies is suspected infection. Radiologists must therefore be
> aware of less common radiographic patterns of pulmonary infection if
> they are to add value in the interpretation of chest radiographs for this in-
> dication. This review uses a case-based format to illustrate a range of
> imaging findings that can be associated with acute pulmonary infection
> and highlight findings that should prompt investigation for diseases other
> than community-acquired pneumonia to prevent misdiagnosis and delays
> in appropriate management.

> Biomarkers are used in the diagnosis, severity determination, and progno-
> sis for patients with community-acquired pneumonia (CAP). Selected bio-
> markers may indicate a bacterial infection and need for antibiotic therapy
> (C-reactive protein, procalcitonin, soluble triggering receptor expressed
> on myeloid cells). Biomarkers can differentiate CAP patients who require
> hospital admission and severe CAP requiring intensive care unit admis-
> sion. Biomarker-guided antibiotic therapy may limit antibiotic exposure
> without compromising outcome and thus improve antibiotic stewardship.

The authors discuss the role of biomarkers in diagnosing, determining severity, defining the prognosis, and limiting antibiotic exposure in CAP and ventilator-associated pneumonia patients.

There are several novel platforms that enhance detection of pathogens that cause common infections in the intensive care unit. These platforms have a sample to answer time of a few hours, are often higher yield than culture, and have the potential to improve antibiotic stewardship.

Ventilator-associated pneumonia (VAP) remains a significant clinical entity with reported incidence rates of 7% to 15%. Given the considerable adverse consequences associated with this infection, VAP prevention became a core measure required in most US hospitals. Many institutions took pride in implementing effective VAP prevention bundles that combined at least head of bed elevation, hand hygiene, chlorhexidine oral care, and subglottic drainage. Spontaneous breathing and awakening trials have also consistently been shown to shorten the duration of mechanical ventilation and secondarily reduce the occurrence of VAP.

Two recent major guidelines on diagnosis and treatment of ventilator-associated pneumonia (VAP) recommend consideration of local antibiotic resistance patterns and individual patient risks for resistant pathogens when formulating an initial empiric antibiotic regimen. One recommends against invasive diagnostic techniques with quantitative cultures to determine the cause of VAP; the other recommends either invasive or noninvasive techniques. Both guidelines recommend short-course therapy be used for most patients with VAP. Although neither guideline recommends use of procalcitonin as an adjunct to clinical judgment when diagnosing VAP, they differ with respect to use of serial procalcitonin to shorten the length of antibiotic treatment.

Infections in heart and lung transplant recipients are complex and heterogeneous. This article reviews the epidemiology, risk factors, specific clinical syndromes, and most frequent opportunistic infections in heart and/or lung transplant recipients that will be encountered in the intensive care unit and will provide a practical approach of empirical management.

Opportunistic infections are a leading cause of lung transplant recipient morbidity and mortality. Risk factors for infection include continuous exposure of the lung allograft to the external environment, high levels of immunosuppression, impaired mucociliary clearance and decreased cough reflex, and impact of the native lung microbiome in single lung transplant recipients. Infection risk is mitigated through careful pretransplant screening of recipients and donors, implementation of antimicrobial prophylaxis strategies, and routine surveillance posttransplant. This review describes common viral, fungal, and mycobacterial infectious after lung transplant and provides recommendations on prevention and treatment.

Patients with cystic fibrosis (CF) often develop respiratory tract infections with pathogenic multidrug-resistant organisms (MDROs) such as methicillin-resistant *Staphylococcus aureus*, and a variety of gram-negative organisms that include *Pseudomonas aeruginosa*, *Burkholderia sp.*, *Stenotrophomonas maltophilia*, *Achromobacter xylosoxidans*, and nontuberculous mycobacteria (NTM). Despite the introduction of new therapies to address underlying cystic fibrosis transmembrane conductance regulator (CFTR) dysfunction, MDRO infections remain a problem and novel antimicrobial interventions are still needed. Therapeutic approaches include improving the efficacy of existing drugs by adjusting the dose based on differences in CF patient pharmacokinetics/pharmacodynamics, the development of inhaled formulations to reduce systemic adverse events, and the use of newer beta-lactam/beta-lactamase combinations. Alternative innovative therapeutic approaches include the use of gallium and bacteriophages to treat MDRO pulmonary infections including those with extreme antibiotic resistance. However, additional clinical trials are required to determine the optimal dosing and efficacy of these different strategies and to identify patients with CF most likely to benefit from these new treatment options.

Viral pneumonia is usually community acquired and caused by influenza, parainfluenza, respiratory syncytial virus, human metapneumovirus, and adenovirus. Many of these infections are airway centric and chest imaging demonstrates bronchiolitis and bronchopneumonia, With the exception of adenovirus infections, the presence of lobar consolidation usually suggests bacterial coinfection. Community-acquired viral pathogens can cause more severe pneumonia in immunocompromised hosts, who are also susceptible to CMV and varicella infection. These latter 2 pathogens are less likely to manifest the striking airway-centric pattern. Airway-centric pattern is distinctly uncommon in Hantavirus pulmonary syndrome, a rare environmentally acquired infection with high mortality.

INFECTIOUS DISEASE CLINICS
OF NORTH AMERICA

Preface

Respiratory Tract Infections in the Postpandemic Era: A Return to Basics and Call to Action

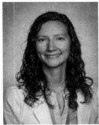

Rachael A. Lee, MD, MSPH, FIDSA   Helen W. Boucher, MD, FACP, FIDSA, Hon. FRCPI
Editors

Respiratory tract infections are a leading cause of death and disability and have remained the world's most deadly communicable disease. Although the burden of respiratory infections decreased over the period of 1990-2019, the world encountered unprecedented challenges due to the COVID-19 pandemic, caused by the SARS-CoV-2 virus. Compared with prepandemic years, the United States experienced higher than usual hospitalizations, numerous shortages in supplies as well as personnel shortages, all of which resulted in increases in patient safety metrics, such as ventilator-associated pneumonia (VAP). Furthermore, advances in medicine, complex patient populations, and antimicrobial resistance have highlighted the continued need in understanding the pathogenesis of lung infections in the twenty-first century.

The guidelines set forth by collaborating societies for the care of respiratory infections have served as an important source of information for the appropriate diagnosis and treatment of pneumonia for the general population. Many respiratory infection guidelines reference traditional diagnosis, such as bacterial culture, antigen detection, and immunologic assays. With the introduction of novel rapid diagnostic tests, guidance is needed for appropriate use in the right patient population; however, traditional guidelines typically require years to update. As we have seen during the COVID-19 pandemic, there remains a need for quick summation of studies to provide high-value care in the face of emerging pathogens.

Infect Dis Clin N Am 38 (2024) xiii–xv
https://doi.org/10.1016/j.idc.2023.11.002
0891-5520/24/© 2023 Published by Elsevier Inc.

In this issue of *Infectious Diseases Clinics of North America*, our expert authors focus on common respiratory infections encountered in the adult inpatient setting. Drs Rafeq and Igneri first discuss broad causes of infectious pulmonary diseases that lead to the diagnosis of community-acquired, hospital-acquired, and VAP, followed by a case-based radiologic review of pneumonia by Dr Washington and colleagues. Drs Sungurlu and Balk describe the importance of biomarkers in the management of patients with pneumonia, assisting clinicians with appropriate diagnosis and therapy duration. Drs Pickens and Wunderink further discuss novel detection methods for identification of the causes of infection in the intensive care unit, highlighting the negative predictive value of many rapid diagnostic tests. Drs Vazquez Guillamet and Kollef illustrate the complexity of VAP diagnosis and outline core practices for VAP prevention, and Drs Metersky and Kalil summarize the most recent VAP guidelines for treatment choice and duration.

Included in this issue is an exploration of host-related factors that may lead to lung infections. Given recent evidence that has identified one out of every ten solid organ transplant recipients may develop bacteremia during the first year following transplant, Drs Alsaeed and Husain describe the epidemiology of heart and lung transplant infections during specific time periods following transplantation, and Dr Magda focuses on opportunistic infections commonly seen in this patient population. Dr Murray and colleagues discuss novel approaches to combat multidrug-resistant bacterial infections in cystic fibrosis, including a discussion of targeting both host immune response and the pathogen with novel drugs with antimicrobial activity.

Along with seasonal influenza virus and respiratory syncytial virus, COVID-19 has become part of the respiratory virus season, and viral infections have accounted for upward of 24% among patients hospitalized with community-acquired pneumonia. Dr Febbo and colleagues review the imaging of community-acquired and hospital-acquired viral pneumonia in both the immunocompetent and the immunocompromised host. Dr Cavallazzi outlines the microbiology, diagnosis, and treatment of influenza and compares other common respiratory viruses, an important topic as we enter the viral respiratory season that is predicted to have higher total hospitalizations than what we experienced prior to the COVID-19 pandemic. Finally, Dr Bertini and colleagues provide an in-depth review of COVID-19 in the immunocompromised host.

We believe that this issue of *Infectious Diseases Clinics of North America* will provide readers with a summary of our knowledge in the diagnosis and management of respiratory infections following the COVID-19 pandemic. As we will continue to see emerging pathogens in a variety of patient populations, we need now more than ever the ability to quickly synthesize data to optimize the use of novel tests, appropriate diagnosis, and use of the right antimicrobial for the right duration to improve care.

DISCLOSURES

No relevant conflicts of interest to disclose.

Rachael A. Lee, MD, MSPH, FIDSA
Department of Medicine
Division of Infectious Diseases
University of Alabama at Birmingham
1900 University Boulevard
THT 229
Birmingham, AL 35294, USA

Helen W. Boucher, MD, FACP, FIDSA, Hon. FRCPI
Department of Medicine
Tufts University School of Medicine
Division of Geographic Medicine and
Infectious Diseases
Tufts Medicine
South Building, 6th Floor
800 Washington Street
Box 238
Boston, MA 02111, USA

E-mail addresses:
ralee@uabmc.edu (R.A. Lee)
Helen.Boucher@tuftsmedicine.org (H.W. Boucher)

Infectious Pulmonary Diseases

Rachel Rafeq, PharmD[a],*, Lauren A. Igneri, PharmD, BCPS, BCCCP[b,1]

KEYWORDS

- Community-acquired pneumonia • Hospital-acquired pneumonia
- Ventilator-associated pneumonia • Antimicrobial stewardship • Allergies
- Cross-sensitivity • Procalcitonin • MRSA nasal screening

KEY POINTS

- Community-acquired pneumonia is most commonly caused by *Streptococcus pneumoniae* and requires various antimicrobial therapy depending on patient disposition and severity of disease.
- Patients with hospital-acquired and ventilator-associated pneumonia are at risk for multidrug-resistant pathogens, especially following exposure to intravenous antibiotics within the last 90 days.
- Immunocompromised populations may require broader spectrum antimicrobial therapy to accommodate additional organisms not typically seen in non-immunocompromised populations.
- Although guidelines serve as an important source for appropriate treatment of pneumonia, a shift in emphasizing individualized approaches to antibiotic therapy is needed to improve patient outcomes.

INTRODUCTION

Pneumonia is a lower respiratory tract infection caused by the inability to clear pathogens from the lower airway and alveoli. Cytokines and local inflammatory markers are released, causing further damage to the lungs through an inflammatory cascade leading to an accumulation of white blood cells and fluid congestion, leading to pus in the parenchyma. The Infectious Diseases Society of America (IDSA) defines pneumonia as the presence of new lung infiltrate with other clinical evidence supporting infection,

This article was previously published in *Emergency Medicine Clinics* 40:3 August 2022.

No commercial or financial conflicts of interest or any funding sources to disclose.

Statement of authorship – both authors contributed equally to this article.

[a] Emergency Medicine, Department of Pharmacy, Cooper University Healthcare, 1 Cooper Plaza, Camden, NJ 08103, USA; [b] Critical Care, Department of Pharmacy, Cooper University Healthcare, 1 Cooper Plaza, Camden, NJ 08103, USA

[1] Author contributed equally to the publication of this article

* Corresponding author.

E-mail address: rafeq-rachel@cooperhealth.edu

including new fever, purulent sputum, leukocytosis, and decline in oxygenation. Importantly, lower respiratory infections remain the deadliest communicable disease. Ranking as the fourth leading cause of death worldwide, 2.6 million lives were claimed from pneumonia in 2019.

COMMUNITY-ACQUIRED PNEUMONIA

Community-acquired pneumonia (CAP) is a leading cause of hospitalization and death in the United States with more than 1.5 million Americans hospitalized annually.[1] It accounts for 4.5 million outpatient and emergency department visits annually. Up to 30% of mortality among intensive care unit (ICU) patients are related to pneumonia, with *S pneumoniae* remaining the most common bacterial pathogen implicated in CAP despite vaccine availability.[2] The understanding of microbiologic studies and inflammatory markers, such as procalcitonin (PCT), can be used to guide management. The American Thoracic Society (ATS) and the IDSA provide antibiotic recommendations, which will vary depending on whether outpatient or inpatient management is required.

Etiology

Several bacterial pathogens and some viral and fungal pathogens are implicated in the cause of CAP including:[3]

Bacterial Pathogen	Characteristics
Streptococcus pneumonia	• Aerobic, gram-positive diplococcus. • The most common cause of CAP; however, the incidence has decreased over the years with the widespread use of pneumococcal vaccine.
Haemophilus influenza	• Aerobic gram-negative coccobacillus. • Spread person to person via airborne droplets or through direct contact with respiratory secretions of an infected or colonized individual.
Legionella pneumophila	• Atypical pathogen • Gram-negative bacilli, classified as an atypical pneumonia. • Implicated in <4% of all CAP cases.
Mycoplasma pneumonia	• Atypical pathogen • Unlike other bacteria, it does not contain a cell wall rendering beta-lactam antimicrobial ineffective. • Unable to be gram stained due to the lack of cell wall.
Chlamydia pneumonia	• Atypical pathogen • Obligate intracellular gram-negative bacteria.
Moraxella catarrhalis	• Gram-negative diplococcus that commonly produces beta-lactamase, rendering it mostly resistant to amoxicillin. • Most frequently found as part of normal flora in infants and children but decreases in adults.
Pseudomonas aeruginosa	• Implicated in up to 8.3% of severe CAP requiring ICU admissions. • Pseudomonal infection is associated with poorer clinical outcomes and multidrug resistance.

• Viruses
  ◦ CAP pathogens include coronaviruses (in 2020, primarily SARS-CoV-2), influenza A, RSV, parainfluenzea, adenovirus, human metapneumovirus, and rhinovirus.
  ◦ The Center for Disease report of 2300 adults hospitalized with CAP showed the most common identified pathogens were rhinovirus (9%), influenza (6%), and *S pneumoniae* (5%). No pathogens were identified in 62% of cases.

- Pathogens to be considered in special circumstances (eg, immunocompromised)
  - *Mycobacterium tuberculosis*
  - *Nocardia* spp.
  - *Pneumocystis jirovecii*
  - *Aspergillus spp.*
  - *Mucorales spp.*
  - *Varicella-zoster virus*
  - *Cytomegalovirus*
  - Group A *Streptococcus*
  - *Neisseria meningitidis*
  - Anaerobes (aspiration pneumonia)

Prognosis Assessment Tools

Clinical comorbidities and social habits (eg, smoking) may worsen or increase the risk of CAP. The pneumonia severity index (PSI) and CURB-65 are assessment tools used to predict 30-day mortality in immunocompetent patients (**Tables 1** and **2**).[4] PSI is recommended over CURB-65 because it has a higher discriminative power in predicting mortality .[5]

Diagnostic Strategies

Microbiologic studies are integral to guiding antimicrobial treatment and vary depending on whether outpatient or inpatient management is required. In the outpatient setting, pretreatment sputum gram stain, the culture of the lower respiratory secretions, and blood cultures are not recommended.[5] However, these studies are crucial in hospital patients, particularly in patients being managed for severe CAP or the patients who are empirically treated for methicillin-resistant *Staphylococcus aureus* (MRSA) or *Pseudomonas aeruginosa*. In addition, these tests should be performed for all patients previously infected with MRSA or *Pseudomonas* spp., or who were hospitalized and received intravenous antibiotics in the last 90 days. In patients with severe CAP, urine *Legionella* and pneumococcal antigen testing are recommended.[5]

The 2019 CAP guidelines address the use of PCT and corticosteroids, which differs from the prior 2007 guideline. PCT, regardless of level, is not recommended to determine the need for empiric antibiotic initiation. Instead, clinical criteria and radiographically confirmed infiltrate should guide the administration of antimicrobials. Although corticosteroids also are not recommended for routine use, they may be considered in patients with septic shock (**Table 3**).[5]

Therapeutic Options

Antimicrobial treatment is initiated on an empiric basis and in hospitalized patients may be streamlined once the causative organism is identified (**Tables 4** and **5**).

The etiology of disease is important for several reasons. As empiric therapy tends to be broad to cover a wide range of possible pathogens, the culture results will allow providers to narrow therapy and determine resistance if applicable.

Risk factors for MRSA or *P aeruginosa:*[5]

- Prior respiratory isolation of MRSA or *P aeruginosa*
- Recent hospitalization plus receipt of parenteral antibiotics in the last 90 days

Table 1
Pneumonia severity index

Patient Characteristics	Points Assigned
Demographic Factors	
Age	1 point per year
Men	Age (y)
Women	Age (y) − 10
Nursing home resident	+ 10
Comorbid Illnesses	
Neoplastic disease	+30
Liver disease	+20
Congestive heart disease	+10
Cerebrovascular disease	+10
Renal disease	+10
Physical examination findings	
Altered mental status	+ 20
Respiratory rate $\geq$ 30 breaths/min	+ 20
Systolic blood pressure <90 mmHg	+ 20
Temperature <30° or $\geq$40° C	+ 15
Pulse $\geq$125 beats/min	+ 10
Laboratory findings	
PH <7.35	+30
blood urea nitrogen >10.7 mmol/L	+20
Sodium <130 meq/L	+20
Glucose >13.9 mmol/L	+10
Hematocrit <30%	+10
PO_2 < 60 mmHg (or SaO_2<90%)	+10
Pleural effusion	+10

Risk Class	Points Total	Mortality Rate	Patient Care Location
I	<51	0.1%	Outpatient
II	51–70	0.6%	Outpatient
III	71–90	2.8%	Observation unit with reevaluation if possible
IV	91–130	8.2%	Inpatient
V	>130	29.2%	Inpatient, likely ICU

Aspiration Pneumonia

In the new 2019 guidelines, the IDSA/ATS suggest not routinely adding anaerobic coverage for suspected aspiration pneumonia unless there is suspicion of or known lung empyema or abscess. Many patients with aspiration pneumonia are found to have self-limiting symptoms that resolve in 24 to 48 hours and only require supportive care without the need for antibiotics. Avoidance of unnecessary antimicrobial therapy has become paramount in light of the growing body of evidence for increased

Table 2 CURB-65 criteria	
Characteristics	**Points Total**
Confusion	1
Increased blood urea nitrogen >20 mg/dL	1
Respiratory rate ≥30 breaths/min	1
Blood pressure (systolic BP <90 mmHg or diastolic ≤60 mmHg)	1
Age >65 y	1

Total Score	Recommendation
0–1	Low risk; outpatient treatment
2	Moderately severe; short inpatient hospitalization or closely supervised outpatient treatment
3–5	Severe pneumonia; hospitalization required; consider intensive care unit admission

Clostridioides difficile infection and multidrug-resistant (MDR) pathogens associated with broad-spectrum antimicrobials (eg, cefepime, ceftriaxone, carbapenems, fluoro-quinolones, clindamycin, and so forth).[5]

Antimicrobial Dosing

Although the CAP guidelines provide clear dosing recommendations for some treatment options, dosing ranges are provided for severe infection treatment options to allow clinicians selection of an optimal dose based on patient-specific characteristics. A systematic review and meta-analysis by Telles *and colleagues* evaluated the efficacy of ceftriaxone 1 g versus 2 g daily for the treatment of CAP based on data pooled from 24 randomized controlled trials. Of note, trials including critically ill patients were excluded: 12 studies evaluated ceftriaxone 1 g and 12 studies evaluated ceftriaxone 2 g. Comparator regimens show similar efficacy ceftriaxone 1 g daily dosing [OR

Table 3 Severe community-acquired pneumonia criteria[5]	
Severe CAP Is Defined as Having Three or More Minor Criteria OR One Major Criteria	
Minor criteria	• Confusion/disorientation • Hypotension requiring aggressive fluid resuscitation • Hypothermia (core temperature <36°C) • Leukopenia from infection along (ie, not related to chemotherapy) defined as white blood cell count <4000 cells/µL • Multilobar infiltrates • PaO_2/FiO_2 ratio ≤250 • Respiratory rate ≥30 breaths/min • Uremia (blood urea nitrogen level ≥20 mg/dL)
Major criteria	• Respiratory failure requiring mechanical ventilation • Septic shock with the need for vasopressors

Table 4
Outpatient community-acquired pneumonia therapeutic options[5]

Patient Characteristics	Antimicrobial Therapy of Choice
No comorbidities or risk factors for MRSA or *P aeruginosa*	• Amoxicillin 1 g oral three times daily OR • Doxycycline 100 mg oral twice daily OR • Azithromycin[a] 500 mg oral on day 1, azithromycin, 250 mg oral on days 2–4 • Clarithromycin[a] 500 mg oral twice daily or clarithromycin ER 1000 mg oral daily
With comorbidities[b]	• Combination therapy with: • Amoxicillin/clavulanate 500 mg/125 mg three times oral daily, amoxicillin/clavulanate 875 mg/125 mg oral twice daily, amoxicillin/clavulanate 2000 mg/125 mg oral twice daily, cefpodoxime 200 mg oral twice daily, or cefuroxime 500 mg oral twice daily AND Azithromycin, 500 mg oral on the first day then 250 mg oral daily, clarithromycin 500 mg oral twice daily, clarithromycin ER 1000 mg oral daily, or doxycycline 100 mg oral twice daily • Monotherapy with respiratory fluoroquinolone levofloxacin 750 mg oral daily, moxifloxacin 400 mg oral daily, or gemifloxacin 320 mg oral daily

[a] Use macrolides only if local pneumococcal resistance is less than 25%.
[b] Chronic heart, liver, lung or renal disease, diabetes mellitus, alcoholism, malignancy, or asplenia.

1.03 (95% CI [0.88–1.20])], and dosages higher than ceftriaxone 1 g daily did not result in improved clinical outcomes for CAP (OR 1.02, 95% CI [0.91–1.14]).[6]

Hasegawa *and colleagues* supported these findings in their evaluation of ceftriaxone 1-g versus 2-g daily dosing. A similar rate of clinical cure was seen with ceftriaxone 1 g (94.6%) versus 2 g (93.1%), risk difference 1.5% (95% CI 3.1–6.0, *P* = .009 for non-inferiority). These studies prove that ceftriaxone 1 g daily is as safe and effective as other CAP regimens, including higher ceftriaxone dosing.[7] This is important as clinicians look to reduce antimicrobial resistance by minimizing excessive antimicrobial exposure.

Treatment Duration

Treatment duration varies based on the resolution of vital sign abnormalities, ability to eat, and normal mentation. IDSA recommends no less than 5 days of therapy in uncomplicated outpatient CAP, and several meta-analysis studies have demonstrated successful efficacy with 5 to 7 day treatment durations.[5,8–10] Inpatient CAP treatment should also be not less than 5 days unless MRSA or *P aeruginosa* is involved, then it is not less than 7 days.

In patients with complicated CAP, such as those with concurrent meningitis or endocarditis, 5 to 7 days of treatment is not sufficient, and longer durations are warranted.[5] PCT may be a useful biomarker to help guide treatment duration and is discussed further in the Antimicrobial Stewardship section.

HOSPITAL-ACQUIRED PNEUMONIA

The IDSA, the ATS, and international guidelines define hospital-acquired pneumonia (HAP) as a nosocomial infection of the lung parenchyma not present at the time of

Table 5
Inpatient community-acquired pneumonia therapeutic options[5]

	NO Risk for *P aeruginosa* or MRSA
Non-severe	Combination therapy with ampicillin–sulbactam 1.5–3 g IV every 6 h, cefotaxime 1–2 g IV every 8 h, ceftriaxone 1–2 g IV daily, or ceftaroline 600 mg IV every 12 h Plus Azithromycin 500 mg oral or IV daily or clarithromycin 500 mg oral twice daily OR monotherapy with levofloxacin 750 mg oral or IV daily or moxifloxacin 400 mg oral or IV daily
Severe	Combination therapy with ampicillin–sulbactam 1.5–3 g IV every 6 h, cefotaxime 1–2 g IV every 8 h, ceftriaxone 1–2 g IV daily, or ceftaroline 600 mg IV every 12 h Plus Azithromycin 500 mg oral or IV daily or clarithromycin 500 mg oral twice daily OR Levofloxacin 750 mg oral or IV daily or moxifloxacin 400 mg oral or IV daily
	WITH Risk Factors for *P aeruginosa* or MRSA
MRSA	If prior respiratory isolation of MRSA, IV antibiotics within the last 90 d, suspected necrotizing pneumonia or empyema regardless of non-severe or severe CAP • MRSA coverage: Vancomycin 15 mg/kg IV every 12 h (adjusted with TDM) or linezolid IV 600 mg every 12 h • Obtain cultures/nasal MRSA PCR to allow for de-escalation or confirmation of the need to continue therapy
P aeruginosa	If prior respiratory isolation of *P aeruginosa*, hospitalization within the last 90 d and receipt of intravenous antibiotics within the last 90 d regardless of non-severe or severe CAP • Piperacillin–tazobactam 4.5 g IV every 6 h, cefepime 2 g IV every 8 h, ceftazidime 2 g IV every 8 h, imipenem 500 mg IV every 6 h, meropenem 1 g IV every 8 h, or aztreonam 2 g IV every 8 h • Obtain cultures to allow for de-escalation or confirmation of the need to continue therapy

hospital admission that develops in patients after 48 hours of hospitalization. A subtype of HAP is ventilator-associated pneumonia (VAP), occurring in patients who have required mechanical ventilation for at least 48 hours.[11,12] Health care-associated pneumonia (HCAP) had previously been included in the HAP and VAP guidelines, but it was removed in the most recent update as new literature demonstrates that patients with HCAP are not at high risk for MDR pathogens as previously thought and are probably better categorized within the CAP guidelines.[11]

Diagnostic Strategies

In nosocomial pneumonia, microbiological studies should be performed before initiation of antimicrobial therapy to guide definitive therapy.

Noninvasive, qualitative, or semiquantitative cultures (eg, spontaneous expectoration, sputum inductions, nasotracheal suctioning, and endotracheal aspiration) are preferred over invasive, quantitative sampling strategies (eg, bronchial-alveolar lavage, protected specimen brush, and blind bronchial sampling) as no statistically significant difference in mortality rates were found between quantitative and qualitative cultures (RR 0.91; 95% CI 0.75–1.11).[13] No difference in other clinical outcomes, including duration of mechanical ventilation, ICU length of stay, and antibiotic change, were seen with the two sampling strategies.[13] In addition, noninvasive sampling can be performed rapidly and avoid delays in the initiation of effective antimicrobial therapy.[11] Blood cultures should be obtained for patients with suspected HAP/VAP as they may provide insight into the severity of illness and direct antimicrobial initiation and ultimately play a role in determining appropriate definitive therapy.

In general, clinical criteria for pneumonia should guide the initiation of empiric antimicrobial therapy in HAP/VAP. Although biomarkers such as PCT, c-reactive protein, or bronchial alveolar fluid soluble triggering receptor expressed on myeloid cells (sTREM-1) have been studied for the initiation of antimicrobial therapy in HAP/VAP, none have been associated with acceptable sensitivity or specificity for the diagnosis of HAP/VAP compared with using clinical criteria alone.[11]

Therapeutic Options

Although prior guidelines differentiated empiric treatment for nosocomial pneumonia based on the bacteriology of disease onset, early (within 4 days) versus late (5 days or more), recent literature indicates that patients with the early-onset disease may still be at risk for MDR pathogens.[12] Therefore, risk stratification for MDR organisms should not be based solely on disease onset. Prior intravenous antibiotic use within the last 90 days is the major risk factor for the development of MDR (eg, MRSA, *Pseudomonas* spp., and so forth), VAP (OR 12.3; 95% CI 6.48–23.35), and HAP (OR 5.17; 95% CI 2.11–12.67).[11] In addition, patients with VAP may be at increased risk of MDR pathogens when infection occurs on hospital day 5 or later or is complicated by septic shock, acute respiratory distress syndrome (ARDS), or need for acute renal replacement therapy.[11]

Empiric antimicrobial therapy selections for HAP and VAP should be stratified based on patient risk factors for MDR pathogens, as outlined in **Tables 6** and **7**. Antipseudomonal beta-lactam therapy is the cornerstone of nosocomial pneumonia treatment. Empiric, dual antipseudomonal coverage from different antibiotic classes is indicated in VAP when the patient has a risk factor for MDR pathogen, greater than 10% of gram-negative isolates are resistant to the antimicrobial being considered for monotherapy or local ICU susceptibilities are unavailable, and in HAP when there is a risk for MDR pathogen, need for mechanical ventilation, or presence of shock.[11] However, dual antipseudomonal therapy is controversial, and ultimately local sensitivities should be taken into consideration when determining empiric therapy. Intensivists should collaborate with antimicrobial stewardship (AMS) to develop local treatment pathways that are based on the national guidelines but are tailored to local data.[14]

Anti-MRSA antimicrobials are indicated for patients with HAP or VAP when there is a risk factor for MDR organisms or if an infection develops in hospital wards whereby greater than 10% to 20% of *Staphylococcus aureus* are methicillin-resistant. Otherwise, empiric treatment for HAP or VAP should target methicillin-sensitive *S aureus*.[11]

Clinical Considerations with Antimicrobial Selection and Dosing

Patient-specific factors including allergy history, organ function, and concomitant medications should be evaluated when selecting empiric antimicrobial regimens. Historically, piperacillin–tazobactam with vancomycin was recommended for empiric HAP/VAP treatment. However, a recent literature shows the odds of acute kidney injury with vancomycin plus piperacillin–tazobactam are significantly increased compared with vancomycin monotherapy (OR 3.40; 95% CI 2.57–4.50), vancomycin plus cefepime or carbapenem therapy (OR 2.68; 95% CI 1.83–3.91), or piperacillin–tazobactam monotherapy (OR 2.70; 95% CI 1.97–3.69).[15] Therefore, the use of cefepime in place of piperacillin–tazobactam may be preferable to avoid potential nephrotoxicity complications.

Table 6
Empiric antimicrobial therapy for hospital-acquired pneumonia[11]

Patient Characteristics	Antimicrobial Therapy Choices	
High risk of mortality[a] or received IV antimicrobials in the past 90 d	Select two of the following, avoid double beta-lactam therapy or same drug class: • Piperacillin–tazobactam 4.5 g IV every 6 h • Cefepime or ceftazidime 2 g IV every 8 h • Levofloxacin, 750 mg IV daily or ciprofloxacin 400 mg IV every 8 h • Imipenem 500 mg IV every 6 h or meropenem 1 g IV every 8 h • Amikacin 15–20 mg/kg IV daily • Gentamicin or tobramycin 5–7 mg/kg IV daily • Aztreonam 2 g IV every 8 h	Plus anti-MRSA therapy: • Vancomycin, 25–30 mg/kg IV once followed by 15 mg/kg IV every 8–12 h with TDM targeting through 15–20 mg/mL, or • Linezolid 600 mg IV every 12 h
Not high risk of mortality, but MRSA risk factor(s) present[b]	Select two of the following, avoid double beta-lactam therapy or same drug class: • Piperacillin–tazobactam 4.5 g IV every 6 h • Cefepime or ceftazidime, 2 g IV every 8 h • Levofloxacin 750 mg IV daily or ciprofloxacin 400 mg IV every 8 h • Imipenem 500 mg IV every 6 h or meropenem 1 g IV every 8 h • Aztreonam 2 g IV every 8 h	Plus anti-MRSA therapy: • Vancomycin 25–30 mg/kg IV once followed by 15 mg/kg IV every 8–12 h with TDM targeting through 15–20 mg/mL or • Linezolid 600 mg IV every 12 h
Not high risk of mortality and no MRSA risk factor(s) present[b]	Select one of the following: • Piperacillin–tazobactam 4.5 g IV every 6 h • Cefepime or ceftazidime 2 g IV every 8 h • Levofloxacin 750 mg IV daily or • Imipenem 500 mg IV every 6 h • Meropenem 1 g IV every 8 h	

[a] High risk for mortality: requiring ventilatory support or presence of septic shock.
[b] MRSA risk factors: prior intravenous antibiotic use within the last 90 d, hospital wards with greater than 10% to 20% MRSA isolates.

Table 7
Empiric antibiotic therapy for ventilator-associated pneumonia[11]

Patient Characteristics	Antimicrobial Therapy Choices	
• Received IV antimicrobials in the past 90 d • Septic shock at onset of VAP • ARDS preceding VAP • Acute renal replacement therapy preceding VAP • VAP onset hospital day 5 or later	Select one agent from each category: β-lactams • Piperacillin–tazobactam 4.5 g IV every 6 h • Cefepime or ceftazidime 2 g IV every 8 h • Imipenem 500 mg IV every 6 h or meropenem 1 g IV every 8 h • Aztreonam 2 g IV every 8 h Non-β-lactams • Levofloxacin 750 mg IV daily or ciprofloxacin 400 mg IV every 8 h • Amikacin 15–20 mg/kg IV daily • Gentamicin or tobramycin 5–7 mg/kg IV daily • Colistin 5 mg/kg IV loading dose followed by maintenance dose (2.5 mg*CrCl + 30) IV every 12 h or polymyxin B 2.5–3.0 mg/kg/d divided twice daily	Plus anti-MRSA therapy: • Vancomycin 25–30 mg/kg IV once followed by 15 mg/kg IV every 8–12 h with TDM targeting through 15–20 mg/mL or • Linezolid 600 mg IV every 12 h

Linezolid may increase the risk of serotonin syndrome when given with serotonergic medications (eg, selective serotonin reuptake inhibitors, serotonin–norepinephrine reuptake inhibitors, serotonin receptor agonists, tricyclic antidepressants, monoamine oxidase inhibitors, and opioid medications.)[11] If linezolid is chosen as either empiric or definitive therapy for HAP/VAP, careful screening for other serotonergic medications is needed. Temporary cessation of concurrent serotonergic medications may be needed if linezolid remains the preferred anti-MRSA therapy.

Pharmacokinetic (PK)-optimized/pharmacodynamic (PD)-optimized antimicrobial dosing should be used when treating serious infections. As antipseudomonal beta-lactam therapy is the backbone of nosocomial pneumonia treatment, the time-free drug concentrations are above the minimum inhibitory concentration (fT > MIC) must be enhanced. Critically ill patients with altered hemodynamics and organ function may benefit from the use of prolonged or continuous infusion dosing strategies and the emerging practice of beta-lactam TDM to ensure PK/PD goals are met.[11,14,16] In addition, vancomycin dosing and monitoring strategies have shifted to targeting an area under the curve to a MIC ratio of $\geq$400.[17] Future nosocomial pneumonia guidelines should be updated to reflect recommended vancomycin PD targets.

Definitive Therapy

Culture data revealing antimicrobial susceptibility testing should guide definitive antimicrobial therapy. In general, empiric regimens should be de-escalated to the most narrow spectrum agent covering the pathogen to avoid complications, such as *Clostridioides difficile* infection.[14] However, in cases whereby pathogens express expanded-spectrum beta-lactamases or carbapenem resistance, antimicrobial therapy should be targeted to treat these organisms.[11] Patients with pneumonia secondary to MDR gram-negative bacilli only sensitive to aminoglycosides or colistin may benefit from the initiation of inhaled antimicrobial therapy in addition to IV systemic therapy.[11]

Treatment Duration

Historically, HAP/VAP were treated for long durations up to 2 weeks, but updated evidence demonstrates that 7 days of therapy is suitable for most patients.[11] One pivotal clinical trial showed that 8 days of VAP treatment was non-inferior to 15 days in that there was no significant difference in mortality (18.8% vs 17.2%, difference 1.6%, 90% CI -3.7%–6.9%) or recurrent infection (28.9% vs 26.0%, difference 2.9%, 90% CI -3.2%–9.1%), but increased mean $\pm$ SD antimicrobial-free days in the 8 days group (13.1 $\pm$ 7.4 vs 8.7 $\pm$ 5.2, P<.001).[18] However, a subgroup of patients with non-lactose fermenting pathogens (eg, *P aeruginosa*) had a higher rate of recurrent infections, which was confirmed in one meta-analysis.[18,19] Updated meta-analyses of HAP/VAP treatment duration did not show a significant difference in recurrent infections with shorter courses regardless of the causative pathogen.[11,20]

Ultimately, clinical criteria should guide HAP/VAP resolution and antimicrobial discontinuation. Select populations may require an individualized duration of treatment, including those with severe immunocompromised state, initially treated with inappropriate antibiotic therapy or highly resistant pathogens, including *P aeruginosa* or carbapenem-resistant *Enterobacteriaceae* or *Acinetobacter* spp.[12]

IMMUNOCOMPROMISED POPULATIONS

Immunocompromised populations are at increased risk of pneumonia from both common pathogens and avirulent or opportunistic organisms.[21] Immunocompromised conditions include, but are not limited to receipt of cancer chemotherapy, solid organ transplantation, hematopoietic stem cell transplantation, HIV infection with a CD4 T-lymphocyte count less than 200 cells/microliter or percentage less than 14%, or receipt of corticosteroid therapy with a dose greater than 20 mg prednisone or equivalent daily for greater than 14 days or a cumulative dose greater than 600 mg of prednisone.[21]

Although immunocompromised patients may develop an infection from the typical CAP respiratory pathogens, they are also at risk for infection due to *Enterobacteriaceae* (including extended-spectrum beta-lactamase and carbapenemase-producing organisms), mycobacteria (eg, *Mycobacterium tuberculosis*), viruses (eg, *Cytomegalovirus*), fungi (eg, *Pneumocystis jirovecii*), and parasites (eg, *Toxoplasma gondii*).[21] Broad-spectrum therapy targeting beyond core respiratory pathogens should be used empirically when risk factors for MDR or opportunistic pathogens exist, and the delay in appropriate therapy will place the patient at increased risk of mortality.

Immunocompromised patients should be managed on a case-by-case basis to ensure pathogen-directed therapy is initiated, as shown **Table 8**.[21] Although a discussion on newer beta-lactam/beta-lactamase inhibitor combinations (eg, ceftolozane/tazobactam, imipenem/relabactam, meropenem/vaborbactam, and so forth) for the treatment of MDR gram-negative bacilli is beyond the scope of this review, there may be a role for these agents in the place of systemic aminoglycoside or colistin when treating highly resistant pathogens (eg, extended-spectrum beta-lactamase producing *Enterobacteriaceae* and carbapenem-resistant *Enterobacteriaceae*) under the direction of an infectious disease specialist.

ANTIMICROBIAL STEWARDSHIP INITIATIVES
Beta-Lactam Allergies

Beta-lactam intolerance (eg, gastrointestinal upset) is often misconstrued as a true allergic reaction and inappropriately documented in the patient chart. This may potentially result in an inferior or unnecessarily broad-spectrum antibiotic prescribing. Although beta-lactam antibiotics are the most common cause of drug-induced delayed rashes, including maculopapular, they infrequently cause true IgE-mediated reactions. Anaphylaxis is rare for penicillin: 0.001% for the parenteral route of administration and 0.0005% for the oral route of administration.[22]

Beta-lactam allergies documented in the medical record should be carefully reviewed to determine if a true allergy exists or whether the allergy is, in fact, a mislabel. Clarification of mislabeled allergies should be made in the medical record to alert other providers of intolerances that may not preclude the use of first-line

Table 8	
Pathogen-directed therapy for immunocompromised patients[21]	
Pathogen	**Empiric Treatment**
P jirovecci	Trimethoprim–sulfamethoxazole 15–20 mg/kg/d divided every 6–8 h
Nocardia spp.	Trimethoprim–sulfamethoxazole 15–20 mg/kg/d divided every 6–8 h
Aspergillus spp.	Preferred: Liposomal amphotericin, 5–7.5 mg/kg/d Alternative: Isavuconazole, 200 mg every 8 h (initial dosing)
Mucorales spp.	Preferred: Liposomal amphotericin 5–7.5 mg/kg/d Alternative: Isavuconazole 200 mg every 8 h (initial dosing)
Varicella-zoster virus	Acyclovir 10–15 mg/kg IV every 8 h
Cytomegalovirus	Ganciclovir 5 mg/kg IV every 12 h

treatment. When a true allergy exists, cross-reactivity between beta-lactam antibiotics must be carefully evaluated to avoid inappropriate exclusion of the entire class in the management of pneumonia.

Cross-reactivity between beta-lactams depends on the R1 side chain of the chemical structure. Therefore, an antibiotic with the same R1 side chain as the drug allergy should not be selected, and an alternative agent should be considered. For example, cephalexin and cefaclor have an identical side chain to amoxicillin.[22]

First generation cephalosporins have a higher cross-reactivity risk with penicillins compared to fourth generation cephalosporins due to similarities in the R1 side chain.[23] The cross-reactivity between penicillins and carbapenems, as well as carbapenems and cephalosporins, is less than 1%.[23] Monobactams do not cross-react with penicillins or carbapenems and could serve as a safe alternative agent in patients with a true risk of IgE reaction. If the R1 side chains are the same or similar, then clinical judgment should be used to determine if the reaction should be challenged.

Procalcitonin

PCT is a precursor hormone of calcitonin that is upregulated by cytokines released in response to bacterial infections. With a half-life of 25 to 30 hours, a rapid rise in PCT levels is seen within 6 to 12 hours of bacterial insult which decline as the infection resolves. Although PCT was first approved by the FDA in 2005 as a diagnostic aid for sepsis, it has proven useful as a tool for antimicrobial de-escalation.[24]

Numerous randomized studies have examined whether PCT-based algorithms can assist clinicians in deciding whether to start or stop antimicrobial therapy without adversely impacting patients through delayed antimicrobial therapy or inadequate treatment courses.[24] Efficacy has been demonstrated in adult patients with suspected respiratory infections. Improving antibiotic use in these scenarios carries the potential for important clinical benefit as respiratory infections are the most common indication for antibiotics in hospitalized patients, and antibiotic use is most prevalent in the ICU.

A systematic review and meta-analysis by Lam *and colleagues* evaluated PCT-guided antibiotic cessation (using PCT drop of 50%–90% from baseline with an absolute value <0.5–1 mcg/L) compared with standard of care in adult critically ill patients was associated with a decrease in 30-day mortality, RR 0.87 (95% CI 0.77–0.98, $P = .02$). However, there was no decrease in short-term mortality when PCT was used for either initiation or initiation and cessation of antibiotics.[25] In addition, they demonstrated that PCT-guided cessation of antibiotics was associated with a significant decrease in antibiotic durations. This finding was confirmed in another meta-analysis, which showed that PCT-guided cessation was associated with a mean antibiotic duration of 7.35 days versus 8.85 days in the control arm −1.49 days (95% CI -2.27–0.71, $P<.001$).[26]

Overall, serial evaluation of PCT in patients with sepsis is associated with significantly reduced 30-day mortality and may allow for a 1 to 3 day shorter duration of antimicrobial therapy with no apparent compromise in clinical outcomes. Of note, there are limitations with PCT as false positives and false negatives may be seen in some patient populations (**Table 9**).[24]

Methicillin-Resistant Staphylococcus aureus Nasal Screening

From 2011 to 2014, *Staphylococcus aureus* was the most prevalent pathogen implicated in VAP.[27] Although there are various methods to detect MRSA colonization, PCR assay has a faster turn-around time (<1 day) than site culture (1–3 days) and a higher sensitivity (92.5%) than culture (86.9%).[28] MRSA PCR testing detects *mecA* genetic sequencing, the gene responsible for methicillin resistance. Therefore, it is more

Table 9
Common causes of false-positive and false-negative procalcitonin results

False-Positive	False-Negative
Burns	Abscesses
Circulatory shock	Empyema
Inhalation injury	Mediastinitis
Pancreatitis	
Severe trauma	
Surgery	

likely to remain positive in patients already receiving antibiotic therapy than culture regardless of bacterial viability.[28]

Anti-MRSA therapy is often prescribed empirically for pneumonia in critically ill patients and de-escalated if MRSA is not isolated in a sputum or blood culture. However, there may be challenges with obtaining adequate respiratory cultures that may result in longer durations of broad-spectrum antimicrobial use, especially in non-intubated patients. Respiratory samples obtained after receipt of empiric antimicrobial therapy may have a lower yield in identifying a causative pathogen and also result in prolonged empiric regimens. Therefore, non-culture-based testing is an important tool for AMS de-escalation strategies.

Several studies have demonstrated high negative predictive values (NPV) of MRSA nares screening for MRSA pneumonia. One study out of the Veterans Affairs system evaluated MRSA nares colonization screening at admission and transfer and data from 561,325 cultures to determine NPV of MRSA screening in determination of subsequent positive MRSA culture. Overall, the NPV of MRSA nares screening for ruling out MRSA infection at any site of infection was 96.5% and 96.1% for respiratory infections.[29] A systematic review and meta-analysis confirmed a high NPV (96.5%) in pneumonia.[30]

Overall, MRSA nares screening has a high specificity and NPV for ruling out MRSA pneumonia. Although many studies used protocols to screen for MRSA in the nares at ICU admission, with some repeating the screening weekly, Mallidi *and colleagues* demonstrated the NPV remained high (98%) even when using nares screens from within 60 days of hospital admission, indicating MRSA nares screening from a recent hospital admission may successfully guide empiric antimicrobial therapy in the ED and ICU settings.[31] When nares screening is negative for MRSA, it is reasonable to withhold or rapidly de-escalate anti-MRSA antimicrobial therapy.

CLINICS CARE POINTS

- Classification of pneumonia as either community-acquired or hospital-acquired will guide selection of empirical antimicrobial therapy.
- 5 to 7 days of treatment is generally sufficient to treat community-acquired pneumonia; however, procalcitonin may be a useful biomarker to support cessation of therapy sooner.
- Patients with hospital-acquired and ventilator-associated pneumonia should be risk-stratified for multidrug-resistant pathogens, with the cornerstone of therapy being a combination of anti-pseudomonal and anti-methicillin-resistant *Staphylococcus aureus* therapy.

- Immunocompromised patients should be managed on a case-by-case basis to ensure appropriate broad-spectrum antibiotics have been initiated to target certain pathogens.
- Collaboration with antimicrobial stewardship programs ensures optimization in overall antibiotic use while minimizing the risk of adverse effects from excessive antibiotic treatment (eg, *Clostridioides difficile* infection, development of antimicrobial resistance, and so forth)

REFERENCES

1. Olson G, Davis AM. Diagnosis and Treatment of Adults with Community-Acquired Pneumonia. JAMA 2020;323(9):885–6.
2. Nair GB, Niederman MS. Updates on community acquired pneumonia management in the ICU. Pharmacol Ther 2021;217:107663.
3. Ticona JH, Zaccone VM, McFarlane IM. Community-Acquired Pneumonia: A Focused Review. Am J Med Case Rep 2021;9(1):45–52.
4. Mandell LA, Wunderink RG, Anzueto A, et al. Infectious Diseases Society of America/American Thoracic Society consensus guidelines on the management of community-acquired pneumonia in adults. Clin Infect Dis 2007;44(suppl 2): S27–72.
5. Metlay JP, Waterer GW, Long AC, et al. Diagnosis and Treatment of Adults with Community-acquired Pneumonia. An Official Clinical Practice Guideline of the American Thoracic Society and Infectious Diseases Society of America. Am J Respir Crit Care Med 2019;200(7):e45–67.
6. Telles JP, Cieslinski J, Gasparetto J, et al. Efficacy of Ceftriaxone 1 g daily Versus 2 g daily for The Treatment of Community Acquired Pneumonia: A Systematic Review with Meta-Analysis. Expert Rev Anti-infective Ther 2019;17(7):501–10.
7. Hasegawa S, Sada R, Yaegashi M, et al. Adult Pneumonia Study Group-Japan. 1g versus 2 g daily intravenous ceftriaxone in the treatment of community onset pneumonia - a propensity score analysis of data from a Japanese multicenter registry. BMC Infect Dis 2019;19(1):1079.
8. Dimopoulos G, Matthaiou DK, Karageorgopoulos DE, et al. Short- versus long-course antibacterial therapy for community-acquired pneumonia: a meta-analysis. Drugs 2008;68:1841–54.
9. Li JZ, Winston LG, Moore DH, et al. Efficacy of short-course antibiotic regimens for community-acquired pneumonia: a meta-analysis. Am J Med 2007;120: 783–90.
10. Tansarli GS, Mylonakis E. Systematic review and meta-analysis of the efficacy of short-course antibiotic treatments for community-acquired pneumonia in adults. Antimicrob Agents Chemother 2018;62. e00635-18.
11. Kalil AC, Metersky ML, Klompas M, et al. Management of Adults With Hospital-acquired and Ventilator-associated Pneumonia: 2016 Clinical Practice Guidelines by the Infectious Diseases Society of America and the American Thoracic Society. Clin Infect Dis 2016;63(5):e61–111.
12. Torres A, Niederman MS, Chastre J, et al. International ERS/ESICM/ESCMID/ALAT guidelines for the management of hospital-acquired pneumonia and ventilator-associated pneumonia: Guidelines for the management of hospital-acquired pneumonia (HAP)/ventilator-associated pneumonia (VAP) of the European Respiratory Society (ERS), European Society of Intensive Care Medicine (ESICM), European Society of Clinical Microbiology and Infectious Diseases

(ESCMID) and Asociación Latinoamericana del Tórax (ALAT). Eur Respir J 2017; 50(3):1700582.

13. Berton DC, Kalil AC, Teixeira PJ. Quantitative versus qualitative cultures of respiratory secretions for clinical outcomes in patients with ventilator-associated pneumonia. Cochrane Database Syst Rev 2014;10:CD006482.

14. Wunderink RG, Srinivasan A, Barie PS, et al. Antibiotic Stewardship in the Intensive Care Unit. An Official American Thoracic Society Workshop Report in Collaboration with the AACN, CHEST, CDC, and SCCM. Ann Am Thorac Soc 2020; 17(5):531–40.

15. Luther MK, Timbrook TT, Caffrey AR, et al. Vancomycin Plus Piperacillin-Tazobactam and Acute Kidney Injury in Adults: A Systematic Review and Meta-Analysis. Crit Care Med 2018;46(1):12–20.

16. Guilhaumou R, Benaboud S, Bennis Y, et al. Optimization of the treatment with beta-lactam antibiotics in critically ill patients - Guidelines from the French Society of Pharmacology and Therapeutics (Société Française de Pharmacologie et Thérapeutique - SFPT) and the French Society of Anaesthesia. Crit Care 2019; 23(1):1–20.

17. Rybak MJ, Le J, Lodise TP, et al. Executive Summary: Therapeutic Monitoring of Vancomycin for Serious Methicillin-Resistant Staphylococcus aureus Infections: A Revised Consensus Guideline and Review of the American Society of Health-System Pharmacists, the Infectious Diseases Society of America, the Pediatric Infectious Diseases Society, and the Society of Infectious Diseases Pharmacists. Pharmacotherapy 2020;40(4):363–7.

18. Chastre J, Wolff M, Fagon JY, et al, PneumA Trial Group. Comparison of 8 vs 15 days of antibiotic therapy for ventilator-associated pneumonia in adults: a randomized trial. JAMA 2003;290(19):2588–98.

19. Pugh R, Grant C, Cooke RP, et al. Short-course versus prolonged-course antibiotic therapy for hospital-acquired pneumonia in critically ill adults. Cochrane Database Syst Rev 2015;2015(8):CD007577.

20. Dimopoulos G, Poulakou G, Pneumatikos IA, et al. Short- vs long-duration antibiotic regimens for ventilator-associated pneumonia: a systematic review and meta-analysis. Chest 2013;144(6):1759–67.

21. Ramirez JA, Musher DM, Evans SE, et al. Treatment of Community-Acquired Pneumonia in Immunocompromised Adults: A Consensus Statement Regarding Initial Strategies. Chest 2020;158(5):1896–911.

22. Blumenthal KG, Peter JG, Trubiano JA, et al. Antibiotic allergy. Lancet 2019; 393(10167):183–98.

23. Zagursky RJ, Pichichero ME. Cross-reactivity in β-Lactam Allergy. J Allergy Clin Immunol Pract 2018;6(1):72–81.e1.

24. Rhee C. Using Procalcitonin to Guide Antibiotic Therapy. Open Forum Infect Dis 2016;7(4):ofw249.

25. Lam SW, Bauer SR, Fowler R, et al. Systematic review and meta-analysis of procalcitonin-guidance versus usual care for antimicrobial management in critically ill patients: focus on subgroups based on antibiotic initiation, cessation, or mixed strategies. Crit Care Med 2018;46:684–90.

26. Iankova I, Thompson-Leduc P, Kirson NY, et al. Efficacy and safety of procalcitonin guidance in patients with suspected or confirmed sepsis: a systematic review and meta-analysis. Crit Care Med 2018;46:691–8.

27. Weiner LM, Webb AK, Limbago B, et al. Antimicrobial-resistant pathogens associated with healthcare-associated infections: summary of data reported to the

National Healthcare Safety Network at the Centers for Disease Control and Prevention, 2011-2014. Infect Control Hosp Epidemiol 2016;37(11):1288–301.

28. Carr AL, Daley MJ, Givens Merkel K, et al. Clinical Utility of Methicillin-Resistant Staphylococcus aureus Nasal Screening for Antimicrobial Stewardship: A Review of Current Literature. Pharmacotherapy 2018;38:1216–28.

29. Mergenhagen KA, Starr KE, Wattengel BA, et al. Determining the Utility of Methicillin-Resistant Staphylococcus aureus Nares Screening in Antimicrobial Stewardship. Clin Infect Dis 2020;71:1142–8.

30. Parente DM, Cunha CB, Mylonakis E, et al. The Clinical Utility of Methicillin-Resistant Staphylococcus aureus (MRSA) Nasal Screening to Rule Out MRSA Pneumonia: A Diagnostic Meta-analysis With Antimicrobial Stewardship Implications. Clin Infect Dis 2018;67:1–7.

31. Mallidi MG, Slocum GW, Peksa GD, et al. Impact of Prior-to-Admission Methicillin-Resistant *Staphylococcus aureus* Nares Screening in Critically Ill Adults With Pneumonia. Ann Pharmacother 2022;56(2):124–30.

Radiographic Imaging of Community-Acquired Pneumonia: A Case-Based Review

Lacey Washington, MD*, Bryan O'Sullivan-Murphy, MD, PhD,
Jared D. Christensen, MD, MBA, H. Page McAdams, MD

KEYWORDS

- Community-acquired pneumonia • Infection • Radiograph • Diagnosis • Differential

KEY POINTS

- Awareness of the multiple chest radiographic patterns of community-acquired pneumonia, including subtle bronchopneumonia and interstitial patterns and round pneumonia, facilitates diagnosis of infection but is not useful in identifying specific infectious agents.
- Pleural fluid and multilobar opacities may influence treatment decisions and should be reported when present.
- Because there are no guidelines that recommend universal follow-up radiography, it is important to correlate with clinical presentation and recommend follow-up radiographs in any patient with a discordant clinical presentation.
- Imaging findings that should prompt immediate consideration of alternative diagnoses include lymphadenopathy visible on radiography and the presence of multiple pulmonary nodules.
- Tuberculosis should be considered in patients with atypical, subacute symptom onset particularly when cavitation is present or when opacities involve the upper lobes.

INTRODUCTION

Chest radiography remains the most common imaging study performed both worldwide and in the United States. Although indications for chest radiography are numerous, many of these studies are performed for the evaluation of suspected infection. According to data from the 2019 Global Burden of Disease from before the coronavirus disease 2019 (COVID-19) pandemic, lower respiratory tract infections are the leading cause of mortality from infectious disease worldwide.[1] These infections are

This article was previously published in *Radiologic Clinics of North America* 60:3 May 2022.
Department of Radiology, Duke University Medical Center, 2301 Erwin Road, DUMC Box 3808, Durham, NC 27710, USA
* Corresponding author.
E-mail address: lacey.washington@duke.edu

Infect Dis Clin N Am 38 (2024) 19–33
https://doi.org/10.1016/j.idc.2023.12.008
0891-5520/24/© 2023 Elsevier Inc. All rights reserved.

divided into community-acquired pneumonia (CAP) and hospital-acquired infections, and also between those in immunocompetent and immunocompromised patients. In the outpatient setting, a single radiograph may be the only imaging study performed and therefore may have a large impact on patient management. Unfortunately, the nonspecific radiographic manifestations of infection lead many radiologists to take a nihilistic approach to the interpretation of radiographs in this setting.

Although it is true that there are limitations of radiographic imaging for CAP, radiologists can still make important contributions to patient care in the setting of suspected acute pulmonary infection. The radiologist who is aware of the broad range of radiographic manifestations of infection may suggest the diagnosis on the basis of findings that are subtle or confusing to clinicians. Radiologic interpretation may identify findings that may alter treatment in the setting of suspected pneumonia. Finally, the radiologist should be alert for findings that are inconsistent with acute CAP or nonspecific enough to call into question a diagnosis of pneumonia in the acute setting, particularly when the clinical presentation is atypical, so as to prevent important misdiagnoses.

This article reviews the indications for radiographic imaging of patients with suspected community-acquired pulmonary infection and discusses the imaging findings that are most important to current clinical guidelines for patient care. The range of radiographic manifestations of acute CAP and principles of image interpretation are presented in a case-based format. COVID-19 is not addressed, because there is an abundance of literature devoted to that specific diagnosis, and coronavirus pneumonias are discussed elsewhere in this issue (see article by Ayushi and colleagues).

INDICATIONS FOR RADIOGRAPHY IN SUSPECTED INFECTION

Very little research has been performed to assess whether obtaining a radiograph has an effect on clinical outcomes of patients with suspected pulmonary infection. A systematic literature review reveals only 2 such studies—one in a pediatric and one in an adult population. In both, the conclusions were confined to an ambulatory population, and neither of these studies showed a demonstrable effect on the primary end points, which were overall clinical outcomes for pediatric patients and length of illness for the adult population, although in the subgroup of adult patients with abnormal radiographs, duration of illness improved, presumably because of a higher rate of antibiotic use.[2]

These findings are in keeping with the results of studies looking at the impact of chest radiographs on patient management. In one series, among 300 patients in whom pneumonia was suspected, clinicians ordered radiographs in only 19%.[3] Radiographs were performed for only 61% of patients in whom a diagnosis of pneumonia was made. The investigators observed that clinicians who have a sufficiently high clinical suspicion of infection will treat patients regardless of imaging findings, making the chest radiograph superfluous. Another study of 2706 patients hospitalized with a diagnosis of pneumonia found that approximately one-third of patients (911) had negative radiographs, indicating that the diagnosis of pneumonia was not made on the basis of radiographic findings alone.[4] There was no difference in the rates of positive sputum or blood cultures between patients with radiographs interpreted as positive or negative for pneumonia, suggesting that significant lower respiratory tract infection may be found in patients with negative radiographs (false negatives). Studies comparing radiography with computed tomography (CT) suggest that radiography is inferior. A multicenter trial of patients in the emergency department observed that radiography was only 43.5% sensitive for the detection of opacities compared with CT,[5] concluding that CT is more accurate in identifying pulmonary infection in this setting. Another study also in the emergency department setting found that almost one-third (29.8%)

of patients with chest radiographs interpreted as positive for pneumonia had subsequently negative CTs, and one-third (33.3%) of patients with radiographs interpreted as negative had subsequently positive CTs.[6]

These studies notwithstanding, the 2007 American Thoracic Society and Infectious Disease Society of America (ATS/IDSA) criteria state that a diagnosis of pneumonia requires a "demonstrable infiltrate by chest radiograph or other imaging technique."[7] The 2019 update to these criteria limits the discussion of pneumonia to "studies that used radiographic criteria for defining CAP, given the known inaccuracy of clinical signs and symptoms alone for CAP diagnosis."[8] British Thoracic Society guidelines recommend radiography in selected outpatients and all patients admitted with CAP.[9] Furthermore, the use of radiography leads to detection of many more cases of pneumonia than clinical judgment alone, with general practitioners' clinical judgment having a sensitivity of only 29% when compared with radiography in one study.[10] Diagnostic radiographs will therefore continue to be performed in this setting, and interpretations should be focused on optimizing the usefulness of these studies.

Clinical guidelines with respect to appropriate radiographic follow-up have varied, with some suggesting that all patients should have follow-up radiographs to establish "a new radiographic baseline,"[11] whereas others implying that radiographic follow-up was unnecessary for patients with a good clinical response to treatment.[12] Major reasons that have been proposed for radiographic follow-up include assessment for improvement, assessment for progression of disease and complications, and the exclusion of malignancy either masquerading as infection or as a cause of postobstructive infection. Lung cancer diagnoses, however, have been reported to be relatively uncommon after a diagnosis of pneumonia.[13,14] As a consequence, the current ATS/IDSA guidelines do not recommend routine follow-up, and the initial radiograph should be interpreted with attention to any findings for which follow-up should be recommended.

Chest radiography may be useful beyond the confirmation of possible infection. Updated ATS/IDSA guidelines give a strong recommendation for the use of the pneumonia severity index (PSI) to identify those patients in need of hospitalization.[8] This index is a scoring system that confers points for parameters on a large number of clinical and laboratory findings; unlike other less well-validated criteria used in assessment of pneumonia severity, PSI includes a radiographic parameter (the presence of a pleural effusion on imaging) as an indicator of severity.[15] The 2007 ATS/IDSA guidelines also set forth additional criteria for severe pneumonia to identify patients early who would ultimately require intensive care unit (ICU) admission, because delayed transfer to the ICU rather than direct ICU admission is associated with increased mortality.[7] In addition to clinical and laboratory values, these criteria include "multilobar infiltrates" as an indication of severe infection (**Fig. 1**). The 2019 ATS/IDSA guidelines expand the use of these criteria, so that the score on this assessment is now one indication for intensive investigation for infectious agents (including sputum gram stain and cultures, blood cultures, and urinary antigen tests for *Legionella* and *Streptococcus pneumoniae*) and in some circumstances the score may influence antibiotic choice (see article by Brixey and colleagues in this issue).[8] Radiography may also be useful to assess for complications of infection, particularly the presence of pleural fluid requiring drainage or the presence of hydropneumothorax.

RADIOGRAPHIC PATTERNS IN ACUTE INFECTION

Classically, the thoracic manifestations of pneumonia are divided into 3 distinct patterns: lobar (also known as focal or airspace) pneumonia, bronchopneumonia, and interstitial pneumonia.[16–18]

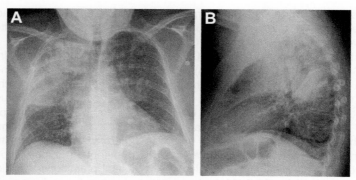

Fig. 1. Infection with findings of severity. Frontal (*A*) and lateral (*B*) views of the chest demonstrating multilobar pneumonia with opacities in the right upper and lower lobes and left lower lobe, and with small bilateral pleural effusions.

Lobar Pneumonia

Lobar or air-space pneumonia (**Fig. 2**) is probably the most familiar of the 3 radiographic patterns of pneumonia. This radiographic abnormality is classically confined to a portion of the lungs subtended by a single lobar or segmental bronchus or group of segmental bronchi and therefore can be described as having an anatomic distribution. The radiographic appearance is a function of the pathophysiology: the acini are filled first with fluid, which spreads easily throughout the collateral ventilatory

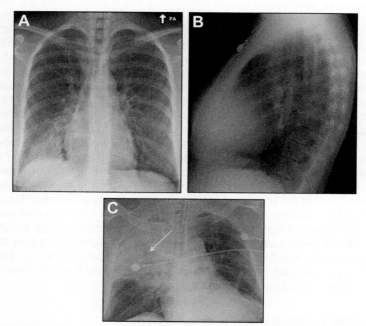

Fig. 2. Lobar pneumonia. (*A, B*) Opacity in a segmental distribution in the right lower lobe. Lateral radiograph shows faint opacity over the lower thoracic spine (spine sign). (*C*) Right upper lobar pneumonia with near-complete opacification of the right upper lobe with air bronchograms (*yellow arrow*).

pathways in the lung, limited only by the pleura of the fissures. Fluid carries organisms throughout the involved portions of the lungs, spreading from the periphery to the more central portions. The large bronchi remain patent, resulting in an air broncho-gram sign. Classically, this radiographic appearance is described in bacterial infec-tions such as those caused by *S pneumoniae*, *Klebsiella pneumoniae*, and *Legionella pneumophila*.

Bronchopneumonia

The second radiographic pattern of pneumonia is the bronchopneumonia pattern (**Fig. 3**). This pattern is characterized by multifocal opacities, predominantly nodules, which tend to become confluent, producing areas of consolidation up to the size of a pulmonary segment. This pattern is thought to be caused by infection originating in the bronchi, with a robust immune response confining the infection to smaller regions of the lungs in the immediate peribronchial parenchyma. The result is a heterogeneous pattern, with areas of opacity interposed with areas of normally aerated lung. The in-fectious agents classically associated with this pattern include *Staphylococcus aureus*, *Haemophilus influenzae*, and anaerobic bacteria. Bronchopneumonia is the pattern classically associated with the development of pulmonary abscesses.

Interstitial Pneumonia

The third, most subtle, radiographic pattern is that of acute infectious interstitial pneu-monia (**Fig. 4**). The primary radiographic features include diffuse reticular opacities corresponding to infection involving the bronchial and bronchiolar walls and the pul-monary interstitium; the alveoli are spared resulting in relatively little air-space abnor-mality. The acute interstitial pneumonia pattern is classically associated with *Mycoplasma*, *Pneumocystis jirovecii*, and a variety of viral pneumonias; due to the as-sociation with *Mycoplasma* infection, this radiographic pattern does not exclude bac-terial pneumonia.

Limitations of the Pattern Approach

Although helpful conceptually in identifying pneumonia on chest radiography, these descriptions cannot reliably diagnose specific infectious pathogens and are therefore limited in directing management. There is little research on the correlation between patterns and infectious agents, perhaps at least in part due to infrequent isolation of a specific infectious pathogen. According to ATS/IDSA guidelines, outpatients and

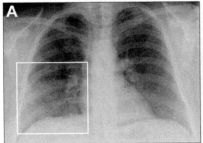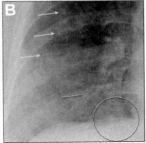

Fig. 3. Bronchopneumonia. (*A*) Nodular opacities with bronchial wall thickening and focal consolidative opacities in the right mid to lower lung, findings associated with broncho-pneumonia. (*B*) Magnified right lower hemithorax (*white box inset* from *A*) highlighting the nodular opacities (*yellow arrows*), bronchial wall thickening (*blue arrow*), and devel-oping confluent opacities (*red circle*).

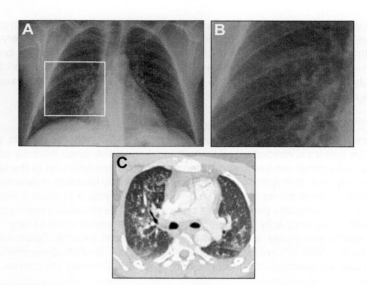

Fig. 4. Interstitial pneumonia. (*A*) Bilateral patchy peribronchovascular and reticular opacities representative of acute interstitial pneumonia. Magnified insert from (*A*) (*B*) and chest CT at the level of the pulmonary artery (*C*) highlight peribronchovascular and centrilobular nodular opacities with limited involvement of intervening parenchyma.

many inpatients who present with pulmonary opacities and symptoms and signs of pulmonary infection are treated empirically rather than being investigated for specific agents.[8] In addition, sputum gram stains and cultures are notoriously often inadequate, with results commonly showing only upper airway flora. Patients are therefore more likely to receive a definitive diagnosis if they have urine antigen test results positive for *S pneumoniae* or *Legionella* or have positive cultures from bronchoscopy, blood, or pleural fluid specimens, leading to a biased distribution of patients who receive definitive diagnoses.

Studies attempting to establish correlations of patterns with agents have met with little success. A study of radiographs in 192 patients with hospital admissions for CAP showed very poor interreader agreement for radiographic pattern (with kappa < 0.4) among 2 radiologists and a pulmonary physician.[19] In this study *Mycoplasma pneumoniae* was not associated with an interstitial pattern (which was seldom described by the observers) but was associated with a "patchy alveolar pattern," and not a lobar pattern. In contrast, in another study of *M pneumoniae*, 48% of patients presented with a pattern of segmental or lobar consolidation.[20] Another study that looked at patients with *Chlamydia pneumoniae* and *S pneumoniae* infections found no radiographic features that distinguished between the 2 agents.[5] For this reason, identifying any possible infection rather than a particular pattern should be the goal of radiographic interpretation.

Principles guiding the interpretation of radiographs in suspected pneumonia are illustrated in a series of cases.

CASES
Case 1

A 50-year-old woman presented to the emergency department with cough and fever. A radiograph showed a moderately well-defined mass in the superior segment of the right lower lobe, measuring approximately 5 cm in diameter (**Fig. 5**A).

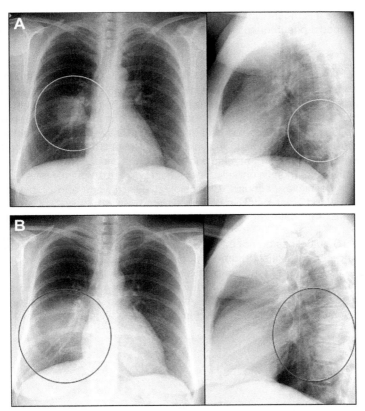

Fig. 5. Case 1. A 50-year-old woman with cough and fever. (*A*) Initial posteroanterior (PA) and lateral chest radiographs reveal mass in the superior segment of the right lower lobe (*yellow circle*). (*B*) Subsequent radiograph 3 days later demonstrates marked enlargement of the opacity.

The radiograph was interpreted as suggestive of malignancy, and the patient's symptoms were attributed to an upper respiratory tract infection. The patient was therefore discharged from the emergency department with a recommendation for follow-up with her primary care provider; antibiotic treatment was not initiated. The patient, however, returned to the emergency department after 3 days with increasing respiratory symptoms. Repeat chest radiograph showed that the mass had nearly doubled in size and the margins were less well defined (**Fig. 5**B).

Diagnosis: Round Pneumonia

The diagnosis of round pneumonia should be considered in any patient who presents with a pulmonary mass at radiography and clinically with symptoms of respiratory tract infection; this is particularly true if the patient is at low risk for lung carcinoma, for example, a young, nonsmoker. If there is a recent normal chest radiograph, the finding of a new mass in a patient with clinical signs of infection is considered "virtually pathognomonic for round pneumonia."[21] Round pneumonia has classically been thought to occur primarily in children and attributed to incomplete development of collateral ventilation pathways. However, round pneumonia is also found occasionally in adults, where it is most commonly a manifestation of bacterial pneumonia, particularly streptococcal pneumonia.

Case 2

A 63-year-old male patient presented with nonproductive cough, and a chest radiograph demonstrated a right middle lobe opacity with mild volume loss (**Fig. 6**A). The patient was thought to have CAP based on the radiographic findings; however, 3 weeks after antibiotic treatment, the opacity was unchanged. The degree of middle lobe volume loss was less pronounced than is usually seen in nonobstructive middle lobe atelectasis, that is, middle lobe syndrome.[22] Chest CT was performed (**Fig. 6**B) and demonstrated a patent right middle lobe bronchus and air bronchograms, making postobstructive pneumonitis unlikely. The patient was subsequently referred for bronchoscopy for definitive diagnosis. Bronchioloalveolar lavage and biopsy were performed and yielded an atypical lymphoid infiltrate.

Diagnosis: Extranodal marginal B-cell lymphoma of mucosa-associated lymphoid tissue.

Current ATS guidelines do not call for routine radiographic follow-up for suspected infection, and current British Thoracic Society guidelines call for follow-up imaging only in patients with persistent symptoms at 6 weeks or those at high risk for malignancy. A survey of the Society of Thoracic Radiology membership indicated that thoracic radiology subspecialists were most influenced by the age of the patient and the appearance of the abnormality in deciding whether to recommend follow-

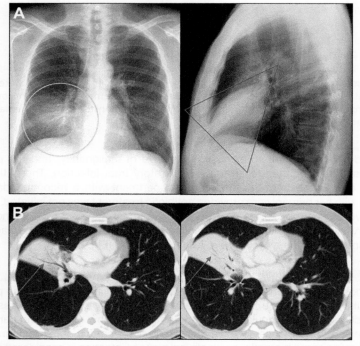

Fig. 6. Case 2. A 63-year-old male with nonproductive cough. (*A*) Initial diagnostic PA and lateral chest radiographs reveal right middle lobar opacity and mild volume loss (*yellow circle* and *blue triangle*). (*B*) Subsequent chest CT demonstrates consolidative opacities in the right middle lobe with patent right middle lobe bronchi and air bronchograms (*red arrows*).

up.[23] In addition, follow-up imaging or further investigation should be recommended when the clinical presentation is atypical. Any nonresolving area of pulmonary consolidation suggests a diagnosis other than CAP, and one of the major concerns is malignancy. "Air-space" opacities on radiographs may result from malignancy with postobstructive pneumonitis or from infiltrative neoplasms, such as adenocarcinoma with lepidic growth and lymphoproliferative disorders. Other possible causes of a nonresolving pulmonary opacity include postobstructive pneumonitis from benign processes including benign neoplasms and aspirated foreign bodies, atypical infections (such as mycobacterial infections, blastomycosis, or cryptococcosis), lipoid pneumonia, and inflammatory processes including organizing pneumonia and vasculitis. In all cases, detection depends on correlating with clinical presentation so that follow-up imaging or more careful immediate investigation is performed.

Case 3

A 72-year-old man who was visiting the United States from his home in Nigeria presented with fever, nausea, and vomiting. A chest radiograph was performed, which showed a masslike area of consolidation with cavitation in the anterior segment of the left upper lobe (**Fig. 7**). An initial diagnosis of pneumonia was made, possibly related to aspiration, given the history of vomiting; however, there was no report of acute cough or sputum production.

The differential diagnosis for cavitary disease does include a wide array of bacterial infections including multiple streptococcal species and *K pneumoniae*[24] sometimes in the form of a cavitary mass or abscess. Additional differential diagnoses include noninfectious diseases such as granulomatosis with polyangiitis and malignancy. The finding of cavitation in the mid and upper lung zones should also raise the possibility of tuberculosis; this is particularly true in any patient who, as in this case, has risk factors such as time spent in an endemic region, and in a patient without acute respiratory symptoms.

Diagnosis: Postprimary Tuberculosis

Tuberculosis is not a common disease in the United States. However, in 2019 it remained the leading cause of infectious disease death among adults worldwide,

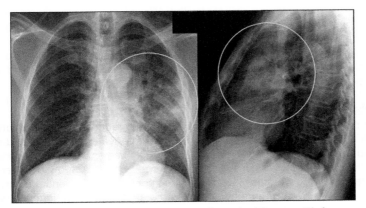

Fig. 7. Case 3. A 72-year-old Nigerian man visiting the United States, with fever, nausea, and vomiting. PA and lateral chest radiographs reveal masslike consolidation with cavitation in the left upper lobe (*yellow circles*).

with the World Health Organization estimating that there were 10 million new cases that year.[25] Tuberculosis is most prevalent in Southeast Asia and Africa, and the 20 countries with the highest disease burden, predominantly in Asia and Africa, accounted for 84% of cases in 2019 (see articles by Teo and colleagues and Ryzdak and colleagues in this issue). In patients without travel history outside the United States, residence in communal living facilities, such as homeless shelters, nursing homes, and prisons, is also a risk factor for tuberculosis.

Approximately 90% of patients with an initial tuberculosis infection have an immune response that sequesters the disease such that it never becomes symptomatic, resulting in "latent" tuberculosis. Almost 5% of patients will have an initial uncontained infection, or "primary tuberculosis," and another 5% will initially contain the infection but will later develop active "postprimary tuberculosis."[26] These patients classically develop cavitary disease in the apical and posterior segments of the upper lobes and the superior segments of the lower lobes, possibly because of high oxygen tension and poor lymphatic drainage in those regions. However, the absence of cavitation should not cause a radiologist to exclude tuberculosis. Cavitation is only seen in roughly 20% to 45% of radiographs of patients with active postprimary tuberculosis.[26] In an appropriate clinical setting, any upper lobe opacities should suggest the possibility of tuberculosis. CT increases the sensitivity for the detection of cavitation, identifying smaller and more subtle cavities, but cavitation is still not seen in all patients with active postprimary disease.

In the United States, nontuberculous mycobacterial infection is substantially more common than tuberculosis. Nontuberculous mycobacterial infection has a variety of radiographic presentations, including the "classic" presentation, described as a mimic of tuberculosis, presenting with apical, frequently cavitary, opacities.[26] This manifestation of nontuberculous mycobacterial infection is usually seen in older patients, predominantly those with chronic obstructive pulmonary disease and should be considered in a patient from the United States with radiographic findings like those illustrated in this case.

Case 4

A 19-year-old male presented with symptoms of cough and fever. A chest radiograph (**Fig. 8**) demonstrates opacities in the right mid and lower lung zones with minimal blunting of the right costophrenic angle suggesting a small pleural effusion. These findings in isolation would be consistent with CAP with parapneumonic effusion; however, additional findings include a right paratracheal opacity and enlargement of the right hilum, suggesting lymphadenopathy (see **Fig. 8**, arrows). Radiographically evident lymphadenopathy in the setting of lung opacities should lead to investigation for diseases other than bacterial pneumonia, including malignancy and primary tuberculosis.

Diagnosis: Primary Tuberculosis

Hilar and mediastinal lymph nodes may be enlarged in the setting of infection, but studies in *S pneumoniae* infection and in bacterial empyema demonstrate only mild lymph node enlargement at CT in this setting,[27–29] in keeping with conventional wisdom that lymph nodes that are sufficiently enlarged that they are evident on radiographs are rare in conventional bacterial pneumonia. The differential diagnosis for radiographically evident lymphadenopathy in the setting of acute infection includes infection by atypical pathogens, including fungal infections. Another potential consideration is acute infection in the setting of an underlying disease, such as neoplasm or sarcoidosis. Neoplasm is also a differential consideration for pulmonary opacities with

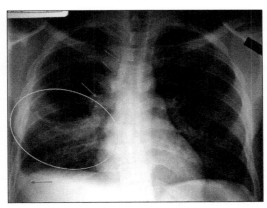

Fig. 8. Case 4. A 19-year-old man presenting with cough and fever. Chest radiograph demonstrates right mid to lower lung heterogeneous opacities (*yellow oval*) with a small right pleural effusion (*blue arrow*). Additional right paratracheal opacities and right hilar enlargement (*red arrows*) are evident.

lymphadenopathy, particularly lymphoma in a young patient such as this one, and also lung carcinoma.

Tuberculosis initially infects the lungs by inhalation of droplet particles, which do not have a strong predilection for specific pulmonary zones but may cause lower lung infection because they are relatively heavy. Primary tuberculosis generally causes nonspecific radiographic opacities that usually are not cavitary and enlargement of ipsilateral hilar and mediastinal lymph nodes, which at CT have low attenuation centrally due to caseation necrosis. These findings usually heal over time as a result of host immune response, frequently although not always leaving calcified nodules and/or calcifications in hilar and mediastinal lymph nodes.

In approximately 5% of patients, the primary infection is not contained; these patients are considered to have progressive primary tuberculosis. Primary tuberculosis has historically been a disease of children, but in the developed world because tuberculosis is less prevalent, it is now the pattern seen in approximately 23% to 34% of cases of tuberculosis in adults.[26]

Case 5

A young woman presented to the emergency department with fever. Clinically, the patient had an acute onset of infectious symptoms, and a radiograph was performed (**Fig. 9**A), which demonstrated bilateral pulmonary opacities. A diagnosis of pulmonary infection was suggested, and the patient was discharged from the emergency department with a prescription for oral antibiotics.

Closer review of the radiograph reveals that the opacities represent scattered bilateral pulmonary nodules, measuring between a centimeter and approximately 3 cm in diameter. Potential causes of multiple pulmonary nodules include metastases; sarcoidosis; vasculitides, particularly granulomatosis with polyangiitis; rheumatoid arthritis; and a few infections. Fungal infections may present with multiple pulmonary nodules; those that are most likely to present this way would be coccidioidomycosis or paracoccidioidomycosis in patients with appropriate travel history or opportunistic fungi such as aspergillosis in immunocompromised patients. In an immunocompetent patient, a common infectious cause of multiple nodules is hematogenous spread of bacterial infection, or septic emboli.

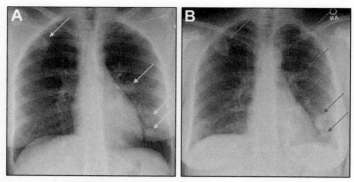

Fig. 9. Case 5. Young woman with fever. (*A*) Initial chest radiograph depicts bilateral nodular opacities (*yellow arrows*) suggesting multifocal community-acquired pneumonia. (*B*) Subsequent chest radiograph 5 days later shows increasing size and number of nodular opacities (*blue arrows*) with more definite cavitation of the right upper lobar nodule (*red arrow*).

Diagnosis: Pulmonary Septic Emboli

This patient returned to the emergency department 5 days later, and, as demonstrated in **Fig. 9**B, the nodules had increased in size and number with a more evident area of cavitation in the nodule at the right lung apex. These findings are consistent with evolution of pulmonary septic emboli. The patient was found to be bacteremic and required intravenous antibiotics as well as echocardiography to exclude endocarditis.

Septic embolism is commonly thought of as occurring in patients with a history of intravenous drug abuse but has also been described in patients with septic thrombophlebitis, classically in the internal jugular vein (Lemierre syndrome); indwelling catheters and other hardware; and other infections, including periodontal infections, pyomyositis, sinusitis and orbital abscess, and abdominal infections.[30] These are severe infections with a reported mortality in some series of approximately 10%. A growing clinical concern is septic emboli from community-acquired infections with methicillin-resistant *S aureus*.

SUMMARY

In conclusion, chest radiography for the investigation of possible CAP remains a common part of radiologic practice. Given this, even in a setting apart from the COVID-19 pandemic, the radiologist can contribute to the care of these patients beyond the simple identification of lobar pneumonia. Radiographs should always be interpreted in light of the clinical setting; subtle findings may correlate with acute interstitial or bronchopneumonia patterns in patients with infectious symptoms, and a masslike presentation that may suggest neoplasm to the untrained observer may also raise the possibility of acute infection. The radiologist should assess for pleural fluid and multilobar involvement, because these may affect clinical decisions about hospital and ICU admission and microbiologic assessment. In contrast, alternative diagnoses should always be considered in patients with a clinical presentation that is discordant from the radiographic finding of apparent pneumonia, at least with follow-up to assess for resolution. When upper lobe cavitation is present, further investigation for tuberculosis should ensue if the onset of symptoms is not acute. Lymphadenopathy evident on a radiograph or multiple pulmonary nodules, particularly when cavitary, should always suggest additional clinical evaluation rather than empirical treatment of CAP. Keeping these principles in mind will allow the radiologist to be a valuable contributor to patient care in the setting of suspected CAP.

CLINICS CARE POINTS

- Chest radiographs in patients with clinical signs and symptoms of pneumonia should be assessed for subtle bronchopneumonia and interstitial patterns of infection and masslike "round pneumonia" in addition to more classic lobar or segmental pneumonia patterns.

- When pneumonia is diagnosed on chest radiographs, reports should always describe pleural fluid and multilobar involvement if present, as these findings may alter management.

- If pneumonia is suspected in patients without classic clinical signs and symptoms of pneumonia, follow-up radiographs should be recommended to confirm the diagnosis based on treatment response and exclude an alternative or underlying process.

- When lymphadenopathy is evident on chest radiographs, atypical infections or neoplasm should be considered as possible diagnoses and, if no immediate further investigation is planned, follow-up radiographs should be obtained.

- If multiple pulmonary nodules are seen in a patient with symptoms of acute respiratory infection, there is a broad differential diagnosis, but septic emboli should be considered.

- Predominantly upper lobe opacities and indolent or subacute presentation should raise the possibility of tuberculosis or nontuberculous mycobacterial infection, particularly when cavitation is present.

DISCLOSURE

None of the authors has a relationship with a commercial company that has a direct financial interest in the subject matter or materials discussed in this article, or with a company making a competing product.

REFERENCES

1. Torres A, Cilloniz C, Niederman MS, et al. Pneumonia. Nat Rev Dis Prim 2021. https://doi.org/10.1038/s41572-021-00259-0.
2. Cao AMY, Choy JP, Mohanakrishnan LN, et al. Chest radiographs for acute lower respiratory tract infections. Cochrane Database Syst Rev 2013;2013(12). https://doi.org/10.1002/14651858.CD009119.pub2.
3. Aagaard E, Maselli J, Gonzales R. Physician practice patterns: chest x-ray ordering for the evaluation of acute cough illness in adults. Med Decis Making 2006;26(6):599–605.
4. Basi SK, Marrie TJ, Huang JQ, et al. Patients admitted to hospital with suspected pneumonia and normal chest radiographs: Epidemiology, microbiology, and outcomes. Am J Med 2004;117(5):305–11.
5. Self WH, Courtney DM, McNaughton CD, et al. High discordance of chest x-ray and computed tomography for detection of pulmonary opacities in ED patients: Implications for diagnosing pneumonia. Am J Emerg Med 2013;31(2):401–5.
6. Claessens Y, Debray M, Tubach F, et al. Early Chest Computed Tomography Scan to Assist Diagnosis and Guide Treatment Decision for Suspected Community-acquired Pneumonia. Am J Respir Crit Care Med 2015;192(8):974–82.

7. Mandell LA, Wunderink RG, Anzueto A, et al. Infectious Diseases Society of America/American Thoracic Society Consensus Guidelines on the management of community-acquired pneumonia in adults. Clin Infect Dis 2007;44(SUPPL. 2).
8. Metlay JP, Waterer GW, Long AC, et al. American thoracic society documents Diagnosis and Treatment of Adults with Community-acquired Pneumonia. Am J Respir Crit Care Med 2019;200(7). https://doi.org/10.1164/rccm.201908-1581ST.
9. Lim W, Baudouin S, George R, et al. BTS guidelines for the management of community acquired pneumonia in adults: update 2009. Thorax 2009;64(Suppl 3). https://doi.org/10.1136/THX.2009.121434.
10. Van Vugt SF, Verheij TJM, De Jong PA, et al. Diagnosing pneumonia in patients with acute cough: Clinical judgment compared to chest radiography. Eur Respir J 2013;42(4):1076–82.
11. Niederman M, Mandell L, Anzueto A, et al. Guidelines for the management of adults with community-acquired pneumonia. Diagnosis, assessment of severity, antimicrobial therapy, and prevention. Am J Respir Crit Care Med 2001;163(7): 1730–54.
12. Bartlett J, Dowell S, Mandell L, et al. Practice guidelines for the management of community-acquired pneumonia in adults. Infectious Diseases Society of America. Clin Infect Dis 2000;31(2):347–82.
13. Tang KL, Eurich DT, Minhas-Sandhu JK, et al. Incidence, correlates,and chest radiographic yield of new lung cancer diagnosis in 3398 patients with pneumonia. Arch Intern Med 2011;171(13):1193–8.
14. Macdonald C, Jayathissa S, Leadbetter M. Is post-pneumonia chest X-ray for lung malignancy useful? Results of an audit of current practice. Intern Med J 2015;45(3):329–34.
15. Fine MJ, Auble TE, Yealy DM, et al. A prediction rule to identify low-risk patients with community-acquired pneumonia. Pneumologie 1997;51(8):834.
16. Hansell DM, McAdams HP. Imaging of diseases of the chest. Mosby, 2010; 2010 [Edinburgh?
17. Fraser RS, Muller NL, Colman N, et al. Fraser and Paré's diagnosis of diseases of the chest. 4th edition. Philadelphia: Saunders, c1999; 1999.
18. Gharib AM, Stern EJ. Radiology of pneumonia. Med Clin North Am 2001;85(6): 1461–91.
19. Boersma WG, Daniels JMA, Löwenberg A, et al. Reliability of radiographic findings and the relation to etiologic agents in community-acquired pneumonia. Respir Med 2006;100(5):926–32.
20. Putman CE, Curtis AM, Simeone JF, et al. Mycoplasma pneumonia. Clinical and roentgenographic patterns. Amerjroentgenol 1975;124(3):417–22.
21. Durning SJ, Sweet JM, Chambers SL. Pulmonary Mass in Tachypneic, Febrile Adult*. Chest 2003;124(1):372–5.
22. Gudbjartsson T, Gudmundsson G. Middle lobe syndrome: a review of clinico-pathological features, diagnosis and treatment. Respiration 2012;84(1):80–6.
23. Humphrey K, Gilman M, Little B, et al. Radiographic follow-up of suspected pneumonia: survey of Society of Thoracic Radiology membership. J Thorac Imaging 2013;28(4):240–3.
24. Gafoor K, Patel S, Girvin F, et al. Cavitary Lung Diseases: A Clinical-Radiologic Algorithmic Approach. Chest 2018;153(6):1443–65.
25. World Health Organization. GLOBAL TUBERCULOSIS REPORT 2020. Published online 2020.
26. Nachiappan A, Rahbar K, Shi X, et al. Pulmonary Tuberculosis: Role of Radiology in Diagnosis and Management. Radiographics 2017;37(1):52–72.

27. Haramati L, Alterman D, White C, et al. Intrathoracic lymphadenopathy in patients with empyema. J Comput Assist Tomogr 1997;21(4):608–11.
28. Stein DL, Haramati LB, Spindola-Franco H, et al. Intrathoracic lymphadenopathy in hospitalized patients with pneumococcal pneumonia. Chest 2005;127(4): 1271–5.
29. Chopra A, Modi A, Chaudhry H, et al. Assessment of Mediastinal Lymph Node Size in Pneumococcal Pneumonia with Bacteremia. Lung 2018;196(1):43–8.
30. Ye R, Zhao L, Wang C, et al. Clinical characteristics of septic pulmonary embolism in adults: A systematic review. Respir Med 2014;108(1):1–8.

The Role of Biomarkers in the Diagnosis and Management of Pneumonia

Sarah Sungurlu, DO, Robert A. Balk, MD*

KEYWORDS

- Biomarkers • Pneumonia diagnosis • Procalcitonin • Scoring systems • Prognosis

KEY POINTS

- Objective criteria and severity scoring system should be supplemented by clinical judgment and evaluation of outside factors, including patient resources, in the diagnosis and management of pneumonia.
- Presently, the diagnosis of pneumonia and the initiation of antibiotics are based on chest radiograph, clinical judgment with guideline-directed antibiotic management not based on the presence or absence of a biomarker.
- Antibiotic stewardship may be enhanced by using biomarkers, specifically procalcitonin, to limit duration of therapy.
- When procalcitonin level is less than 80% of the first peak concentration, or if it reaches an absolute concentration of less than 0.5 ng/mL, a physician is encouraged to stop antibiotics in the treatment of pneumonia as long as this decision is also supported by patient improvement and clinical judgment.
- Biomarkers such as the neutrophil-to-lymphocyte ratio, lactate, and serial procalcitonin clearance, along with severity scoring systems, may be useful in the prognostication of pneumonia.

INTRODUCTION

According to the US Centers for Disease Control and Prevention in 2014, pneumonia and influenza were the eighth leading cause of death in the United States accounting

---

This article was previously published in *Clinics in Chest Medicine* 39:4 December 2018.
Disclosure Statement: Dr S. Sungurlu has no conflicts of interest to disclose. Dr R.A. Balk has received research support and honoraria and participated in advisory boards for BioMerieux, Roche Scientific, and ThermoFisher. He also represented the American College of Chest Physicians in the Multi-Society Panel to the CDC on the definition of Ventilator-Associated Events and Ventilator-Associated Pneumonia.
Division of Pulmonary, Critical Care, and Sleep Medicine, Rush University Medical Center, Rush Medical College, 1725 West Harrison Street Suite 054, Chicago, IL 60612, USA
* Corresponding author.
E-mail address: robert_balk@rush.edu

Infect Dis Clin N Am 38 (2024) 35–49
https://doi.org/10.1016/j.idc.2023.12.005
0891-5520/24/© 2023 Elsevier Inc. All rights reserved.

id.theclinics.com

for 15.9 deaths per 100,000 population. Community-acquired pneumonia (CAP) is diagnosed in approximately 4 million adults in the United States annually and accounts for $10 billion in costs in the United States and €10 billion in Europe.[1] Hospital-acquired pneumonia (HAP) and ventilator-associated pneumonia (VAP) have been associated with increased mortalities, length of hospital stay, and cost of care.[2] Pneumonia is also a frequent cause of sepsis, and sepsis guidelines have emphasized the importance of early initiation of the "correct" antibiotic in order to produce improved outcomes.[3] Guidelines have been published and are widely used to aid the clinician in the initiation of antibiotic treatment of CAP, HAP, and VAP.[2] However, a consequence of early initiation of potent antibiotic treatment to patients suspected of having pneumonia is the potential overtreatment of some non-bacterial-infected patients in order to prevent delayed antibiotic administration to those who do have a bacterial pulmonary infection. Overtreatment with antibiotics and unnecessary antibiotic treatment can give rise to selected pressure on bacteria, result in multidrug-resistant organisms, and give rise to resistant infections, such as *Clostridium difficile*, methicillin-resistant *Staphylococcus aureus*, and fungal superinfections.[4] Balancing appropriate antibiotic use is part of antibiotic stewardship. This process has been aided by rapid assays to detect resistant organisms and sensitivity patterns as well as by the proposed use of biomarkers to help identify selected populations of pneumonia patients who may have more severe disease requiring intensive care unit (ICU) treatment and/or those who more likely have a bacterial pathogen as the cause of the pneumonia.

As defined by the World Health Organization, a biomarker is "any substance, structure, or process that can be measured in the body and influence or predict the incidence or outcome of disease."[5] Several investigations have sought to identify a biomarker or group of biomarkers that can be easily and reliably measured and that will have a high sensitivity, specificity, positive and negative predictive value and demonstrate benefit in the management of patients with pneumonia. Biomarkers have been used to aid in the diagnosis, decision to start antibiotic therapy, assist with triage decisions, determine the duration of antibiotic treatment, and assist with prognostication for patients with pneumonia. Some biomarkers have had greater acceptance compared with others. This article reviews some of the common biomarkers (**Box 1**) used in the diagnosis, management, and treatment of patients with both CAP and HAP. **Box 2** describes some of the ways various biomarkers may be used to assist in the management of patients with pneumonia. The list includes using biomarkers to assist with the diagnosis of pneumonia, severity of illness scoring, risk stratification and triage decisions, initiation of antibiotic therapy, continuation of antibiotic therapy, duration, and/or discontinuation of antibiotic therapy, and with determining the prognosis of patients with suspected pneumonia.

BIOMARKER DIAGNOSIS OF PNEUMONIA

Presently, the diagnosis of pneumonia remains a clinical one and includes an abnormal chest radiograph or chest computed tomographic (CT) scan coupled with clinical criteria that include fever, cough, purulent sputum, chest pain, and often evidence of decrease in oxygen saturation.[4,6] VAP can include similar criteria, but can be more difficult to diagnose because the patients often have preexisting pulmonary infiltrates that account for the reason the patient was on a ventilator in the first place.[2] To aid in the surveillance diagnosis of VAP, a multisociety task force has recently proposed a new diagnostic strategy that includes ventilator-associated events, ventilator-associated conditions, infectious ventilator-associated complications, and possible or

---

Box 1
Common biomarkers used in the diagnosis, management, and treatment of community and/or hospital-acquired pneumonia

Severity scoring systems for severe community-acquired pneumonia

British Thoracic Society (BTS) guideline

CURB-65

CUROX-80

Pneumonia Severity Index (PSI)

IDSA/ATS major and minor criteria to define SCAP

Clinical Pulmonary Infection Score (CPIS)

Selected blood biomarkers

Procalcitonin

C-reactive protein

White blood cell count

Lactate

Soluble triggering receptor expressed on myeloid cells (sTREM)

Pro-adrenomedullin (Pro-ADM)

B-natriuretic peptide (BNP)

Troponin I

Thrombocytopenia

---

probableVAP.[7,8] Several investigators have proposed the use of biomarkers to help establish a diagnosis of VAP and distinguish it from airway colonization or ventilator-associated tracheobronchitis.[9–12] Unfortunately, as of this time, there is no uniformly agreed on biomarker or diagnostic test that on its own will establish the diagnosis of VAP or CAP.

SEVERITY SCORING SYSTEMS

There are several scoring systems to identify patients appropriate for outpatient versus inpatient care, to prognosticate risk of death, and to potentially aid in the

---

Box 2
Biomarker use in pneumonia

Diagnosis of pneumonia

Determining severity of pneumonia with scoring systems

Risk stratification and triage of pneumonia

Initiation of antibiotic therapy

Continuation of antibiotic therapy

Duration/discontinuation of antibiotic therapy (antibiotic stewardship)

Determining prognosis

decision of initiating antibiotics. The Infectious Disease Society of America (IDSA)/ American Thoracic Society (ATS) guidelines suggest that objective criteria or scores should always be supplemented with physician judgment and factors including the ability to take medications and access support resources.[4] Proper triage of CAP patients has been associated with improved survival in comparison to those patients who are initially admitted to a general medical floor and then require transfer to an ICU.[13,14] To aid in the decision of hospital admission as well as the classification of SCAP, there have been several severity of illness scoring systems, some of which are easier to use than others. The authors describe some of the more common severity of pneumonia scoring systems in use today.

British Thoracic Society Guidelines

The original British Thoracic Society (BTS) guidelines, developed in 1987, were based on the finding that the risk of death was increased 21-fold if a patient had 2 of the following 3 criteria on admission: tachypnea (respiratory rate ≥30 breaths per minute), diastolic hypotension (diastolic blood pressure ≤60 mm Hg), elevated blood urea nitrogen (BUN >7 mmol/L).[4] The BTS tool stratified patients into a severe or nonsevere category and had an overall sensitivity and specificity in predicting death of approximately 80%. Lim and colleagues[15] performed a multivariate analysis of 1068 patients in 2003, which expanded on the BTS guidelines and led to the concept of CURB-65 as a tool to define SCAP.

CURB-65

The CURB-65 pneumonia severity score incorporates the BTS guidelines (respiratory rate, hypotension, and BUN) with mental status and age to create a scoring system to aid patient disposition when diagnosed with pneumonia.[15] One point per category is assigned for confusion (based on mental test score <8 or disorientation to person, place or time), urea >7 mmol/L (20 mg/dL), respiratory rate ≥30 breaths per minute, hypotension (systolic blood pressure <90 mm Hg or diastolic ≤60 mm Hg), and age ≥65 years. If the score is 0 to 1, mortality is 1.5%, and therefore, the patient is suitable for home treatment. If the score is 2, the mortality is 9.2% and the physician should consider hospital-supervised treatment (short-stay inpatient or intensive in-home health care services). Finally, if score is ≥3, then mortality is approximately 22%, and in-hospital management for severe pneumonia is recommended with the additional recommendation of assessment for ICU admission (especially if score is >3).[15] This scoring system is rated as a moderate recommendation (level III evidence) in the updated IDSA recommendations based on a validation study, which found that a score of 4 had a mortality of 40% and a score of 5 had a mortality of 57%.[4,16] Of note, for community physicians who do not have access to rapid blood work to obtain a BUN, the simplified CRB-65 was found to also correlate with risk of mortality and need for ventilatory support. For this system, a score of 0 is associated with low mortality (1.2%) and therefore suitable for home; a score of 1 to 2 is intermediate mortality (8.15%) and should have hospital referral and assessment, and a score of ≥3 has a high mortality (31%) and needs urgent hospitalization.[15,16]

CUROX-80

Spanish investigators have developed a severe community-acquired pneumonia (SCAP) prediction rule to aid patient disposition and triage.[17] In their study, 1057 emergency room patients with presumed pneumonia underwent multivariate analyses of 8 predictive factors for SCAP. They included 2 major criteria (1 needed): arterial pH less than 7.30 or systolic blood pressure less than 90 mm Hg, and 6 minor criteria abbreviated CUROX-80 (>2 needed): confusion/altered mental status, urea (BUN >30 mg/dL), respiratory rate greater than 30 breaths per minute, partial pressure of oxygen in arterial blood (P_aO_2) less than 54 mm Hg, or ratio of arterial oxygen tension to fraction of inspired oxygen (P_aO_2/F_iO_2) less than 250, multilobar/bilateral infiltrates on chest radiograph, and age $\geq$80 years old. The SCAP prediction score had a sensitivity and specificity for predicting SCAP of 92.1% and 73.8%, respectively. In comparison, the sensitivity and specificity for CURB-65 in diagnosing SCAP were 68.4% and 86.4%, and Pneumonia Severity Index (PSI) were 94.7% and 68.1%, respectively. The investigators concluded that the SCAP prediction score was more sensitive than CURB-65, but less than PSI, in identifying severe pneumonia.[17]

Pneumonia Severity Index

The PSI is another prognostic model that is based on weighting several comorbidities, clinical findings, and age rather than solely the severity of illness.[4] It has been used as a mortality prediction model and to help determine the need for inpatient admission versus outpatient management as well as to identify the population with a high risk for mortality that should be cared for in the ICU.[4,13] The prediction rule was derived from data on 14,199 adult inpatients with CAP and validated with data on 38,039 inpatients and 2287 mixed inpatients and outpatients with CAP. Patients are stratified into 5 mortality classes according to total points from 20 different variables, including age, presence of coexisting disease, abnormal physical findings (respiratory rate, temperature), and abnormal laboratory findings (pH, BUN, sodium) on presentation. Based on the associated mortality, class I and II should be considered for treatment as an outpatient, class III as a short hospitalization, and class IV and V as an inpatient admission.[4] There are several limitations to PSI, primarily related to the complexity of the tool that necessitates the use of scoring sheets, thereby creating a time constraint and limiting its practice utility.

Infectious Disease Society of America/American Thoracic Society Definition for Severe versus Nonsevere Pneumonia

The 2007 IDSA/ATS CAP guideline established major and minor criteria to diagnose SCAP that required ICU admission with a goal to avoid delayed admission to the ICU.[4] The investigators recognized that there is increased mortality (up to 45%) for patients with CAP that have such delayed transfers to the ICU. A retrospective study of CAP patients admitted to the ICU who were categorized by CURB-65 and PSI led to the observation that both were overly sensitive and nonspecific in comparison to clinical decision, which prompted the IDSA/ATS guideline committee to suggest the following major and minor criteria to define SCAP that should be cared for in the ICU.[13] Both of the 2 major criteria (need for invasive mechanical ventilation or septic shock with need for vasopressors) are absolute indications for admission to the ICU, independently. The presence of 3 or more of the minor criteria is a moderate recommendation for admission to the ICU. The minor criteria include respiratory rate of greater than 30 breaths per minute, P_aO_2/F_iO_2 ratio of less than 250 (or need for noninvasive ventilation), multilobar infiltrates, confusion/disorientation, uremia (BUN >20 mg/dL), leukopenia (<4000 cells/mm^3 caused by infection), thrombocytopenia (<100,000 cells/mm^3), hypothermia (<36°C), and hypotension requiring aggressive fluid resuscitation.[4]

Clinical Pulmonary Infection Score

Unlike the other scoring systems, the Clinical Pulmonary Infection Score (CPIS) was developed as a diagnostic tool for VAP. The score is calculated based on several clinical factors (temperature, white blood cell [WBC] count, oxygenation [$P_{a}O_2/F_iO_2$ ratio], radiographic findings, radiographic progression, tracheal secretions, and culture of tracheal aspirate). Each factor can be scored from 0 to 2 points. If the total is >6 points, this is suggestive of VAP. The 2016 IDSA/ATS guidelines recommend not using the CPIS to aid in the decision to initiate antibiotics based on a meta-analysis of 13 studies, which found a sensitivity of 65% and specificity of 64% to confirm or exclude VAP. Likewise, the IDSA/ATS guidelines do not recommend for the CPIS to be used as an aid in discontinuation of antibiotics after a review of 3 studies had inconsistent evidence, suggesting it does not reliably discriminate patients who can have their antibiotics safely discontinued.[2]

SELECTED BIOMARKERS AND THEIR ROLE
Procalcitonin

Arguably, the most commonly used biomarker in the diagnosis and management of pneumonia is procalcitonin (PCT), which is a 116-amino-acid peptide produced by the liver as an acute phase reactant as well as by thyroid C cells and lung K cells.[11,18] PCT is then cleaved into the hormone calcitonin, katacalcin, and an N-terminal fragment. Bacterium-specific proinflammatory cytokines (interleukin-1beta [IL-1β], tumor necrosis factor-alpha [TNF-α], IL6) as well as microbial toxins (endotoxins) stimulate nonneuroendocrine calcitonin gene expression and release of PCT from parenchymal tissue, such as the liver. For this reason, the circulating PCT level elevates without a corresponding increase in the circulating calcitonin level during this inflammatory response. In contrast, viral infections stimulate release of interferon-γ, which along with other cytokines downregulates this pathway. Therefore, although PCT may have some increase in response to sterile inflammation or viral infection, it is less profound than other biomarkers.[11] However, PCT can be falsely low in some localized infections, such as abscesses or empyema.[19] Because the cleavage of PCT occurs before release of calcitonin, healthy individuals normally have a very low circulating level (<0.1 ng/mL).[11] It is released into the circulation within 6 to 12 hours of infection, and the half-life is approximately 25 to 30 hours.[20]

C-Reactive Protein

C-reactive protein (CRP) is a pentameric protein, with 5 identical noncovalently bound subunits, synthesized by hepatocytes (molecular mass 118,000 Da). Infection or inflammation can generate cytokine release (IL-6, IL-1, and TNF-α), which then stimulates CRP synthesis. As a nonspecific acute phase reactant, it cannot accurately differentiate potential sources of tissue destruction.[21] However, there is a reasonable correlation between the severity of sepsis and degree of organ failure with CRP concentrations.[22]

White Blood Cell

Both the elevation and the depression of white blood cell (WBC) count are used to aid in the diagnosis of infection. In addition, the differential of WBCs (neutrophil to lymphocyte count ratio) can provide information on the type of response. For example, leukopenia has been associated with an increased mortality.[20]

Lactate

Normal healthy patients have a circulating blood lactate level of 0.5 to 1 mmol/L, and patients with critical illness can have normal concentrations up to 2 mmol/L. Lactate production by anaerobic metabolism (type A lactic acidosis) is used as a marker for tissue hypoperfusion and sepsis. It is clinically necessary to distinguish type B lactic acidosis (B1, liver failure; B2, drug or toxins; B3, errors of metabolism). In addition, decreased lactate clearance (primarily liver and to some extent kidney) can contribute to increased concentration of lactate not correlated with tissue hypoxia.[23]

Soluble Triggering Receptor Expressed on Myeloid Cells

An activating receptor that is expressed on the surface of neutrophils, mature monocytes, and macrophages, which amplifies the inflammatory response synergistically with the toll-like receptor signaling pathway when stimulated by bacteria or fungi.[5,24] As opposed to the membranous form, soluble triggering receptor expressed on myeloid cells (sTREM) is known to be specifically released during infectious processes.[25]

Pro-Adrenomedullin

Adrenomedullin is also a member of the calcitonin family. It acts as a vasodilating agent with immune modulating, metabolic, and bactericidal activity. However, with its rapid degradation and clearance, it is not stable, and therefore, for improved reliability, the midregional fragment Pro-Adrenomedullin (Pro-ADM) is measured.[19] The midregional fragment Pro-ADM seems to correlate with the severity of pneumonia and the intensity of the inflammatory cytokine response to the infection, but may also be elevated in heart failure and/or renal dysfunction (**Box 3**).[26]

USE OF BIOMARKERS FOR DIAGNOSIS

The diagnosis of pneumonia is predominantly based on an abnormal chest radiograph or chest CT scan coupled with clinical manifestations of cough, fever, purulent sputum, elevated WBC count, in addition to absence of another likely explanation for the clinical findings and radiographic abnormalities.[4,6] With the recognition that most of the time the cause of CAP is undetermined or viral, it has been advocated that use of biomarkers specific for bacterial infection would be beneficial in defining the patient population that would benefit from antibiotic administration.[4,27,28] In the era of rapidly advancing antibiotic resistance and a greater number of infections with multiple drug-resistant organisms, it would be beneficial to have either rapid determination of the causative organism and/or the availability of a biomarker or biomarkers that would signify a bacterial infection that requires antibiotic treatment. Of the currently used biomarkers, PCT has shown the most promise in aiding in the diagnosis of bacterial infections, including pneumonia.[19] However, there still are several limitations. Localized infections, such as empyema, may have no systemic release of PCT (only localized synthesis). ICU patients often suffer from sepsis, shock, or multiorgan failure, or can have the systemic inflammatory response syndrome (SIRS) from surgery and/or trauma, all of which can raise the PCT without the presence of a bacterial infection. Finally, a time lag of 24 to 48 hours can exist between bacterial infection onset and peak PCT, and therefore, at the time of diagnosis, there may be a false low PCT level.[11] PCT levels were helpful in diagnosing bacterial infection in immunosuppressed organ transplant recipients, even in the setting of acute rejection.[29–31] The PCT elevations in the setting of infection are not influenced by the use of corticosteroids, immunosuppressants, or leukopenia.[29–31] In a prospective study of postoperative infections in adult patients who underwent vascular surgery, significant elevations in PCT levels were found in those patients who had renal dysfunction in comparison to normal renal function.[32] Although the diagnostic accuracy of PCT to detect bacterial infection was still present, the threshold for determining bacterial infection needed to be adjusted upward.[32]

Box 3
Use of selected biomarkers in pneumonia management

Procalcitonin (PCT)
   Diagnosis of bacterial versus nonbacterial infection
   Need for antibiotic therapy
   Prediction of severity of CAP (ICU admission/triaging emergency room patients)
   Prognosis of pneumonia patients
   Duration of antibiotic treatment

C-reactive protein (CRP)
   Prediction of severity of CAP
   Diagnosis of bacterial versus nonbacterial infection

Pro-adrenomedullin (Pro-ADM)
   Severity of CAP

B-natriuretic peptide (BNP)
   Severity of CAP

Troponin I
   Degree of hypoxemia: severity of illness

Soluble triggering receptor expressed on myeloid cells (sTREM)
   Diagnosis of VAP

Lactate
   Severity of pneumonia
   Prognosis and mortality prediction

White blood cells
   Severity of pneumonia

Thrombocytopenia
   Severity of pneumonia

P_aO_2/F_iO_2 Ratio
   Degree of oxygenation abnormality

Most of the data in support of using initial PCT levels to determine which patients with a presumed lower respiratory tract infection (LRTI) require antibiotic treatment has come from European studies, predominantly conducted in Switzerland and Germany.[33–35] ProHosp, a large multicenter trial conducted in Switzerland with 1825 patients, found that in patients with LRTI PCT guidance compared with standard guidelines reduced antibiotic exposure and adverse effects associated with antibiotic use without adversely affecting patient outcomes.[35] Schuetz and colleagues[27] included acute bronchitis, acute exacerbations of chronic obstructive pulmonary disease, and pneumonia in their definition of LRTI, noting that 75% of LRTIs are treated with antibiotics despite a predominant viral cause. However, for the creation of the IDSA/ATS guideline, a meta-analysis looking at 6 studies (665 participants) found a low sensitivity of 67% and specificity of 83% for PCT in the diagnosis of HAP/VAP. Therefore, the IDSA/ATS guideline has a strong recommendation against use of PCT with clinical criteria to decide when to initiate antibiotics.[2]

Many of the previously mentioned biomarkers have been studied as potential tools for the diagnosis of pneumonia, but have thus far failed to show reproducible benefit. Systemic sTREM levels, along with the presence of 2 of the SIRS criteria, have been used to help differentiate patients with and without underlying infection.[24] However, there have been contradictory findings for measuring sTREM in bronchoalveolar lavage (BAL) fluid for the diagnosis of VAP.[12,36] In a meta-analysis of 6 studies, including 2008 patients with clinically suspected pneumonia, the sensitivity for sTREM was 84% and specificity was 49% for the diagnosis of HAP/VAP. Therefore, The IDSA/ATS guidelines give a strong recommendation against use of BAL fluid sTREM level plus clinical criteria to decide when to start antibiotic therapy.[2]

In a study of 48 patients, using the CRP threshold level of greater than 9.6 mg/dL, the sensitivity was 87.5% and the specificity was 86.1% for the diagnosis of VAP.[22] In addition, a meta-analysis of 3 studies found that in critically ill patients with and without pneumonia, the CRP levels were the same. Therefore, like sTREM, the IDSA/ATS guidelines give a strong recommendation against use of serum CRP plus clinical criteria to decide when to start antibiotics.[2]

USE OF BIOMARKERS FOR RISK STRATIFICATION

Another role for biomarkers is to aid in risk stratification for patients with pneumonia, including inpatient versus outpatient treatment and ICU versus general medical floor (GMF) admission.[4,13,15] As previously discussed, many of the severity scoring indices are used for this purpose. A systematic review and meta-analysis compared the performance of PSI, CURB-65, CRB-65, and CURB. The sensitivity and specificity for differentiating survivors versus nonsurvivors were 90% and 53% for PSI, 62% and 79% for CURB-65, 33% and 92% for CRB-65, and 63% and 77% for CURB, respectively.[37] For the identification of SCAP, the SCAP prediction score (CUROX-80) had a sensitivity and specificity of 92.1% and 73.8%, compared with 68.4% and 86.4% for CURB-65, and 94.7% and 68.1% for PSI.[17] The IDSA/ATS guidelines created severe versus nonsevere pneumonia major and minor criteria due to concerns that the PSI and CURB-65 were overly sensitive and not specific enough for clinical decision making.[13] The accuracy of the minor severity criteria of the IDSA/ATS guidelines was better than biomarkers alone in predicting ICU admission. In a secondary analysis of 453 CAP patients admitted to the ICU within 3 days of emergency room presentation, there was a decreased mortality (11.7% versus 23.4% [odds ratio, OR, 2.31, confidence interval, CI, 1.11–4.77, $P<.02$]) and shorter length of stay (7 versus 13 days [OR 0.55, CI 0.40–0.76, $P<.001$]) when the patient was initially admitted to the ICU compared with delayed ICU admission.[14] Biomarkers and scoring systems can improve clinical decision-making and triaging ability so that patients are admitted to the best unit for care. For example, a patient who has severe pneumonia, defined by the IDSA/ATS minor criteria, but a low level of PCT may be safely admitted to GMF.[38] The addition of biomarkers, such as CRP or PCT, to pneumonia severity scores will assist with the identification of those patients with greater need for hospital or even ICU management.[26] Much of the focus on the addition of biomarkers to pneumonia severity scores has been directed toward determining which patients will benefit from antibiotic therapy and which patients do not require antibiotic therapy. In the United States, antibiotic decisions are primarily based on guidelines that classify patients based on clinical presentation, risk factors, and assessment of severity of their clinical illness. All agree that serum PCT or CRP levels on their own should not be used as a stand-alone tool to identify those patients with bacterial pneumonia or to determine the type of bacterial infection.[39] There are data that suggest that atypical bacteria may not generate the same degree of PCT increase as is seen with other bacterial infections.[39] In a study of 1770 adult CAP patients, the degree of PCT elevation on initial presentation was strongly associated with the risk of requiring invasive respiratory and/or vasopressor support during the ensuing 72 hours.[40]

USE OF BIOMARKERS FOR INITIATION, CONTINUATION, AND DURATION OF ANTIBIOTIC THERAPY

Promoting antibiotic stewardship, and thereby decreasing costs and side effects, is where biomarkers have shown the most promise. The PNEUMA trial compared 401 patients with VAP who received antibiotics for 15 days versus 8 days and found the shorter duration did not have poorer outcomes.[41] They did have a slightly higher rate of recurrent pulmonary infections, however. PCT-guided algorithms for antibiotic stewardship in critically ill patients with VAP had similar mortalities, ICU length of stay, and comparable superinfection and relapsed infection rates.[41] The PRORATA trial looked at a PCT-based algorithm wherein physicians were encouraged to start antibiotics if PCT level was greater than 0.5 ng/mL and discouraged from starting antibiotics if it was less, although their clinical judgment overruled any level. Six hundred twenty-one patients were randomized to receive treatment based on physician judgment versus the PCT level guided algorithm. If a patient did receive antibiotics, a daily PCT was drawn, and when the level was less than 80% of the first peak concentration, or if it reached an absolute concentration of less than 0.5 ng/mL, the physician was encouraged to stop the antibiotics (again physician clinical judgment overruled any level). The PCT-guided algorithm had significantly more antibiotic-free days than the control (absolute difference of 2.7 days) without an increase in adverse outcomes (comparable day 28 and day 60 mortalities).[11]

PCT-guided antibiotic treatment versus usual care for septic patients was evaluated in a prospective, multicenter, randomized, controlled, open-label trial conducted in 15 hospitals in the Netherlands.[42] There was nonbinding advice given to the PCT-guided clinicians when the PCT level decreased by greater than 80% from the peak level or to a level of $\leq$0.5 μg/L to discontinue antibiotic therapy, whereas the usual care patients were managed according to the local standard of care for antibiotic use and duration. The PCT guidance was associated with a reduction in the duration of antibiotic treatment and decreased daily defined doses of antibiotic therapy. In addition to the reduced antibiotic therapy, the PCT-guided therapy was also associated with a significant decrease in 28-day (20% vs 25% [between group absolute difference 5.4%, 95% CI 1.2–9.5, $P = .0122$]) and 1-year mortality (36% vs 43% [between groups absolute difference 7.4, 95% CI 1.3-13.8, $P = .0188$]) rates in comparison to usual care.[42] Schuetz and colleagues[43] reviewed 14 clinical trials involving more than 4200 patients and concluded that using PCT to guide antibiotic discontinuation was not associated with increased mortality or treatment failure. Multiple meta-analyses have also supported a beneficial role for the use of serial PCT to decrease the duration of antibiotic therapy and potentially improve antibiotic stewardship.[27,44,45]

Lam and colleagues[46] conducted a systematic review and meta-analysis of the use of PCT versus usual care to guide the antimicrobial management (initiation, cessation, or mixed approach) in critically ill patients. Their analysis of the 15 studies that met the inclusion and exclusion criteria was that overall PCT guidance did not decrease short-term mortality. However, studies of PCT-guided antibiotic cessation were associated with decreased antibiotic duration and decreased mortality. The use of PCT to guide antibiotic initiation or using PCT in a mixed approach for initiation and cessation did not decrease mortality. There was also no difference in ICU length of stay, hospital length of stay, or recurrent infection.[46] Iankova and coworkers[47] conducted a systematic review and meta-analysis of the efficacy and safety of PCT guidance of antibiotic therapy in patients with suspected or confirmed sepsis. They included 10 randomized controlled trials that included 3489 patients and found that PCT guidance decreased antibiotic duration and there was no adverse impact on mortality or length of stay in the ICU.[47] Presently, there is a weak recommendation by the IDSA/ATS guidelines for the use of PCT levels plus clinical criteria to guide discontinuation of antibiotics in VAP patients. This recommendation is based on a systematic review of 14 randomized trials (4221 patients), which concluded that PCT-based decision making was able decrease the antibiotic exposure (adjusted mean difference of 3.47 days) and was not associated with increased treatment failure or mortality.[2]

USE OF BIOMARKERS FOR PROGNOSIS

The PSI and CURB-65, as previously discussed, are key scoring systems that have demonstrated utility in prognostication of pneumonia. Individual biomarkers have also been studied in their prognostic utility. There has been evidence suggesting that neutrophil to lymphocyte ratio (NTLR) can be used as a prognostic marker. During systemic inflammation, the demargination of neutrophils and stimulation of stem cells by granulocyte colony stimulating factor lead to neutrophilia, whereas accelerated apoptosis and margination and redistribution of lymphocytes cause lymphocytopenia. A prospective study with 195 CAP elderly patients looked at the NTLR as a predictor for mortality. The area under the curve (AUC) for NTLR was 0.95, higher compared with CRP (0.49), WBC count (0.55), PSI (0.87), and CURB-65 (0.61).[48]

In a multicenter prospective cohort study of 1653 emergency department patients, pro-ADM levels increased in correlation with increasing severity of illness and death.[49] The median pro-ADM level in 30-day nonsurvivors was 1.6 mmol/L versus 0.9 mmol/L in survivors. The optimal prognostic cutoff with maximum combined sensitivity and specificity for pro-ADM was determined to be 1.3 mmol/L with a sensitivity of 68% and specificity of 73% for 30-day mortality. However, high pro-ADM levels did not alter PSI risk assessment in most CAP patients and had no additional stratification benefit in high-risk CAP patients.[49]

Lactate and lactate clearance are other commonly used biomarkers for prognostication.[3,50] In normotensive patients with sepsis, lactate is closely monitored because it is independently correlated with a higher mortality if it remains greater than 4 mmol/L.[23] A retrospective observational study of 553 CAP patients calculated a national early warning score-lactate score (NEWS-L score) based on systolic blood pressure, heart rate, respiratory rate, temperature, pulse oximetry, supplemental oxygen use, and lactate level. This study found that the mean lactate level was 1.6 and was significantly higher in nonsurvivors versus survivors (2.5 vs 1.5). In addition, the NEWS-L score was comparable to PSI and CURB-65 in predicting inpatient mortality in adult CAP patients.[51]

PCT levels have been shown to increase with severity of pneumonia, unlike WBC or CRP.[52] In a prospective observational cohort study, looking at 472 patients admitted to the ICU, daily PCT measurements were followed. A high maximum PCT level and a PCT increase for 1 day were found to be independent predictors of 90-day mortality, with a relative risk after 1-day increase of 1.8, after 2-day increase of 2.2, and 3-day increase of 2.8.[52,53] The German multicenter CAPNETZ trial looked at 1671 patients with CAP (66.6% of whom were hospitalized, whereas the remainder were treated as outpatients) and followed their PCT, CRP, WBC, and CRB-65 for 28 days.[33] The PCT level on admission had a similar prognostic accuracy (looking at severity and outcome) to CRB-65 and a higher prognostic accuracy than CRP and leukocyte count. PCT on admission in nonsurvivors (median of 0.88) was significantly higher than that of survivors (median of 0.13). The optimal prognostic accuracy for mortality prediction with PCT was with a cutoff of 0.228 ng/mL (sensitivity of 84.3% and specificity of 66.6%). The AUC for PCT was 0.80, which was not significantly different than CRB-

65 (0.79), but significantly higher than CRP (0.62) or WBC (0.61). By combining PCT and CRB-65, the AUC improved to 0.83.[33]

Another large prospective randomized trial by Schuetz and colleagues[53] demonstrated that PCT on admission had only a moderate prognostic ability to predict 30-day mortality, but follow-up PCT measurements did show better prognostic performance. Specifically, the increase in PCT from day 0 to day 3, with a less pronounced PCT decrease thereafter, was identified in nonsurvivors. In addition, the risk of adverse events significantly increased by 3-fold from 6% in the lowest PCT tier to 19% in the highest tier. These data support the idea that a serial PCT increase accurately prognosticates the potential for adverse events associated with CAP, including ICU admission and empyema.[53] Another prospective observational study performed on 63 patients with VAP measured PCT and CRP on days 1 and 7 and likewise found that using a PCT threshold of 0.5 ng/mL on day 7, PCT had a 90% sensitivity and 88% specificity for unfavorable outcomes (including death, VAP recurrence, and extrapulmonary infections).[41]

The MOSES study was a large prospective, multicenter, US trial that evaluated the ability of serial PCT levels to predict mortality in 858 patients admitted to the ICU for treatment of severe sepsis. The patients who were not able to decrease their PCT level by greater than 80% by day 4 were found to have an increase in their 28-day mortality compared with the patients who were able to achieve a greater than 80% reduction in PCT by day 4.[34]

SUMMARY

The use of various biomarkers in the management of pneumonia patients can help identify those patients who should be admitted to the hospital, cared for in the ICU, and may help with decisions related to duration of antibiotic therapy and/or patient prognosis. At this time, there is not a biomarker that on its own will establish a diagnosis of pneumonia. Current US standard of care supports the decision on initiation of antibiotic therapy and the type of antibiotic therapy based on guidelines and a clinical assessment of the patient, which is typically aided by severity guidelines with or without the use of additional biomarkers. As more sensitive and specific biomarkers are found and greater experience is obtained with the use of biomarkers, there may be an expanded use for biomarkers in the diagnosis, management, and treatment of pneumonia in the future.

REFERENCES

1. Fine MJ, Auble TE, Yealy DM, et al. A prediction rule to identify low-risk patients with community-acquired pneumonia. N Engl J Med 1997;336(4):243–50.
2. Kalil AC, Metersky ML, Klompas M, et al. Management of adults with hospital-acquired and ventilator-associated pneumonia: 2016 clinical practice guidelines by the infectious diseases society of America and the American Thoracic Society. Clin Infect Dis 2016;63(5):e61–111.
3. Dellinger RP, Levy MM, Rhodes A, et al. Surviving sepsis campaign: international guidelines for management of severe sepsis and septic shock: 2012. Crit Care Med 2013;41(2):580–637.
4. Mandell LA, Wunderink RG, Anzueto A, et al. Infectious Diseases Society of America/American Thoracic Society consensus guidelines on the management of community-acquired pneumonia in adults. Clin Infect Dis 2007;44(Suppl 2): S27–72.

5. Kaziani K, Sotiriou A, Dimopoulos G. Duration of pneumonia therapy and the role of biomarkers. Curr Opin Infect Dis 2017;30(2):221–5.
6. Musher DM, Thorner AR. Community-acquired pneumonia. N Engl J Med 2014; 371(17):1619–28.
7. Klompas M. Ventilator-associated conditions versus ventilator-associated pneumonia: different by design. Curr Infect Dis Rep 2014;16(10):430.
8. Magill SS, Klompas M, Balk R, et al. Developing a new, national approach to surveillance for ventilator-associated events*. Crit Care Med 2013;41(11):2467–75.
9. Craven DE, Chroneou A, Zias N, et al. Ventilator-associated tracheobronchitis: the impact of targeted antibiotic therapy on patient outcomes. Chest 2009;135(2): 521–8.
10. Nseir S, Favory R, Jozefowicz E, et al. Antimicrobial treatment for ventilator-associated tracheobronchitis: a randomized, controlled, multicenter study. Crit Care 2008;12(3):R62.
11. Brechot N, Hekimian G, Chastre J, et al. Procalcitonin to guide antibiotic therapy in the ICU. Int J Antimicrob Agents 2015;46(Suppl 1):S19–24.
12. Gibot S, Cravoisy A, Levy B, et al. Soluble triggering receptor expressed on myeloid cells and the diagnosis of pneumonia. N Engl J Med 2004;350(5):451–8.
13. Angus DC, Marrie TJ, Obrosky DS, et al. Severe community-acquired pneumonia: use of intensive care services and evaluation of American and British Thoracic Society Diagnostic criteria. Am J Respir Crit Care Med 2002;166(5): 717–23.
14. Renaud B, Santin A, Coma E, et al. Association between timing of intensive care unit admission and outcomes for emergency department patients with community-acquired pneumonia. Crit Care Med 2009;37(11):2867–74.
15. Lim WS, van der Eerden MM, Laing R, et al. Defining community acquired pneumonia severity on presentation to hospital: an international derivation and validation study. Thorax 2003;58(5):377–82.
16. Capelastegui A, Espana PP, Quintana JM, et al. Validation of a predictive rule for the management of community-acquired pneumonia. Eur Respir J 2006;27(1): 151–7.
17. Espana PP, Capelastegui A, Gorordo I, et al. Development and validation of a clinical prediction rule for severe community-acquired pneumonia. Am J Respir Crit Care Med 2006;174(11):1249–56.
18. Gilbert DN. Use of plasma procalcitonin levels as an adjunct to clinical microbiology. J Clin Microbiol 2010;48(7):2325–9.
19. Christ-Crain M, Schuetz P, Muller B. Biomarkers in the management of pneumonia. Expert Rev Respir Med 2008;2(5):565–72.
20. Nair GB, Niederman MS. Pneumonia: considerations for the critically ill patient. In: Parrillo JE, Dellinger RP, editors. Critical care medicine: principles of diagnosis and management in the adult. 4h edition. Philadelphia: Elsevier/Saunders; 2013. p. 1, online resource (xx, 1447 pages).
21. Lee JH, Kim J, Kim K, et al. Albumin and C-reactive protein have prognostic significance in patients with community-acquired pneumonia. J Crit Care Jun 2011; 26(3):287–94.
22. Povoa P, Coelho L, Almeida E, et al. C-reactive protein as a marker of infection in critically ill patients. Clin Microbiol Infect 2005;11(2):101–8.
23. Suetrong B, Walley KR. Lactic acidosis in sepsis: it's not all anaerobic: implications for diagnosis and management. Chest 2016;149(1):252–61.
24. Ewig S, Welte T. Biomarkers in the diagnosis of pneumonia in the critically ill: don't shoot the piano player. Intensive Care Med 2008;34(6):981–4.

25. Kopterides P, Siempos II, Tsangaris I, et al. Procalcitonin-guided algorithms of antibiotic therapy in the intensive care unit: a systematic review and meta-analysis of randomized controlled trials. Crit Care Med 2010;38(11):2229–41.
26. Schuetz P, Christ-Crain M, Muller B. Biomarkers to improve diagnostic and prognostic accuracy in systemic infections. Curr Opin Crit Care 2007;13:578–85.
27. Schuetz P, Christ-Crain M, Thomann R, et al. Effect of procalcitonin-based guidelines vs standard guidelines on antibiotic use in lower respiratory tract infections: the ProHOSP randomized controlled trial. JAMA 2009;302(10):1059–66.
28. Schuetz P, Albrich W, Christ-Crain M, et al. Procalcitonin for guidance of antibiotic therapy. Expert Rev Anti Infect Ther 2010;8(5):575–87.
29. Delevaux I, Andre M, Colombier M, et al. Can Procalcitonin measurement help in differentiating between bacterial infection and other kinds of inflammatory processes? Ann Rheum Dis 2003;62:337–40.
30. Staehler M, Hammer C, Meiser B, et al. Differential Diagnosis of acute rejection and infection with procalcitonin and cytokines. Langenbecks Arch Chir 1997;1: 205–9.
31. Al Nawas B, Shah PM. Procalcitonin in patients with and without immunosuppression and sepsis. Infection 1996;24:434–6.
32. Amour J, Birenbaum A, Langeron O, et al. Influence of renal dysfunction on the accuracy of procalcitonin for the diagnosis of postoperative infection after vascular surgery. Crit Care Med 2008;36:1147–54.
33. Kruger S, Ewig S, Marre R, et al. Procalcitonin predicts patients at low risk of death from community-acquired pneumonia across all CRB-65 classes. The Eur Respir J 2008;31(2):349–55.
34. Schuetz P, Birkhahn R, Sherwin R, et al. Serial procalcitonin predicts mortality in severe sepsis patients: results from the multicenter procalcitonin MOnitoring SEpsis (MOSES) study. Crit Care Med 2017;45(5):781–9.
35. Schuetz P, Wirz Y, Sager R, et al. Effect of procalcitonin-guided antibiotic treatment on mortality in acute respiratory infections: a patient level meta-analysis. Lancet Infect Dis 2018;18(1):95–107.
36. Phua J, Koay ES, Zhang D, et al. Soluble triggering receptor expressed on myeloid cells-1 in acute respiratory infections. The Eur Respir J 2006;28(4): 695–702.
37. Loke YK, Kwok CS, Niruban A, et al. Value of severity scales in predicting mortality from community-acquired pneumonia: systematic review and meta-analysis. Thorax 2010;65(10):884–90.
38. Ramirez P, Ferrer M, Marti V, et al. Inflammatory biomarkers and prediction for intensive care unit admission in severe community-acquired pneumonia. Crit Care Med 2011;39(10):2211–7.
39. Schuetz P, Amin DN, Greenwalkd JL. Role of procalcitonin in managing adult patients with respiratory tract infections. Chest 2012;141:1063–73.
40. Self WH, Grijalva CG, Williams DJ, et al. Procalcitonin as an early marker of the need for invasive respiratory or vasopressor support in adults with community-acquired pneumonia. Chest 2016;150:819–28.
41. Luyt CE, Guerin V, Combes A, et al. Procalcitonin kinetics as a prognostic marker of ventilator-associated pneumonia. Am J Respir Crit Care Med 2005;171(1): 48–53.
42. de Jong E, van Oers JA, Beishuizen A, et al. Efficacy and safety of procalcitonin guidance in reducing the duration of antibiotic treatment in critically ill patients: a randomised, controlled, open-label trial. The Lancet Infect Dis 2016;16(7): 819–27.

43. Schuetz P, Briel M, Mueller B. Clinical outcomes associated with procalcitonin algorithms to guide antibiotic therapy in respiratory tract infections. JAMA 2013; 309(7):717–8.
44. Huang HB, Peng JM, Weng L, et al. Procalcitonin-guided antibiotic therapy in intensive care unit patients: a systematic review and meta-analysis. Ann Intensive Care 2017;7(1):114.
45. Schuetz P, Wirz Y, Sager R, et al. Procalcitonin to initiate or discontinue antibiotics in acute respiratory tract infections. Cochrane Database Syst Rev 2017;(10):CD007498.
46. Lam SW, Bauer SR, Fowler R, et al. Systematic review and meta-analysis of procalcitonin-guidance versus usual care for antimicrobial management in critically ill patients: focus on subgroups based on antibiotic initiation, cessation, or mixed strategies. Crit Care Med 2018;46:684–90.
47. Iankova I, Thompson-Leduc P, Kirson NY, et al. Efficacy and safety of procalcitonin guidance in patients with suspected or confirmed sepsis: a systematic review and meta-analysis. Crit Care Med 2018;46:691–8.
48. Cataudella E, Giraffa CM, Di Marca S, et al. Neutrophil-to-lymphocyte ratio: an emerging marker predicting prognosis in elderly adults with community-acquired pneumonia. J Am Geriatr Soc 2017;65(8):1796–801.
49. Huang DT, Angus DC, Kellum JA, et al. Midregional proadrenomedullin as a prognostic tool in community-acquired pneumonia. Chest 2009;136(3):823–31.
50. Gu WJ, Zhang Z, Bakker J. Early lactate clearance-guided therapy in patients with sepsis: a meta-analysis with trial sequential analysis of randomized controlled trials. Intensive Care Med 2015;41(10):1862–3.
51. Jo S, Jeong T, Lee JB, et al. Validation of modified early warning score using serum lactate level in community-acquired pneumonia patients. The National Early Warning Score-Lactate score. Am J Emerg Med 2016;34(3):536–41.
52. Jensen JU, Heslet L, Jensen TH, et al. Procalcitonin increase in early identification of critically ill patients at high risk of mortality. Crit Care Med 2006;34(10): 2596–602.
53. Schuetz P, Suter-Widmer I, Chaudri A, et al. Prognostic value of procalcitonin in community-acquired pneumonia. Eur Respir J 2011;37(2):384–92.

Novel and Rapid Diagnostics for Common Infections in the Critically Ill Patient

Chiagozie I. Pickens, MD[a],*, Richard G. Wunderink, MD[a]

KEYWORDS

- Rapid diagnostic • Molecular • Antibiotic stewardship • Infection • Critical care

KEY POINTS

- Diagnosing infection in critically ill patients is complex and can be limited by the long turn-around time and poor sensitivity of standard culture.
- Some advantages of rapid diagnostic tests include semiautomated protocols, short turn-around times, and high sensitivity and specificity.
- There are multiple single-target and multiplex culture-independent assays to rapidly detect organisms from respiratory samples.
- Some novel diagnostics for bloodstream infection can be direct from whole blood, by-passing the need for a positive culture.
- Rapid diagnostics for intraabdominal, genitourinary, and neurologic infection exist; however, the impact on clinically important outcomes is unclear.

INTRODUCTION

Infection associated with sepsis is the most common immediate cause of death in the intensive care unit (ICU).[1,2] The ICU mortality rate of critically ill patients with infection ranges from 25% to 60%, more than twice the mortality rate of noninfected critically ill patients.[3,4] Infection in critically ill patients is also an independent risk factor for delirium, acute renal failure, and increased hospital length of stay.[5] The economic burden of hospital-acquired infections in the United States is estimated to be $9.8 billion dollars yearly with infections common in the critically ill, such as ventilator-associated pneumonia (VAP), making up a significant proportion of the cost.[6] For these reasons, a comprehensive understanding of diagnostic tools for common infections in ICU patients is important for clinicians.

This article was previously published in *Clinics in Chest Medicine* 43:3 September 2022.
[a] Department of Medicine, Pulmonary and Critical Care Division, Northwestern University Feinberg School of Medicine, 303 E. Superior Street Simpson Querrey 5th Floor, Suite 5-406, Chicago, IL 60611-2909, USA
* Corresponding author.
E-mail address: chiagozie-ononye@northwestern.edu

Infect Dis Clin N Am 38 (2024) 51–63
https://doi.org/10.1016/j.idc.2023.12.003
0891-5520/24/© 2023 Elsevier Inc. All rights reserved.

id.theclinics.com

Detection of infection in critically ill patients is complex. First, a history localizing infectious symptoms is often difficult to obtain because patients are unable to communicate due to pain, agitation, encephalopathy, and/or intubation. Second, typical signs of infection such as tachypnea, leukocytosis, or tachycardia may not be present in critically ill patients with sepsis.[7] Conversely, these signs may be present in noninfected critically ill patients, often leading to excessive antibiotic use in this population.[8] Third, infection is a continuous threat to a critically ill patient and thus a negative diagnostic workup is only valid for a limited amount of time. The risk of infection increases as ICU length of stay increases, particularly for infection with drug-resistant organisms.[3] This increase creates the challenge of deciding when to repeat an infectious workup and when to initiate or deescalate antibiotic therapy. Fourth, critically ill patients are subject to atypical and opportunistic pathogens that are often difficult to detect with standard diagnostic tests. And lastly, the tenuous status of many critically ill patients due to the underlying disease that caused ICU admission often creates a sense of urgency regarding "missing" an infection, leading to greater reliance on empirical antibiotic use. These factors contribute to the challenge of identifying infection in the ICU. Unfortunately, the complexity of detecting infection in critically ill patients is further heightened by the limitations of current diagnostic tools. This review discusses the advantages and disadvantages of current diagnostics tools and describe some of the available novel rapid diagnostic tests (RDT) for evaluating infection in an ICU population.

Traditional Diagnostic Techniques

In the clinical setting, semiquantitative culture is perhaps the test most commonly used to diagnose infection. Culture is prepared by using aseptic technique to inoculate growth media with a tissue or body fluid sample. The sample is then incubated at a specific temperature for 24 to 48 hours. If growth is present, traditionally Gram stain is performed for morphology, and subcultures may be prepared to maintain bacterial growth. Identification of bacteria occurs using a combination of stains, motility testing, rapid biochemical tests, and commercial identification assays. Only after sufficient growth to allow subculturing is antibiotic susceptibility testing performed. The process to culture other pathogens, including viruses, fungi, and *Mycobacterium*, is different.

Quantitative culture remains the gold standard for detecting infection and has several strengths as a diagnostic tool. The unsupervised approach of the test allows many organisms to be identified without the requirement for the clinician to indicate a pathogen of interest *a priori*. Culture is versatile; pertinent pathogens can be cultured from almost any tissue of body fluid specimen as long as the clinical team is able to obtain a sample. Importantly, culture is low cost relative to other diagnostic tests, allowing its use in almost any clinical setting.

However, several limitations of culture exist. The prolonged turnaround time is a significant disadvantage in the ICU setting where delay in appropriate antibiotic therapy directly translates to increases in mortality.[9] The median turnaround time from initial culture preparation to bacterial identification and antibiotic sensitivities ranges from 48 to 72 hours.[10] Any error or delay in the multiple steps from sample collection to final report may prolong the turnaround time.[11–13] The insensitivity of culture is also an important weakness. A culture may be negative for multiple reasons: delay in transport to the microbiology laboratory, errors in preparation, receipt of antibiotics before the sample being cultured, suboptimal growth media, and metabolic impairment of growth of certain bacteria in polymicrobial infections. For fastidious or uncommon organisms, additional subcultures and/or molecular studies for identification may be required.[14] These disadvantages highlight the need for more rapid and sensitive diagnostic tests for common infections in the ICU.

Novel Diagnostics for Pulmonary Infections

Pulmonary infections are the most common infection in the ICU.[15] In a point prevalence study of more than 13,000 ICU patients, the lung was the source of infection 64% of the time.[3] In patients who are admitted to the ICU, the incidence rate of nosocomial pneumonia is 6% to 27%.[16] The mortality associated with pneumonia requiring ICU admission ranges from 15% to 50%.[17] Empirical treatment choices are determined by multiple factors including whether the patient meets criteria for community-acquired pneumonia (CAP), hospital-acquired pneumonia (HAP), or VAP.[18,19] Definitive treatment is determined by the cause of the infection.

Multiplex nucleic amplification tests (NAAT) are an example of a novel, RDT uniquely positioned to improve the diagnosis and management of pneumonia in the ICU. These tests address many of the shortcomings of culture with their rapid turnaround time and excellent sensitivity for the detection of certain pathogens. The operating characteristics of both multiplex and single-target polymerase chain reaction (PCR) assays vary based on the platform but generally have a sensitivity and specificity greater than 90%.[20] However, no test is completely accurate, and the performance characteristics of both single-target and multiplex platforms should be interpreted in the context of disease prevalence; for example, a positive test for influenza is more likely to be a false positive during periods of low influenza infection frequency compared with seasons of high disease prevalence.

Rapid diagnostic tests for viral respiratory infection

Multiplex NAATs for detection of respiratory viruses gained widespread acceptance over the past decade and have largely replaced viral culture. More than 15 NAATs are dedicated to the detection of individual respiratory viruses. The comprehensive list can be found on the Food and Drug Administration (FDA) Web site (https://www.fda.gov/medical-devices/in-vitro-diagnostics/nucleic-acid-based-tests). These tests are semiautomated and can be run on samples obtained by minimally invasive methods, such as nasopharyngeal swab, with a turnaround time less than 2 hours.

Viral pneumonia requiring ICU admission has a mortality rate comparable to severe bacterial pneumonia. Yet no prospective studies report superior clinical outcomes from either earlier or more specific detection of viruses in the lower respiratory tract (LRT) of patients with severe pneumonia. The major limitation is the small armamentarium of antivirals. However, avoidance of empirical antibiotic therapy is also an important therapeutic result. Thus, the decision to test lower respiratory tract (LRT) samples for viruses remains controversial. Multiple studies demonstrate discordance between viral test results from nasopharyngeal swabs and LRT samples.[21–23] Studies also indicate that patients with respiratory failure from nonviral causes may still test positive for a virus.[24,25] Importantly, upper respiratory tract testing is not sufficient to diagnose LRT viral infection in critically ill patients. However, except for the FilmArray Respiratory Panel, most multiplex NAATs for viruses are not FDA approved for use on BAL fluid. Conversely, bacterial superinfection is a major concern for severe viral pneumonia, and distinguishing between the primary viral pneumonia and bacterial superinfection is difficult. The ATS Consensus Statement recommends nucleic-acid-based testing for patients with severe CAP and/or immunocompromised status.[26,27] This recommendation is based on low-quality evidence that suggests a positive NAAT result may reduce antibiotic duration.[28,29]

Rapid diagnostic tests for bacterial pneumonia

The clinical utility of multiplex molecular diagnostic assays for the detection of a bacterial pneumonia is evolving. The BioFire FilmArray Pneumonia Panel and the Unyvero LRT are 2 FDA-approved molecular diagnostic platforms for detection of multiple bacterial pathogens from respiratory samples. **Table 1** compares the 2 platforms.[30,31] The Unyvero LRT panel includes *Pneumocystis jirovecii* and *Stenotrophomonas maltophilia*, which are not present on the FilmArray. Operating characteristics of these tests should be interpreted with the understanding that culture was used as the gold standard. Thus, a high positive predictive value could indicate that the test is generating false-positive results or that the test is accurately detecting a pathogen that did not grow on culture. Independent validation suggests that most discrepant results are false-negative cultures, rather than false-positive NAATs. However, prospective, randomized trials are needed to determine the impact of multiplex bacterial NAATs on antibiotic management, especially the safety of test-based antibiotic deescalation/discontinuation. Current studies suggest significant opportunities for antibiotic deescalation using NAATs on LRT specimens.[32,33]

The ability of an NAAT to specifically exclude methicillin-resistant *Staphylococcus aureus* (MRSA) pneumonia has unique implications for antibiotic stewardship. Empirical antibiotic regimens for CAP with risk factors or HAP/VAP include anti-MRSA antibiotics because of the increased mortality associated with this infection. The prolonged turnaround time of culture leads to critically ill patients often being exposed to several days of empirical anti-MRSA therapy while awaiting culture results. Use of multiplex or single-target PCR assays for detection of the *mec*A gene, which confers methicillin resistance, can effectively rule out the presence of MRSA pneumonia. Nasal swabs that screen for MRSA colonization have been studied as tools to rule out MRSA pneumonia. The negative predictive value of an MRSA nasal swab for the detection of culture-proven MRSA pneumonia is as high as 99.2%.[34] This excellent negative predictive value suggests that nasal swabs can be used to rule out MRSA pneumonia. Note that the studies investigating MRSA nasal swabs as tools to detect MRSA pneumonia are retrospective. However, the assay used for detecting MRSA from nasopharyngeal samples has been prospectively validated for use on bronchoalveolar lavage samples. In a randomized controlled trial of antibiotic deescalation based on the results of MRSA PCR tests on BAL samples compared with usual care, MRSA PCR tests run on BAL samples had a sensitivity of 95.7%, specificity of 98.2%, and negative predictive value of 99.6% for the detection of culture-positive MRSA pneumonia. In this trial there was a trend toward decreased mortality in patients randomized to antibiotic deescalation based on PCR. Thus, if MRSA is not detected in a respiratory sample, and no suspicion for extrapulmonary MRSA infection exists, clinicians can safely discontinue anti-MRSA antibiotics in critically ill patients without risk of adverse outcomes.[35,36] It is important for clinicians to know that nasopharyngeal colonization with MRSA is a risk factor for MRSA pneumonia, but the positive predictive value of an MRSA nasal swab is still is low, ranging from 17% to 35%. Therefore, a positive test cannot be use to rule-in MRSA pneumonia.[37]

In addition to methicillin resistance, the 2 major multiplex NAATs for bacterial pneumonia also include carbapenem resistance genes. Because many mechanisms of carbapenem resistance other than resistance genes occur, including efflux pumps, enzymatic deactivation (acquired carbapenemases), and target site mutations,[38] multiplex NAATs cannot reliably exclude carbapenem resistance. However, detection of these carbapenem resistance genes is highly predictive of phenotypic carbapenem resistance. The same is true of detection of the *ctx*M mutation, leading to extended spectrum beta-lactamase resistance in Enterobacterales.

Rapid Diagnosis of Bloodstream Infection

Bloodstream infections (BSI) are common in the ICU. Risk factors for BSI include disruption of anatomic barriers, presence of central venous catheters,

Table 1
Comparison of Two Multiplex PCR Panels for Pneumonia

	BioFire FilmArray Pneumonia Panel	Unyvero Lower Respiratory Tract Panel
Specimen	Bronchoalveolar lavage Sputum Endotracheal aspirate	Bronchoalveolar lavage Sputum Endotracheal aspirate
Bacterial Targets	18	20 (includes *Pneumocystis jirovecii* and *Stenotrophomonas maltophilia*)
Viral Targets	8	0
Resistance Markers	7	10
Quantitation	Semiquantitative	No quantitation
Overall Weighted Sensitivity	96.2% (96.3% for sputum)	94.7%
Specificity	98.3% (97.2% for sputum)	98.4%
Turnaround Time	1.5 h	4.5 h
Technology	Multiplex PCR	Multiplex PCR followed by probe array
Clinical Application	Could allow for antibiotic deescalation in hospitalized patients, could save 6.2 antibiotic days per patient[32]	Could allow for antibiotic deescalation in hospitalized patients[33]

immunosuppression, dialysis, and parenteral nutrition.[39] Development of BSI is associated with longer hospital stays, increased in-hospital mortality, and increased hospital expenditures.[40–42] Blood culture is the standard diagnostic tool for the identification of BSI; however, the yield of blood cultures is notoriously low. Two blood cultures can typically detect 80% of BSIs but sensitivity may be lower if antibiotics are administered before collection.[43] Over that past decade multiple RDTs have been developed to improve detection of BSI. Because critically ill patients have multiple risk factors for BSI, these novel diagnostic tools may be particularly useful in the ICU.

Mechanisms by which the novel diagnostics tests detect BSI vary. The first mechanism is matrix-assisted laser desorption ionization–time-of-flight mass spectrometry (MALDI-TOF). With MALDI-TOF, a sample is placed into a mass spectrometer and then ionized to become electrically charged. The charged molecule is accelerated through a tube and lands on a detector. The time taken for the molecule to accelerate, known as "time of flight," is recorded by the detector and compared with a calibrated standard of peptide mass fingerprints to provide identification of the bacteria.[44] Two commercial kits use MALDI-TOF technology for detection of BSI—Vitek MS and Sepsityper. MALDI-TOF has been reported to decrease time to organism identification by 1.5 days and decrease time to appropriate antibiotic therapy.[45] This technology has the advantage of identifying known and unknown organisms, unlike PCR where primers are required to identify an organism. However, MALDI-TOF is only clinically applicable for positive culture samples. Thus, MALDI-TOF is useful for organism identification but not for baseline detection of infection. MALDI-TOF is also unable to reliably differentiate bacteria in a polymicrobial infection because of overlap in spectra.[46–49]

Another technique used by newer diagnostic tools for BSI is gel electrofiltration and fluorescent in-situ hybridization. The Accelerate Pheno system is a fully automated assay that uses this technique to identify bacteria within 2 hours and antimicrobial susceptibility within 7 hours.[50] Accelerate has a reported overall sensitivity and specificity of 95.6% and 99.5%, respectively.[50] When combined with an antibiotic stewardship program, the Accelerate PhenoTest was shown to lead to earlier deescalation of unnecessary antibiotics in greater than 50% of patients.[51] As MALDI-TOF, the major limitation of the Accelerate PhenoTest is current availability only for positive blood cultures.

Several novel diagnostic tools for BSI use standard nucleic acid amplification to detect infection. These assays are either fully automated or semiautomated, have a turnaround time less than 3 hours, and can detect multiple pathogens. Commercially available NAATs for BSI from positive blood cultures include the BioFire FilmArray BCID, Unyvero System, and Verigene BC-GN. Similar to NAATs for LRT infection, randomized controlled trials of NAATs for BSI are lacking in an ICU population. Available data for the BioFire FilmArray BCID demonstrated a decrease in duration of piperacillin-tazobactam therapy when hospitalized patients with BSI were randomized to use of the FilmArray BCID plus an antimicrobial stewardship intervention versus usual care.[52]

Unlike the aforementioned tests for BSI, the T2 Biosystems NAATs can diagnose infection direct from blood and do not require a positive blood culture. The T2 Biosystems platform is also unique in that it uses T2-magnetic resonance biosensing capabilities to detect cellular and nucleic acid targets in whole blood. The instrument concentrates the microbial cells and cellular debris, amplifies DNA using target-specific primers, and detects amplified product by amplicon-induced aggregation of magnetic particles with a turnaround time of 3 to 5 hours. The T2Bacteria Panel is FDA approved for the detection of *Pseudomonas aeruginosa*, *Escherichia coli*, *Klebsiella pneumoniae*, *S aureus*, and *Enterococcus faecium*. The T2Candida Panel NAAT detects 5 *Candida* species with an overall sensitivity of 91% and specificity of 94%.

Next-generation sequencing (NGS) takes an unbiased approach to sequencing DNA or RNA present in a given sample. The Karius test is a commercially available NGS platform approved for use on whole blood samples. The assay is capable of detecting more than 1000 bacteria, viruses, and fungi by sequencing of cell-free DNA, with results potentially available within 24 hours. Clinically, the Karius test has a reported agreement of 100% when the identified organism is compared with conventional diagnostic methods. In addition, Karius testing has been applied to diagnostically challenging scenarios such as febrile neutropenia and culture-negative endocarditis. Clinical trials on the effect of Karius testing on clinical outcomes in critically ill patients are ongoing.

Rapid Diagnosis of Intraabdominal Infections

Intraabdominal infections are the third most common cause of sepsis in the ICU.[53] Many intraabdominal infections can be the primary reason for ICU admission, but other infections such as peritonitis, acalculous cholecystitis, and *Clostridioides* (formerly *Clostridium*) *difficile* infection (CDI) are often acquired during hospitalization. Radiographic imaging and culture of a fluid sample from the site of infection with or without blood culture is the current standard for diagnosis of cholecystitis, cholangitis, intraabdominal fluid collections, and/or peritonitis, with the limitations of culture discussed earlier. No commercially available multiplex molecular diagnostic assays are designed specifically for intraabdominal fluid collections. However, several small studies report use of 16s rRNA sequencing and/or metagenomic shotgun sequencing on intraabdominal fluid samples to detect infection.

Commercially available multiplex NAATs for intraabdominal infection are only applicable to acute diarrheal syndromes. These multiplex gastrointestinal NAATs contrast to the current method of diagnosis, which includes fecal culture, ova and parasite stains, and single-target PCRs. Bacteria on the panels include enteric pathogens such as E coli, Salmonella, and Campylobacter with a turnaround time of 2 to 5 hours depending on the platform. Some platforms also test for parasites and/or viruses, whereas others do not. The comprehensive list of pathogens can be found on the FDA Web site. In the clinical setting, the BioFire FilmArray Gastrointestinal panel detected pathogens in 54% of cases compared with an 18% detection rate with conventional culture. Importantly, the CDC has emphasized that multiplex NAAT for enteric pathogens may negatively affect public health foodborne disease surveillance. This concern was raised because, once C difficile has been excluded, diagnosing the exact cause of acute diarrheal illness may have little impact on clinical course (many acute illnesses self-resolve) and the cost of multiplex NAATs can be substantial.

Although multiplex PCR testing for diarrheal pathogens is controversial, specific testing for C difficile is widely accepted as important for critically ill patients. CDI is the most common infectious cause of diarrhea in the ICU.[54] About 20% of patients with symptomatic CDI will develop fulminant infection, which is associated with a mortality of greater than 50%.[55] The diagnosis of C difficile can be particularly challenging in the ICU setting. Severe CDI may not present with a classic diarrheal illness but with signs and symptoms of shock indistinguishable from other causes of shock. A variety of diagnostic tools are currently available to detect CDI. Importantly, these tests must be sent in the appropriate clinical setting, as they do not differentiate between asymptomatic colonization and true infection. The gold standard for C difficile diagnosis is a culture that first detects growth of C difficile, followed by testing to detect toxin production. A second test also considered to be the gold standard is a cell cytotoxicity test to detect toxin A or B. Although both gold-standard tests have excellent sensitivity, they are no longer used in clinical laboratories due to long turnaround time and have been replaced by novel RDTs.

NAATs for C difficile may be single-target or part of a multiplex enteropathogen panel with a sensitivity ranging from 87% to 95% and a specificity up to 98% based on multiple systematic analyses.[56] Enzyme immunoassay (EIA) is another RDT currently used by many clinical laboratories. EIA can detect the presence of toxin A or B or the presence of glutamate dehydrogenase (GDH). Note that GDH is an enzyme produced by both toxigenic and nontoxigenic strains of C difficile, and thus, GDH testing should be paired with testing for toxins. Many society guidelines recommend a combination of EIA and PCR testing to confirm C difficile diagnosis in symptomatic patients. RDTs for C difficile in hospitalized patients can significantly decrease empirical antibiotic therapy and decrease duration of isolation.[57,58]

Rapid Detection of Meningitis

Although an uncommon infection, meningitis affects a disproportionate number of ICU admissions. The potential spectrum is very broad, and empirical therapy is usually a complex regimen of multiple antibiotics, antivirals, and occasionally antifungals. Delays in treatment are associated with adverse neurologic outcomes, so empirical therapy is commonly given even before a diagnostic lumbar puncture, markedly compromising the yield of bacterial cultures. This infection is therefore a prime candidate for use of RDTs.

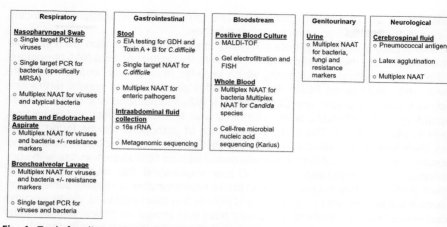

Fig. 1. Tools for diagnosis of common infections in the ICU.

The BinaxNOW test is an immunochromatographic test for rapid detection of the *S pneumoniae* antigen in cerebrospinal fluid (CSF). The sensitivity of the test ranges from 85% to 95% with a specificity of 95% to 100%.[59,60] Clinically, this test has demonstrated enhanced detection of pneumococcal meningitis in culture-negative cases.[60] Latex agglutination (LA) is another rapid test commonly used in bacterial meningitis.[61] This test uses latex beads coated with antibodies to bacterial antigens, and if the antigen is present the beads will agglutinate. Results of the test are typically available in less than 30 minutes. The commercially available LA assays detect *S pneumoniae*, *Haemophilus influenzae*, and *Neisseria meningitidis* with a sensitivity greater than 90%. There are also multiplex NAATs to diagnose meningitis.[62,63] The FilmArray Meningitis/Encephalitis Panel is an example of a multiplex PCR for CSF. The 14 targets included in this panel cover the spectrum of major viral, bacterial, and fungal pathogens. Clinical application of this test has shown enhanced detection of a pathogen compared with standard diagnostic tools.[61,64] The impact on antibiotic stewardship is unknown.

Rapid Diagnosis of Urinary Tract Infections

Genitourinary tract infection (UTI) is among the most common causes of sepsis and septic shock in critically ill patients. The incidence of nosocomial UTI increases with hospital length of stay, and patients with ICU-acquired UTI have increased mortality. The gold standard for diagnosis of UTI is urine quantitative culture with an organism growing at least 10^5 CFU from a clean catch specimen or 10^3 from a catheterized specimen. Urine cultures have the same limitations as cultures from other fluids, especially inability to distinguish between true infection and colonization or contamination.[65,66] Some single-center studies report multiplex PCR-enhanced detection of polymicrobial infection in symptomatic patients with UTI. 16s rRNA sequencing has also been used as a method of identifying the cause of culture-negative UTIs.[66,67]

DISCUSSION

Fig. 1 lists some commercially available tools for diagnosis of common infections in the ICU. Although there are clear advantages of RDTs in critically ill patients, areas of uncertainty are also present. A positive result from an NAAT may not translate into true infection, given the high sensitivity of many tests. Furthermore, interpretation of a persistently positive test when a patient is clinically improving is unclear. Many

PROCESS TO IMPLEMENT A NOVEL DIAGNOSTIC TEST IN THE ICU   *EXAMPLE*

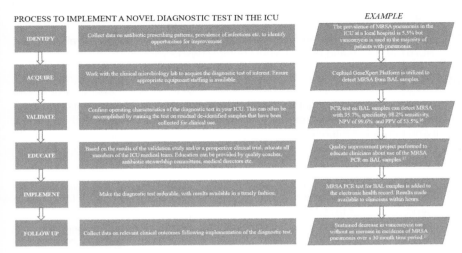

Fig. 2. Novel diagnostics review.

NAATs have a limited panel of pathogens they detect, and thus a negative test does not completely exclude infection. These tests should be used in conjunction with culture, not as a replacement for culture. In addition, many NAATs provide limited or no information on resistance patterns, making it difficult to definitively deescalate antibiotics. Finally, the cost-benefit of RDTs in critically ill patients is unclear.

SUMMARY

Our approach to incorporating RDTs into clinical practice is as follows (**Fig. 2**). The platform of choice should be locally validated before implementing the test into routine clinical care. Education on test result interpretation and antibiotic stewardship should be provided to critical care physicians and staff to maximize the potential benefit of the test. We encourage the use of tests that have an excellent negative predictive value and can safely lead to antimicrobial deescalation. Examples of this would be using an RDT to rule out influenza and discontinue empirical oseltamivir or using a rapid test to rule out MRSA pneumonia to avoid or discontinue empirical vancomycin. As with any diagnostic test, the results of rapid diagnostic platforms must be interpreted in the clinical context. Although there are no large, multicenter, prospective, randomized controlled trials on use of RDTs compared with standard of care to determine their effect on important clinical outcomes, we believe novel diagnostics could have the potential to be a powerful adjunct to culture and improve the management of infection in critically ill patients.

CLINICS CARE POINTS

- The negative predictive value of many RDTs, particularly nucleic acid amplification tests, is high. A clinician can reliably exclude infection by a pathogen on panel if the test is negative.
- The yield of a culture-independent test is generally higher than standard culture. Thus, molecular testing should be considered in culture-negative cases.
- Studies demonstrate RDTs may improve antibiotic stewardship but the impact on other clinically important outcomes remains unclear.

FUNDING

This work is supported by the National Institute of Health Institutional Training grant (3T32HL76139–13S2) and by NIH/NIAID grant U19AI135964.

DISCLOSURE

R.G. Wunderink is a consultant for bioMerieux and Accelerate Diagnostics. His institution has received research grants from bioMérieux and Curetis. All other authors declare no conflict of interest.

REFERENCES

1. Rhee C, Jones TM, Hamad Y, et al. Prevalence, underlying causes, and preventability of sepsis-associated mortality in US acute care hospitals. JAMA Netw Open 2019;2(2):e187571.
2. Perner A, Gordon AC, De Backer D, et al. Sepsis: frontiers in diagnosis, resuscitation and antibiotic therapy. Intensive Care Med 2016;42(12):1958–69.
3. Vincent J-L, Rello J, Marshall J, et al. International study of the prevalence and outcomes of infection in intensive care units. JAMA 2009;302(21):2323–9.
4. Angus DC, Linde-Zwirble WT, Lidicker J, et al. Epidemiology of severe sepsis in the United States: analysis of incidence, outcome, and associated costs of care. Crit Care Med 2001;29(7):1303–10.
5. Aldemir M, Özen S, Kara IH, et al. Predisposing factors for delirium in the surgical intensive care unit. Crit Care 2001;5(5):265.
6. Zimlichman E, Henderson D, Tamir O, et al. Health care–associated infections: a meta-analysis of costs and financial impact on the US health care system. JAMA Intern Med 2013;173(22):2039–46.
7. Kaukonen KM, Bailey M, Pilcher D, et al. Systemic inflammatory response syndrome criteria in defining severe sepsis. N Engl J Med 2015;372(17):1629–38.
8. Vincent JL, Opal SM, Marshall JC, et al. Sepsis definitions: time for change. Lancet 2013;381(9868):774–5.
9. Kumar A, Roberts D, Wood KE, et al. Duration of hypotension before initiation of effective antimicrobial therapy is the critical determinant of survival in human septic shock. Crit Care Med 2006;34(6):1589–96.
10. Lagier JC, Edouard S, Pagnier I, et al. Current and past strategies for bacterial culture in clinical microbiology. Clin Microbiol Rev 2015;28(1):208–36.
11. Tabak YP, Vankeepuram L, Ye G, et al. Blood culture turnaround time in U.S. acute care hospitals and implications for laboratory process optimization. J Clin Microbiol 2018;56(12).
12. MacVane SH, Oppermann N, Humphries RM. Time to result for pathogen identification and antimicrobial susceptibility testing of bronchoalveolar lavage and endotracheal aspirate specimens in U.S. acute care hospitals. J Clin Microbiol 2020;58(11):e01468.
13. Fernandes CM, Walker R, Price A, et al. Root cause analysis of laboratory delays to an emergency department. J Emerg Med 1997;15(5):735–9.
14. Srinivasan R, Karaoz U, Volegova M, et al. Use of 16S rRNA gene for identification of a broad range of clinically relevant bacterial pathogens. PloS One 2015;10(2):e0117617.
15. Spencer RC. Epidemiology of infection in ICUs. Intensive Care Med 1994;20(Suppl 4):S2–6.

16. Koenig SM, Truwit JD. Ventilator-associated pneumonia: diagnosis, treatment, and prevention. Clin Microbiol Rev 2006;19(4):637–57.
17. Li G, Cook DJ, Thabane L, et al. Risk factors for mortality in patients admitted to intensive care units with pneumonia. Respir Res 2016;17(1):80.
18. Kalil AC, Metersky ML, Klompas M, et al. Executive summary: management of adults with hospital-acquired and ventilator-associated pneumonia: 2016 clinical practice guidelines by the infectious diseases society of America and the American thoracic society. Clin Infect Dis 2016;63(5):575–82.
19. Metlay JP, Waterer GW, Long AC, et al. Diagnosis and treatment of adults with community-acquired pneumonia. an official clinical practice guideline of the American thoracic society and infectious diseases society of America. Am J Respir Crit Care Med 2019;200(7):e45–67.
20. Mahony JB. Detection of respiratory viruses by molecular methods. Clin Microbiol Rev 2008;21(4):716–47.
21. Boonyaratanakornkit J, Vivek M, Xie H, et al. Predictive value of respiratory viral detection in the upper respiratory tract for infection of the lower respiratory tract with hematopoietic stem cell transplantation. J Infect Dis 2019;221(3):379–88.
22. Walter JM, Wunderink RG. Testing for respiratory viruses in adults with severe lower respiratory infection. Chest 2018;154(5):1213–22.
23. Luyt C-E. Virus diseases in ICU patients: a long time underestimated; but be aware of overestimation. Intensive Care Med 2006;32(7):968–70.
24. Legoff J, Zucman N, Lemiale V, et al. Clinical significance of upper airway virus detection in critically Ill hematology patients. Am J Respir Crit Care Med 2019; 199(4):518–28.
25. Martino R, Porras RP, Rabella N, et al. Prospective study of the incidence, clinical features, and outcome of symptomatic upper and lower respiratory tract infections by respiratory viruses in adult recipients of hematopoietic stem cell transplants for hematologic malignancies. Biol Blood Marrow Transplant 2005; 11(10):781–96.
26. Evans SE, Jennerich AL, Azar MM, et al. Nucleic acid-based testing for noninfluenza viral pathogens in adults with suspected community-acquired pneumonia. an official American thoracic society clinical practice guideline. Am J Respir Crit Care Med 2021;203(9):1070–87.
27. Choi SH, Hong SB, Ko GB, et al. Viral infection in patients with severe pneumonia requiring intensive care unit admission. Am J Respir Crit Care Med 2012;186(4): 325–32.
28. Afzal Z, Minard CG, Stager CE, et al. Clinical diagnosis, viral PCR, and antibiotic utilization in community-acquired pneumonia. Am J Ther 2016;23(3):e766–72.
29. Gelfer G, Leggett J, Myers J, et al. The clinical impact of the detection of potential etiologic pathogens of community-acquired pneumonia. Diagn Microbiol Infect Dis 2015;83(4):400–6.
30. Webber DM, Wallace MA, Burnham C-AD, et al. Evaluation of the biofire filmarray pneumonia panel for detection of viral and bacterial pathogens in lower respiratory tract specimens in the setting of a tertiary care academic medical center. J Clin Microbiol 2020;58(7):00320–e00343.
31. Klein M, Bacher J, Barth S, et al. Multicenter evaluation of the unyvero platform for testing bronchoalveolar lavage fluid. J Clin Microbiol 2021;59(3).
32. Buchan BW, Windham S, Balada-Llasat JM, et al. Practical comparison of the biofire filmarray pneumonia panel to routine diagnostic methods and potential impact on antimicrobial stewardship in adult hospitalized patients with lower respiratory tract infections. J Clin Microbiol 2020;58(7).

33. Pickens C, Wunderink RG, Qi C, et al. A multiplex polymerase chain reaction assay for antibiotic stewardship in suspected pneumonia. Diagn Microbiol Infect Dis 2020;98(4):115179.
34. Dangerfield B, Chung A, Webb B, et al. Predictive value of methicillin-resistant Staphylococcus aureus (MRSA) nasal swab PCR assay for MRSA pneumonia. Antimicrob Agents Chemother 2014;58(2):859–64.
35. Paonessa JR, Shah RD, Pickens CI, et al. Rapid detection of methicillin-resistant staphylococcus aureus in BAL: a pilot randomized controlled trial. Chest 2019; 155(5):999–1007.
36. Pickens CI, Qi C, Postelnick M, et al. Association between a rapid diagnostic test to detect methicillin-resistant Staphylococcus Aureus pneumonia and decreased vancomycin use in a medical intensive care unit over a 30-month period. Infect Control Hosp Epidemiol 2021;42(11):1–3.
37. Sarikonda KV, Micek ST, Doherty JA, et al. Methicillin-resistant Staphylococcus aureus nasal colonization is a poor predictor of intensive care unit-acquired methicillin-resistant Staphylococcus aureus infections requiring antibiotic treatment. Crit Care Med 2010;38(10):1991–5.
38. Bush K, Fisher JF. Epidemiological expansion, structural studies, and clinical challenges of new β-lactamases from gram-negative bacteria. Annu Rev Microbiol 2011;65(1):455–78.
39. Bassetti M, Righi E, Carnelutti A. Bloodstream infections in the intensive care unit. Virulence 2016;7(3):267–79.
40. Barnett AG, Page K, Campbell M, et al. The increased risks of death and extra lengths of hospital and ICU stay from hospital-acquired bloodstream infections: a case–control study. BMJ Open 2013;3(10):e003587.
41. Laupland KB, Zygun DA, Davies HD, et al. Population-based assessment of intensive care unit-acquired bloodstream infections in adults: incidence, risk factors, and associated mortality rate. Crit Care Med 2002;30(11):2462–7.
42. Kaye KS, Marchaim D, Chen T-Y, et al. Effect of nosocomial bloodstream infections on mortality, length of stay, and hospital costs in older adults. J Am Geriatr Soc 2014;62(2):306–11.
43. Shafazand S, Weinacker AB. Blood cultures in the critical care unit: improving utilization and yield. Chest 2002;122(5):1727–36.
44. Tuma RSP. MALDI-TOF mass spectrometry: getting a feel for how it works. Oncol Times 2003;25(19):26.
45. French K, Evans J, Tanner H, et al. The clinical impact of rapid, direct MALDI-ToF identification of bacteria from positive blood cultures. PLoS One 2016;11(12): e0169332.
46. Faron ML, Buchan BW, Samra H, et al. Evaluation of WASPLab software to automatically read chromID CPS elite agar for reporting of urine cultures. J Clin Microbiol 2019;58(1).
47. Ferreira L, Sánchez-Juanes F, Porras-Guerra I, et al. Microorganisms direct identification from blood culture by matrix-assisted laser desorption/ionization time-of-flight mass spectrometry. Clin Microbiol Infect 2011;17(4):546–51.
48. Vlek AL, Bonten MJ, Boel CH. Direct matrix-assisted laser desorption ionization time-of-flight mass spectrometry improves appropriateness of antibiotic treatment of bacteremia. PLoS One 2012;7(3):e32589.
49. Tan KE, Ellis BC, Lee R, et al. Prospective evaluation of a matrix-assisted laser desorption ionization-time of flight mass spectrometry system in a hospital clinical microbiology laboratory for identification of bacteria and yeasts: a bench-by-

bench study for assessing the impact on time to identification and cost-effective-ness. J Clin Microbiol 2012;50(10):3301–8.

50. Charnot-Katsikas A, Tesic V, Love N, et al. Use of the accelerate pheno system for identification and antimicrobial susceptibility testing of pathogens in positive blood cultures and impact on time to results and workflow. J Clin Microbiol 2018;56(1):e01166.

51. Humphries R, Di Martino T. Effective implementation of the Accelerate Pheno™ system for positive blood cultures. J Antimicrob Chemother 2019; 74(Supplement_1):i40–3.

52. Banerjee R, Teng CB, Cunningham SA, et al. Randomized trial of rapid multiplex polymerase chain reaction-based blood culture identification and susceptibility testing. Clin Infect Dis 2015;61(7):1071–80.

53. Friedrich AK, Cahan M. Intraabdominal infections in the intensive care unit. J Intensive Care Med 2014;29(5):247–54.

54. Bagdasarian N, Rao K, Malani PN. Diagnosis and treatment of Clostridium diffi-cile in adults: a systematic review. JAMA 2015;313(4):398–408.

55. Riddle DJ, Dubberke ER. Clostridium difficile infection in the intensive care unit. Infect Dis Clin North America 2009;23(3):727–43.

56. Spina A, Kerr KG, Cormican M, et al. Spectrum of enteropathogens detected by the FilmArray GI Panel in a multicentre study of community-acquired gastroenter-itis. Clin Microbiol Infect 2015;21(8):719–28.

57. Debast SB, Bauer MP, Kuijper EJ. European Society of Clinical Microbiology and Infectious Diseases: update of the treatment guidance document for Clostridium difficile infection. Clin Microbiol Infect 2014;20(Suppl 2):1–26.

58. Barbut F, Surgers L, Eckert C, et al. Does a rapid diagnosis of Clostridium difficile infection impact on quality of patient management? Clin Microbiol Infect 2014; 20(2):136–44.

59. Marcos MA, Martínez E, Almela M, et al. New rapid antigen test for diagnosis of pneumococcal meningitis. Lancet 2001;357(9267):1499–500.

60. Moïsi JC, Saha SK, Falade AG, et al. Enhanced diagnosis of pneumococcal men-ingitis with use of the binax NOW immunochromatographic test of streptococcus pneumoniae antigen: a multisite study. Clin Infect Dis 2009;48(Supplement_2): S49–56.

61. Leber AL, Everhart K, Balada-Llasat JM, et al. Multicenter evaluation of biofire fil-marray meningitis/encephalitis panel for detection of bacteria, viruses, and yeast in cerebrospinal fluid specimens. J Clin Microbiol 2016;54(9):2251–61.

62. Fleischer E, Aronson PL. Rapid diagnostic tests for meningitis and encephalitis—biofire. Pediatr Emerg Care 2020;36(8):397–401.

63. Poplin V, Boulware DR, Bahr NC. Methods for rapid diagnosis of meningitis etiol-ogy in adults. Biomark Med 2020;14(6):459–79.

64. Domingues RB, Santos MVd, Leite FBVdM, et al. FilmArray Meningitis/Encepha-litis (ME) panel in the diagnosis of bacterial meningitis. Braz J Infect Dis 2019; 23(6):468–70.

65. Laupland KB, Bagshaw SM, Gregson DB, et al. Intensive care unit-acquired uri-nary tract infections in a regional critical care system. Crit Care 2005;9(2):R60–5.

66. Xu R, Deebel N, Casals R, et al. A new gold rush: a review of current and devel-oping diagnostic tools for urinary tract infections. Diagnostics (Basel) 2021;11(3).

67. García LT, Cristancho LM, Vera EP, et al. A new multiplex-PCR for urinary tract pathogen detection using primer design based on an evolutionary computation method. J Microbiol Biotechnol 2015;25(10):1714–27.

Is Zero Ventilator-Associated Pneumonia Achievable? Updated Practical Approaches to Ventilator-Associated Pneumonia Prevention

Cristina Vazquez Guillamet, MD[a], Marin H. Kollef, MD[b],*

KEYWORDS

- Ventilator-associated pneumonia • Prevention bundle • Antimicrobial resistance
- Compliance • Effectiveness

KEY POINTS

- Ventilator-associated pneumonia (VAP) rates remain relatively high across the world including North America. These are predicated on long durations of mechanical ventilation and increasing rates of antimicrobial resistance as occurred during the coronavirus 2 (SARS-CoV-2) pandemic.
- VAP prevention is a worthwhile goal, and using an efficient prevention bundle is a core measure for both governmental agencies and hospitals alike.
- Local VAP prevention bundle measures should be supported by national guidelines, recent clinical data, and local resource availability.

INTRODUCTION

Ventilator-associated pneumonia (VAP) accounts for approximately half of all nosocomial pneumonia cases and remains the most common infection in patients requiring mechanical ventilation (**Table 1**).[1,2] European prevalence of infection in intensive care (EPIC) III, a 24-hour point prevalence study conducted at 1150 centers in 88 countries on September 13, 2017, found that 54% of patients in the intensive care unit (ICU) had suspected or proven infection.[3] The most common site of infection

Portions of this article were previously published in Clinics in Chest Medicine 39:4 December 2018.

[a] Division of Infectious Diseases, Washington University School of Medicine, St. Louis, MO, USA;
[b] Division of Pulmonary and Critical Care Medicine, Washington University School of Medicine, St. Louis, MO, USA
* Corresponding author. Washington University School of Medicine, 4523 Clayton Avenue, Campus Box 8052, St. Louis, MO 63110.
E-mail address: kollefm@wustl.edu

Infect Dis Clin N Am 38 (2024) 65–86
https://doi.org/10.1016/j.idc.2023.11.001
0891-5520/24/© 2023 Elsevier Inc. All rights reserved.

Table 1
Recommendations for prevention of ventilator-associated pneumonia and applicable patient populations

Mechanism	Recommendation	Level of Support	Patient Population	Cons/Observations
Decrease duration/avoid mechanical ventilation	Consider NIPPV in certain types of respiratory failure, pre-intubation or as weaning modalities	RCT[123,124]	COPD, certain types of hypoxemic respiratory failure	Delaying intubation when clinically indicated may jeopardize patient's stability
Decrease colonization with resistant pathogens	Optimal hand hygiene practices	Observational studies	All patients	Very low compliance rates[57]
Decrease colonization with resistant pathogens	Gown/glove isolation for patients with resistant bacteria	Observational studies	All patients	Universal gown/glove precautions only decreased MRSA acquisition rates as a secondary outcome[125]
Reduce duration of mechanical ventilation	Spontaneous breathing trials	RCT[48-51]	All patients	Low compliance rates
Reduce duration of mechanical ventilation	Spontaneous awakening trials	RCT[42-45]	All patients	None
Reduce duration of mechanical ventilation	Early mobilization	RCT[53-55]	All stable patients	Larger resources needed
Reduce aspiration	Head of bed elevation to 30°–45°	RCT[33-37]	All stable patients	Hemodynamic instability
Reduce aspiration	Avoid unnecessary suctioning and ventilatory circuit changes	RCT[60,61]	All patients	Safe practice, decreased costs when tubes changed only as needed
Decrease aspiration, reduce bacterial load to the airways	Orogastric tubes	Observational studies[126]	All patients	Lower rates of nosocomial sinusitis
Decrease oral bacterial load	Administer chlorhexidine-based oral care	RCT[100-102]	Postsurgical patients with short intubation	Recent trials showed increased mortality in medical intubated patients[38,104,105]

Decrease oral bacterial load	Administer topical oral antibiotics (selective oral decontamination)	RCT[96]	ICUs with low antimicrobial resistance rates and low antibiotic utilization[a]	Unclear long-term impact on antimicrobial resistance in ICUs with moderate, high resistance rates
Decrease oral and gastric bacterial load	Selective digestive decontamination	RCT[87,88]	unclear	Unclear long-term impact on antimicrobial resistance in ICUs with moderate, high resistance rates
Decrease bacterial load in the airways	Subglottic drainage	RCT[62–64,66]	All patients	New data questioning benefit
Decrease bacterial load in the airways	Silver-impregnated endotracheal tubes	RCT[77]	All patients especially at high risk for VAP	May not be cost-effective
Reduce bacterial load/Improve dysbiosis	Probiotics	RCT[112]	None	Avoid usage based on recent RCT

Abbreviations: COPD, chronic obstructive pulmonary disease; MRSA, methicillin-resistant *Staphylococcus aureus*; NIPPV, noninvasive positive pressure ventilation; RCT, randomized controlled trial; VAP, ventilator-associated pneumonia.

[a] Less than 5% and daily antibiotic doses less than 1000 per 1000 d of admission.

was the respiratory tract in 60% of patients, the abdomen in 18%, and the bloodstream in 15%, and among respiratory tract infections 56% were either hospital acquired or ICU acquired.[3] Before the coronavirus 2 (severe acute respiratory syndrome [SARS]-CoV-2) pandemic, VAP was associated with additive mortality, prolonged length of stay both in the ICU and the hospital, greater antimicrobial use, and significant health care costs.[4,5] Therefore, the prevention of VAP was considered a cornerstone quality improvement program for most governing bodies and ICUs.[6] Despite advances in microbiologic diagnostics and ICU-specific therapies, such as new antibiotics, the epidemiology and definition of VAP are still debated and have been influenced by the SARS-CoV-2 pandemic rendering efforts aimed at VAP prevention and outcome data interpretation to be inconclusive.

The initial center for disease control and prevention (CDC) VAP definition relied heavily on radiographic criteria for establishing this diagnosis. This was shown to add unwanted subjectivity to the already subjective nature of symptoms and physical signs interpretation within the VAP criteria.[7,8] Data reported to the CDC more than the two decades before the SARS-CoV-2 pandemic suggested a dramatic decrease in VAP rates in US hospitals, with some hospitals achieving an impressive and unthinkable rate of zero episodes.[9,10] However, clinical data showed a different pattern with VAP still being diagnosed by ICU clinicians and treated with antibiotics.[11,12] Although US rates reportedly were dropping, VAP rates remained consistently higher (approximately 3–5 fold greater) in Western Europe and middle-income countries across four continents.[10–12] To balance this discrepancy between the rates of VAP reported by US hospitals and the rest of the world, as well as between hospital surveillance data and clinician-diagnosed VAP, attempts were made at redefining VAP as part of the ventilator-associated events (VAEs) criteria.[13] The main changes from the old definition were excluding the radiographic criteria and adding a significant change in oxygenation that followed a period of 48 hours of clinical stability.

VAEs, along with infection-related ventilator-associated complications (IVACs) and the possible and probable VAP criteria, have been proposed by the CDC as a methodology for improving the evaluation of medical care quality rendered in the ICU setting. Unfortunately, these new definitions do not seem to correlate well with the clinical understanding and incidence of VAP. It is reasonable to think that not all VAEs are VAPs but it also seems that not all VAPs are VAEs which leads to underestimating current rates of VAP.[14,15] Moreover, PROPHETIC, a prospective cohort study among adults hospitalized for more than 48 hours and considered high risk for pneumonia (defined as treatment with invasive or noninvasive ventilatory support or high levels of supplemental oxygen), identified 32% of patients being treated for possible nosocomial pneumonia with 37% of those meeting the study pneumonia definition.[16] PROPHETIC, along with prospective identification of pneumonia in hospitalized patients in the intensive care unit in Europe (PROPHETIC EU),[17] demonstrated that rates of lung infection are likely higher than what US surveillance data suggest and accounting for the majority of antibiotic administration in the ICU setting.

The SARS-CoV-2 pandemic saw rates of VAP, and other nosocomial infections dramatically increase along with increasing emergence of antimicrobial resistance.[18] This was likely the result of patients being treated for prolonged time periods in the ICU on mechanical ventilation and the uncertainty in excluding concomitant bacterial infections leading to excessive empirical antibiotic use. The French REA-REZO surveillance network conducted a comparative study with three groups of adult medical ICU patients: control group (64,816 patients admitted between 2016 and 2019; prepandemic patients), 7442 pandemic non-COVID-19 patients, and 1687 pandemic COVID-19 positive patients admitted during 2020.[19] The incidence of VAP was

14.2%, 18.3%, and 31.9%, respectively, with attributable mortality being 3.2%, 2.9%, and 8.1%, respectively.[19] Similarly, the US study found that more than 40% of mechanically ventilated COVID-19 positive patients developed at least one episode of VAP and that the emergence of infection with antibiotic-resistant bacteria increased with longer duration of mechanical ventilation.[20] Thus, the SARS-CoV-2 pandemic was associated with a greater overall prevalence of VAP and increased infections due to multidrug-resistant bacteria.

Diagnostic uncertainty and confusion around the diagnosis of VAP represents the first layer of complexity in VAP prevention. How do we define and assess VAP prevention in the context of fluctuating VAP definitions? Despite previous overly optimistic reports, available data suggest that VAP is still prevalent in US ICUs at constant and predictable rates. When Medicare reviewers analyzed randomly selected postsurgical and medical patients admitted with acute myocardial infarction and congestive heart failure between 2006 and 2010, they discovered a constant VAP rate of approximately 10 cases per 100 ventilated patients.[21] In addition, ventilated hospital-acquired pneumonia has been shown to be common with a greater mortality than VAP, adding a significant burden to patients' risk of mortality and prolonged hospital stays.[22,23]

The second layer of complexity in understanding VAP prevention stems from the inherent limitations of before–after time series studies that examined the impact of prevention bundles on VAP rates. Randomized controlled double-blinded trials are ideally suited to minimize the subjectivity and inherent observer bias in assessing patient outcomes. This is not the case with before–after studies where observers' biases are likely to be prevalent. Also, with frequent implementation and reinforcement, a cultural shift, similar to the acceptance of rapid response team initiatives, may have occurred resulting in the routine acceptance of VAP prevention interventions. Health care providers have seemingly become more aware of the importance of preventing VAP, as well as implementing prevention strategies that may or may not be part of the bundle components, potentially biasing any assessment of the true occurrence of VAP and the impact of VAP on patient outcomes. The contextual effect whereby multiple levels of variability (hospital population, type of ICU, patient characteristics) contribute to the outcome of interest may also weigh significantly on the interpretation of VAP prevention studies, especially those using before–after study designs.

Because VAP definitions are in flux, determining the benefits of VAP prevention may need to focus on other objective outcomes besides incidence rates. However, VAP-attributable mortality is also difficult to discern with various studies citing a varying impact of attributable mortality from VAP ranging between 0% and 50%.[24,25] Mechanical ventilation-free days, length of stay, and antibiotic utilization may serve as more accurate and objective outcomes of interest to gauge the success of VAP prevention programs. Given the difficulties in adequately assessing the impact of VAP prevention strategies on patient outcomes, it is important to question whether it is really possible to achieve zero rates for this infection. This seems highly unlikely, nevertheless hospitals should attempt to reduce their VAP rates to the lowest degree possible to improve patient outcomes and reduce the use of antimicrobial agents. This review focuses on reviewing the practical evidence-based approaches for the prevention of VAP.

POTENTIAL STRATEGIES IN VENTILATOR-ASSOCIATED PNEUMONIA PREVENTION

VAP represents a heterogeneous disease affecting both medical and surgical ICU patients with different predisposing conditions thus resulting in variable incidence rates.

The microbiology of VAP and resultant antibacterial treatment are dependent on host factors but also the duration of ventilation, hospital length of stay before pneumonia onset, and the spectrum of antibiotic-resistant microbes present within the hospital. The cost of VAP prevention strategies is also a relevant issue whereby more expensive prevention strategies or devices should be reserved for patients at the highest risk for developing VAP or for ICUs demonstrating a higher prevalence of infection attributed to antibiotic-resistant pathogens. The most useful and cost-effective strategies should generally be applied to all at-risk patients in the ICU according to the availability of such resources at the local hospital level. Therefore, a multilevel practical approach may be more beneficial in thinking about how VAP prevention programs should be implemented in various patient populations, although such an approach could limit acceptance by health care providers.[26,27]

Many elements considered to have a significant impact on reducing the incidence of VAP have been investigated either solely or as part of a ventilator bundle. The most robust prevention bundles attempt to account for the dual pathogenesis of VAP, colonization with pathogenic bacteria, and aspiration of contaminated secretions, when designing the individual component elements included within the prevention bundle. However, the duration of mechanical ventilation is one of the most important determinants for the occurrence of VAP as well as emergence of antibiotic resistance.[20] Thus, preventing the need for intubation and mechanical ventilation in the first place and shortening the duration of mechanical ventilation should be key components of all prevention bundles. It has also been established that hospitalized patients become colonized with nosocomial microbes as early as 48 hours after admission, especially in the ICU setting. The implication of this is that clinicians should have a keen understanding of the predominant antibiotic-resistant microbes present within their hospitals when designing prevention strategies. Moreover, numerous host factors have been described increasing the likelihood of VAP attributed to antibiotic-resistant bacteria including immune suppression, previous hospitalizations and antibiotic courses, and admission from nursing homes or long-term acute care facilities where infection control practices may not be as rigorous as in acute care hospitals. These antibiotic-resistant infections are the VAPs that are most likely to impact patient outcomes due to the administration of ineffective antibiotic therapy and thus the ones that should be targeted for prevention.[28,29]

Aspiration of contaminated oropharyngeal secretions or stomach contents refluxing into the oropharynx and then into the airways plays a paramount role in VAP pathogenesis and likely represents one of the most preventable factors that should be factored into the design of VAP prevention strategies. Radiolabeling studies clearly described passage of contaminated gastric contents into the airways via the pharynx in supine mechanically ventilated patients.[30] Similarly, other studies have shown the frequent occurrence of bacterial-laden oral secretions being aspirated into the bronchial tree as a potential starting point for VAP.[31,32] Therefore, the most likely successful strategy for the prevention of VAP should be one that emphasizes shorter durations of mechanical ventilation, prevention of colonization of the aerodigestive tract with pathogenic bacteria, and prevention of the subsequent aspiration of bacterial contaminated secretions.

PRACTICAL APPROACHES TO VENTILATOR-ASSOCIATED PNEUMONIA PREVENTION

In designing a prevention bundle, clinicians must first consider the sine-qua-non elements that have been proven to impact VAP rates and ideally other objective outcomes. Easy application and cost-effectiveness may be desirable attributes but additional considerations should include the potential for future changes in either patient population, staffing, predominant bacterial pathogens and occurrence of pandemics. Secondary elements can then be added to the baseline prevention bundle depending on the hospital's resources while also avoiding overburdening the health care teams. Sometimes less may be more effective as indiscriminate use of multiple interventions not tied to improved outcomes may lead to unnecessary workload increases and decreased compliance with the bundle elements.

Core Measures

Some prevention measures have strong evidence to support their routine use, whereas others have been proven to be associated with decreased transmission and propagation of resistant microbes. Intuitively, all measures that shorten the duration of intubation and decrease the transmission of resistant microbes should positively impact rates of complications associated with mechanical ventilation including VAP. Although many interventions have been tested as part of a prevention bundle making it difficult to ascertain the relative weight or importance of the individual element, we will present potential bundle elements with the best supporting evidence.

1. Head of bed elevation to 30° to 45°

This is probably one of the oldest and simplest prevention measures used after gastroesophageal reflux was shown to worsen in supine-positioned patients.[30] However, one can also argue that semirecumbent positioning favors gravitational pulling of oropharyngeal secretions into the airways making aspiration around endotracheal tube (ETT) cuffs more likely. A trial in 86 patients showed that semirecumbent positioning reduced the rates of clinically suspected and microbiologically proven nosocomial pneumonia by fourfold.[33] However, subsequent studies showed poor compliance with head of bed elevation,[34] but easy solutions such as visual cues and small bedside devices are now available to improve compliance.[35,36] A Cochrane literature review based on small and potentially biased studies found an overall benefit in reducing VAP rates when patients were positioned at 30°-60° versus 0°-10° but there was no significant difference in the occurrence of microbiologically confirmed episodes of VAP.[37]

Although trying to discern the relative contribution of individual VAP bundle components, Klompas and colleagues found that the head of bed elevation was associated with relatively high rates of compliance (>85%) and faster times to extubation, but it did not significantly impact rates of possible VAP, IVACs, or VAEs.[38] Trying to counteract the gravitational disadvantage of the semirecumbent positioning, a large multicenter trial randomized patients to semirecumbent positioning versus the lateral Trendelenburg position.[39] Overall, the VAP incidence was very low in this trial at 0.5%, and even though there were fewer microbiologically confirmed cases of VAP in the lateral Trendelenburg group, none of the primary or secondary outcomes reached statistical significance. Moreover, greater numbers of adverse events were reported with lateral Trendelenburg positioning including vomiting, intracranial hemorrhage, and brachial plexus injury making this an unacceptable component of any prevention bundle. Similarly, studies examining the use of prone positioning have failed to demonstrate reduced rates of VAP.[40]

To date, we believe that head of bed elevation to 30° to 45° provides the safest positioning for the prevention of VAP in hemodynamically stable patients. The availability of ETTs with subglottic suctioning also mitigates the gravitational pull of oropharyngeal secretions that might occur in the semirecumbent position. The simplicity and minimal risk of semirecumbent positioning, as well as its ability to facilitate patient mobility and weaning from mechanical ventilation compared with supine positioning, makes it a core element within prevention bundles.[41]

2. Decrease sedation: daily awakening trials

In general, daily awakening trials have been associated with shortening the duration of mechanical ventilation by 2 to 4 days.[42] This has been extrapolated to result in decreased risk for VAP and has become part of the society of healthcare epidemiology of america (SHEA) guidelines for VAP prevention. Analgesia alone without accompanying sedation may also provide the same benefit of shorter durations of mechanical ventilation based on a Danish study,[43] although both the control and intervention groups had longer durations of mechanical ventilation compared with patients in the study by Kress and colleagues. When coupled with daily spontaneous breathing trials (SBTs), the use of sedation interruption was associated with a larger number of ventilator-free days (14.7 vs 11.6, $P=.02$) and faster discharge from the ICU and the hospital as demonstrated in a multicenter trial of 336 patients.[44] Daily interruption in sedation was one of the strongest measures associated with higher likelihood of extubation, shorter hospital stay, and even lower ventilator mortality in the study by Klompas and colleagues analyzing the association between individual bundle components and outcomes.[38] A multicenter trial in 16 Canadian hospitals that relied on benzodiazepines as the main sedatives found no difference in duration of intubation between a nursing-driven protocol targeting light sedation and daily interruptions in sedation.[45] However, the total daily doses and boluses used in the interruption group were also higher than those used in the comparator group and those reported in previous studies. Taken together, the evidence in support of minimizing sedation to achieve more timely liberation from mechanical ventilation should be seen as a fundamental element of any VAP prevention bundle.

A recent analysis of a US multicenter cohort of critically ill patients found in multivariable models, controlling for admitting patient characteristics, factors independently associated with higher odds of a next-day spontaneous awakening trial (SAT) and SBT including physical restraint use, documented target sedation level, more frequent level of arousal assessments, and dexmedetomidine administration.[46] Factors independently associated with lower odds of a next-day SAT and SBT included deep sedation/coma and benzodiazepine or ketamine administration.[46] Moreover, a recent meta-analysis showed that implementation of ICU bundles that include SATs may reduce length of ICU stay, mechanical ventilation time, delirium, ICU and hospital mortality, and promoted early mobilization in critically ill patients.[47] Thus, SBTs and avoidance of excess sedation should be part of all VAP prevention bundles.

3. Spontaneous breathing trials

Many studies have described the positive impact of readiness assessment and SBTs in shortening the duration of mechanical ventilation, reducing ICU length of stay, and costs associated with ICU hospitalization.[47,48] Subsequently, these interventions became protocolized making their applicability more facile.[49,50] Heterogenous meta-analyses grouping randomized and quasi-randomized trials obtained the same results.[51] Now, daily SATs and SBTs are performed synchronously. Unfortunately, daily breathing trials have been shown to have among the lowest compliance rates[38] compared with other prevention bundle elements and have primarily been associated with the prevention of VAEs but without a significant impact on possible VAP rates (odds ratio [OR] 0.7, 95%CI 0.4–1.6, $P = .5$). Nevertheless, given the strong evidence linking VAP to more prolonged episodes of mechanical ventilation, we favor using SBTs as part of all ventilator bundles and VAP prevention bundles. The type of SBT, T-piece versus pressure support ventilation, does not seem to influence patient outcomes including pneumonia occurrence.[52] The key factor is performing SBTs systematically to shorten the duration of mechanical ventilation.

4. Early mobilization

Along the same lines, physical therapy and early mobilization have been proven to be safe, even in high-risk patients including those with acute respiratory distress syndrome, continuous renal replacement therapy, shock requiring vasopressors, and BMIs greater than 30, to shorten the length of mechanical ventilation.[53] When applied to patients already benefiting from daily sedation interruptions, the benefit of early mobilization resulted in further shortening of mechanical ventilation duration (ventilator-free days 23.5 vs 21.1, $P = .05$).[54] Compared with control patients, a strategy of whole-body rehabilitation, consisting of interruption of sedation and physical and occupational therapy in the earliest days of critical illness, was found to be safe and well tolerated and resulted in better functional outcomes at hospital discharge, a shorter duration of delirium, and more ventilator-free days.[55]

5. Hand hygiene

Hand hygiene with either soap or alcohol-based solutions has been repeatedly linked to decreased transmission of nosocomial pathogens and the occurrence of nosocomial infections. In a quasi-experimental study with interrupted time series analysis, a simple ventilator bundle that consisted only of hand hygiene, oral care with chlorhexidine, and health care provider education decreased VAP rates by 59%.[56] Yet, hand hygiene remains the measure with the lowest compliance rates across prevention bundle components even as low as 10% to 15%.[57] The use of protective gloves and gowns when necessary for contact with individuals infected or colonized with highly resistant bacteria can also decrease the rate of transmission of multidrug-resistant pathogens. Overall, enhanced hand hygiene may have an effect on the prevention of VAP. However, the reliability of this conclusion is limited because of the quality of available studies.[58,59]

6. Ventilator circuit manipulation

Maintenance of the ventilator circuit without needless disconnections and manipulation is safe and may decrease entry of bacteria into the trachea even though no impact on VAP rates has been noted.[60,61] Avoiding unnecessary suctioning may also protect against unneeded contamination of the bronchial tree with pathogenic bacteria.

Additional Adjunctive Prevention Measures

1. Subglottic drainage/suctioning, cuff pressure monitoring, and ETT cuff design

Subglottic drainage refers to specially designed ETTs that allow suctioning of contaminated oropharyngeal secretions that accumulate above the ETT cuff. By decreasing the quantity of these secretions and therefore the bacterial load that trickles in the lower airway, VAP may presumably be avoided. Many studies, including meta-analyses examining subglottic drainage, have shown a reduction in early-onset VAP by approximately 50%.[62–64] Randomized controlled trials have varied in terms of pneumonia definitions, expected durations of mechanical ventilation cutoffs, and suctioning techniques (continuous vs intermittent). The earliest meta-analysis by Dezfulian and colleagues included five randomized trials and demonstrated shorter mechanical ventilation and also ICU length of stay with the use of subglottic drainage.[62] A subsequent meta-analysis by Muscedere and colleagues included 2442 patients from 13 trials and partially replicated the findings by Dezfulian and colleagues; however, the analyses for duration of mechanical ventilation and length of stay were biased by significant study heterogeneity.[63] Carroff and colleagues included four newer trials but did not find the same benefit in terms of shorter durations of mechanical ventilation and overall length of stay.[64] The findings within that meta-analysis were reinforced after excluding a Chinese study thought to be an outlier.[65] A more recent meta-analysis found that the highest VAP reduction occurred with ICU care bundles adopting the Institute for Healthcare Improvement Ventilator Bundle combined with adequate ETT cuff pressure and subglottic suctioning achieving a greater than 50% reduction in VAP rates.[66]

Ideally, ETT cuff pressures should be maintained at 25 to 30 cm H_2O to allow for optimal closure within the trachea thus avoiding aspiration around the cuff while also minimizing the occurrence of tracheal ischemia. Small, single-center studies have looked at intermittent versus continuous cuff pressure monitoring (pneumatic or electronic devices) with conflicting results in terms of reducing aspiration, tracheal secretion, and bacterial loads and incidence of VAP.[67–69] A trial of two different manual cuff monitoring practices found that more frequent cuff pressure monitoring was not associated with any identifiable clinical outcome benefit, including VAP.[70] A more recent large study in trauma patients found that continuous regulation of cuff pressure of the tracheal tube using a pneumatic device was not superior to routine care in preventing VAP.[71]

It has also been postulated that various tube shapes (eg, tapered cuff) or materials (polyurethane) may help to hold the secretions above the cuff and avert microaspiration. Initial animal and small human studies showed contradictory results. Two randomized controlled trials also failed to find a benefit when using tapered cuffs or polyurethane tubes.[72,73] In a French trial, 326 patients were enrolled across 10 ICUs looking at the advantage of tapered-cuffs on microaspiration of gastric contents.[74] Microaspiration was measured using pepsin and salivary amylase levels in the tracheal aspirates. Although a previous study found tracheal salivary amylase to only moderately correlate with microaspiration events (area under the receiver operating curve [AUROC] 0.56).[75] All outcomes including microaspiration and pneumonia rates were similar, but tracheobronchial bacterial colonization was less in the tapered cuff group.[74] Six randomized trials were included in the most recent meta-analysis that again failed to reveal a reduction in VAP rates in critically ill and postoperative patients receiving tapered ETT cuffs.[76]

A relative risk reduction of 36% for microbiologically confirmed VAP was observed in a large randomized trial using silver-coated ETTs to prevent VAP.[77] However, it is unclear whether the routine use of these coated tubes is cost-effective given their high cost and the relatively low incidence of VAP in many ICUs.[78,79] A small trial using ETT cleaning of silver-coated ETTs using the endOclear catheter found that periodic cleaning maneuvers did not decrease bacterial colonization of the tubes and did not lower respiratory tract colonization compared with standard suctioning.[80] It is unlikely that such cleaning devices would impact VAP rates in patients with standard ETTs. However, large clinical trials are lacking.

2. Gastric distention

Clinically, gastric over distention augments gastroesophageal reflux and can contribute to micro- and macroaspiration events. Naso- or orogastric tubes are routinely inserted in mechanically ventilated patients for both enteral nutrition administration and also decompression of the stomach. However, routine monitoring of gastric residual volumes is not currently recommended based on a large randomized trial and orogastric tubes are preferred to reduce the occurrence of nosocomial sinusitis.[81,82]

3. Selective digestive decontamination

Selective digestive decontamination (SDD) has been a promising strategy in European countries with low incidences of resistant microbes and has been promoted as a core recommendation in the French guidelines on VAP prevention.[83] SDD usually requires the application of an oral paste and administration of a gastric suspension containing colistin, tobramycin, and nystatin for the duration of mechanical ventilation, plus a 4-day course of an intravenous antibiotic with a broad antimicrobial spectrum, usually a third-generation cephalosporin. SDD is not only associated with decreasing VAP rates but also decreasing mortality and other objective outcomes.[84–86] In a large, cluster randomized, crossover Dutch study including close to 6000 ICU patients, SDD was compared with selective oral decontamination (SOD) and regular care.[85] The initial study was retracted and revised after it was discovered that the control and intervention periods were misclassified for one of the 16 participating ICUs. A recent meta-analysis of SDD from 32 trials with 24,389 patients concluded that the use of SDD compared with standard care or placebo was associated with lower hospital mortality and that the evidence regarding the effect of SDD on antimicrobial resistance was of very low certainty.[87] However, a more recent randomized trial of SDD compared with placebo from Australia with 5982 mechanically ventilated participants found no difference in mortality (27.0% vs 29.1%; mean difference −1.7%; 95% CI -4.8%–1.3%).[88] The main concern regarding the routine use of SDD, as well as SOD, is the long-term detrimental effect of these agents on antimicrobial resistance. The routine use of third-generation cephalosporins may increase the rates of methicillin-resistant *Staphylococcus aureus* (MRSA), extended spectrum beta lactamase (ESBL)-*Enterobacteriaceae*, and *Pseudomonas aeruginosa* which usually arise after previous exposure to antibiotics as also supported by the experience during the SARS-CoV-2 pandemic.[20]

No increased resistance to aminoglycosides or colistin was noted among sites using SDD and SOD in prior studies,[89,90] in fact decreased colonization with antibiotic-resistant strains and lower overall rates of resistance to third-generation cephalosporins was described during some of the larger SDD trials.[91,92] Although a transient increase in the rate of susceptible *S aureus* and *Enterococcus fecalis* were reported at the initiation of SDD, these effects reportedly dissolved after 5 years of SDD utilization.[93] Oostdijk and colleagues looked at the ecological effects of SDD and SOD in all ICU patients not only the ones who had received SDD or SOD.[94] Both rectal and respiratory colonization with ceftazidime-resistant strains more than doubled after the end of the SDD period after initially declining during the SDD period (from 5% to 15%, $P = .05$ for the trend of ceftazidime resistance in respiratory samples). Other interesting findings came from a recent Dutch study that followed mechanically ventilated patients receiving SDD between 2011 and 2015.[95] The investigators found that rectal colonization with Gram-negative bacteria correlated with ICU-acquired infections, more than half being respiratory tract infections. The congruence between the rectal colonizing species and respiratory species was low at 35% questioning the role of gastrointestinal bacteria in producing VAP. Most importantly, it remains to be seen which patient populations would benefit the most from the use of SDD and SOD especially in countries with higher rates of patient colonization with antimicrobial-resistant bacteria.

Considering all these aspects from the available clinical trials and the potential impact on bacterial resistance from escalating the routine use of SDD and SOD, we agree with the European guidelines on VAP prevention recommending SOD but not SDD in ICUs with low antimicrobial resistance rates less than 5% and low antibiotic consumption (<1000 daily doses per 1000 admission days).[96] Moreover, SDD has primarily been studied in ICU populations with low antimicrobial prevalence mainly from northern Europe. SDD investigators conducting a narrative review themselves concluded that in settings with low prevalence of antibiotic resistance, SDD is consistently associated with less antibiotic resistance and improved patient outcome.[97] In settings with moderate-to-high prevalence of antibiotic resistance, benefits of SDD on clinically relevant patient outcomes remain to be demonstrated.[97]

4. Oral care/selective oral decontamination

Because aspiration of oropharyngeal secretions seems to be the principal mechanism for the development of VAP, a plethora of modalities trying to curb the oral bacterial load have been tested. These modalities have ranged from brushing teeth with toothpaste to the oral application of antiseptics (chlorhexidine and povidone-iodine) and topical antibiotics such as SOD. Based on four studies, tooth brushing did not reduce the incidence of VAP or other objective outcomes.[98] A more recent systematic review and meta-analysis reviewed 2337 studies of which four were included in the systematic review and three in the meta-analysis comparing tooth brushing combined with oral chlorhexidine to oral chlorhexidine alone.[99] The investigators concluded that more studies with larger sample sizes are needed to draw strong conclusions. However, considering that tooth brushing is a simple intervention, it should be a common practice in mechanically ventilated patients.

Antiseptics were thought to be ideal tools in oral care, and the initial randomized trials in cardiac surgery patients showed a benefit in reducing VAP rates and at times mortality.[100] In subsequent meta-analyses, it seemed that the benefit was not so striking for povidone-iodine as it was for chlorhexidine and that the main achievement was lower VAP rates without significant impact on mortality or duration of ventilation and ICU stays.[101-103] More recent studies have questioned chlorhexidine's positive role. When isolating the impact on mortality using a network meta-analysis methodology, British investigators found chlorhexidine to augment the risk of dying in a general ICU population (OR 1.25, 95% CI 1.05–1.5).[104] However, in the same study, SDD was the most beneficial in terms of improving outcomes with OR 0.73 (0.64–0.84), whereas SOD had OR of 0.85 (0.74–0.97). In a detailed meta-analysis, Klompas and colleagues found that the benefit of VAP reduction with chlorhexidine of approximately 27% was mainly derived from studies in cardiac surgery patients.[105] For noncardiac patients, the OR crossed 1 (OR 0.78, 95% CI 0.6–1.02) and the investigators also discovered that chlorhexidine may increase the risk of dying in these patients, although this finding did not reach statistical significance (respiratory rate [RR] 1.13, 0.99–1.29). The same group found a stronger association between chlorhexidine use and ventilator mortality when analyzing the bundle components separately (heart rate [HR] 1.6, 95% CI 1.2–2.3, $P = .06$).[38] Taking into account these findings, the European Respiratory Society guidelines favored SOD but did not make any recommendation on chlorhexidine use for VAP prevention.[96]

The two most recent meta-analyses concluded that oral chlorhexidine was associated with a reduction in VAP rates and not associated with excess mortality.[106,107] However, these analyses suggested that the quality of the evidence was poor and that more studies are required to determine the overall benefit of oral chlorhexidine administration as well as the optimal drug concentration to be used.

5. Intravenous antibiotics

As noted above, the aspiration of contaminated secretions likely contributes to the occurrence of nosocomial pneumonia. Therefore, intravenous antibiotic prophylaxis has been suggested as a means to prevent these infections in patients with altered mental status at high risk for aspiration. A meta-analysis found identified three studies with 267 patients for analysis with most patients being comatose due to head trauma.[108] Systemic antibiotic administration was associated with decreased incidence of VAP and shorter ICU length of stay, but had no effect on mortality or duration of mechanical ventilation. A large recent trial in almost 200 patients found that a 2-day course of amoxicillin–clavulanate in patients receiving a 32-to-34°C targeted temperature management strategy after out-of-hospital cardiac arrest with initial shockable rhythm resulted in a lower incidence of VAP.[109] No significant between-group differences were observed for other key clinical variables, such as ventilator-free days and mortality at day 28.

6. Probiotics

The use of probiotics has been associated with improved VAP rates but without significant changes in mortality, duration of mechanical ventilation, and length of stay.[110,111] However, a recent randomized trial of 2650 critically ill patients requiring mechanical ventilation found that the administration of the probiotic *Lactobacillus rhamnosus* GG compared with placebo, resulted in no significant difference in the development of VAP.[112] Therefore, the routine use of probiotics in critically ill patients to reduce VAP rates is not recommended.

Bundle Compliance

Just recommending a list of bundled measures will never suffice. Health care providers need to be engaged and be active participants in the quality improvement process. A sustained effort is expected along with auditing, feedback, and continuous education. In general, the higher the compliance rates with the proposed bundles, the better the outcomes, although some studies recorded improved VAP rates even with compliance below 30%.[57] Studies have also shown that a higher level of understanding of VAP among health care providers helps to improve compliance rates.[113] The highest reductions in VAP rates have been achieved with sequential introduction of mandatory measures but it can take up to 1 to 2 years for the full benefit to be seen.[114] Compliance rates also vary across bundle components,[57,113] but it remains unclear which bundle elements should be focused on given the significant interactions between these elements in the available studies. It is expected that compliance with bundle elements will wane over time in the absence of constant reinforcement and that there is a threshold effect beyond which VAP incidence cannot be lowered any further even in the presence of well-constructed and managed prevention programs.[115]

Recent studies provide contradictory findings regarding the relationship between bundle compliance and occurrence of VAP or other adverse events. A study from Vanderbilt University found that ventilator bundle compliance was not associated with a reduced risk for VAEs or VAP.[116] Higher compliance with chlorhexidine oral care was associated with a greater risk for VAE development. Alternatively, a recent retrospective study conducted in a trauma ICU found that reduction in VAP rates could be achieved by implementing a standardized, evidence-based, prevention protocol, at least for the short term.[117] The future application of artificial intelligence methods may help identify patients at high risk for VAP so that the directed interventions can be targeted to those patients.[118,119]

Cost-Effectiveness

With a myriad of available interventions, cost-effectiveness becomes relevant. Unfortunately, cost-effectiveness is a very dynamic process and the medical costs change for interventions that have been accepted over long periods of time. Branch-Elliman and colleagues tried to identify the most cost-effective strategy for VAP prevention from both hospital and societal perspectives.[78] From the hospital standpoint, the Institute for Healthcare Improvement VAP prevention bundle, subglottic suctioning, and probiotics were found to be preferred. The preferred methods from the societal perspective included oral care with chlorhexidine and SDD. Cost-effectiveness goals could also differ between various types of ICUs and types of patients, and they should also consider the impact on longer term outcomes including the emergence of antimicrobial resistance. More recently, a systematic review concluded that effective implementation of VAP care bundles was associated with superior clinical and economic outcomes.[120] However, despite finding a moderate volume of research, study heterogeneity inhibited strong conclusions being drawn regarding the degree of associated cost savings.

SUMMARY

In an era dominated by antimicrobial resistance that defines nosocomial pneumonia, especially VAP in the post-SARS-CoV-19 era, it is unlikely that our vulnerable, immunocompromised patients requiring prolonged hospitalizations for new surgeries or cancer treatments will not be at risk for developing VAP. We need better VAP definitions to truly assess the impact of VAP on patient outcomes and the impact of prevention bundles on VAP incidence. If VAP remains a subjective, elusive diagnosis, the focus should be on more objective improvements such as ventilator-free days, length of stay, and antibiotic use. Prevention bundles should generally be as simple as possible, made up of evidence-based interventions but also taking into account variables that determine long-term compliance rates and workload burden. More research is needed to identify which prevention strategies perform best in hospitals with high rates versus low rates of bacterial resistance, or surgical versus medical ICUs, and to help identify patients at the highest risk for VAP therefore creating a more ICU personalized efficient bundle. Finally, the use of prolonged mechanical ventilation with tracheostomy, and often transfer to special long-term acute care facilities, is increasing in North America despite poor outcomes, or futile care, for many of these patients.[121,122] Given this trend, there is really no hope for attaining zero rates of VAP in the future.

CLINICS CARE POINTS

- Mechanical ventilation weaning protocols that are updated and adhered to are an effective method for reducing the occutrence of ventilator-associated pneumonia.
- Keeping the head of the bed elevated can help reduce aspiration and ventiltor-associated pneumonia.
- Each intensive care unit should have a ventilator-associated pneumonia prevention program in place with compliance montiored on a regular basis.

DISCLOSURES

Dr M.H. Kollef's efforts were supported by the Barnes-Jewish Hospital Foundation, United States. Dr C.V. Guillamet has no conflicts of interest to report.

REFERENCES

1. Kalil AC, Metersky ML, Klompas M, et al. Management of Adults With Hospital-acquired and Ventilator-associated Pneumonia: 2016 Clinical Practice Guidelines by the Infectious Diseases Society of America and the American Thoracic Society. Clin Infect Dis 2016;63:e61–111.
2. Torres A, Niederman MS, Chastre J, et al. International ERS/ESICM/ESCMID/ALAT guidelines for the management of hospital-acquired pneumonia and ventilator-associated pneumonia: Guidelines for the management of hospital-acquired pneumonia (HAP)/ventilator-associated pneumonia (VAP) of the European Respiratory Society (ERS), European Society of Intensive Care Medicine (ESICM), European Society of Clinical Microbiology and Infectious Diseases (ESCMID) and Asociación Latinoamericana del Tórax (ALAT). Eur Respir J 2017;50:1700582.
3. Vincent JL, Sakr Y, Singer M, et al. Prevalence and Outcomes of Infection Among Patients in Intensive Care Units in 2017. JAMA 2020;323:1478–87.
4. Melsen WG, Rovers MM, Groenwold RHH, et al. Attributable mortality of ventilator-associated pneumonia: a meta-analysis of individual patient data from randomised prevention studies. Lancet Infect Dis 2013;13:665–71.
5. Kollef MH, Hamilton CW, Ernst FR. Economic impact of ventilator-associated pneumonia in a large matched cohort. Infect Control Hosp Epidemiol 2012; 33:250–6.
6. Klompas M, Branson R, Eichenwald EC, et al. Strategies to prevent ventilator-associated pneumonia in acute care hospitals: 2014 update. Infect Control Hosp Epidemiol 2014;35:915–36.
7. Wunderink RG, Woldenberg LS, Zeiss J, et al. The radiologic diagnosis of autopsy-proven ventilator-associated pneumonia. Chest 1992;101:458–63.
8. Klompas M. Interobserver variability in ventilator-associated pneumonia surveillance. Am J Infect Control 2010;38:237–9.
9. Dudeck MA, Weiner LM, Allen-Bridson K, et al. National Healthcare Safety Network (NHSN) report, data summary for 2012, Device-associated module. Am J Infect Control 2013;41:1148–66.
10. Rosenthal VD, Al-Abdely HM, El-Kholy AA, et al. International Nosocomial Infection Control Consortium report, data summary of 50 countries for 2010-2015: Device-associated module. Am J Infect Control 2016;44:1495–504.
11. Kollef MH, Chastre J, Fagon J-Y, et al. Global prospective epidemiologic and surveillance study of ventilator-associated pneumonia due to *Pseudomonas aeruginosa*. Crit Care Med 2014;42:2178–87.
12. Skrupky LP, McConnell K, Dallas J, et al. A comparison of ventilator-associated pneumonia rates as identified according to the National Healthcare Safety Network and American College of Chest Physicians criteria. Crit Care Med 2012;40:281–4.
13. Magill SS, Klompas M, Balk R, et al. Developing a new, national approach to surveillance for ventilator-associated events: executive summary. Clin Infect Dis 2013;57:1742–6.
14. Kobayashi H, Uchino S, Takinami M, et al. The Impact of Ventilator-Associated Events in Critically Ill Subjects with Prolonged Mechanical Ventilation. Respir Care 2017;62:1379–86.
15. Fan Y, Gao F, Wu Y, et al. Does ventilator-associated event surveillance detect ventilator-associated pneumonia in intensive care units? A systematic review and meta-analysis. Crit Care 2016;20:338.

16. Bergin SP, Coles A, Calvert SB, et al. PROPHETIC: Prospective Identification of Pneumonia in Hospitalized Patients in the ICU. Chest 2020;158:2370–80.

17. Bergin SP, Calvert SB, Farley J, et al. PROPHETIC EU: Prospective Identification of Pneumonia in Hospitalized Patients in the Intensive Care Unit in European and United States Cohorts. Open Forum Infect Dis 2022;9:ofac231.

18. CDC. COVID-19: U.S. Impact on antimicrobial resistance, special report 2022. Atlanta, GA: U.S. Department of Health and Human Services, CDC; 2022. Available at: https://www.cdc.gov/drugresistance/covid19.html. (Accessed 19 June 2023).

19. Vacheron C-H, Lepape A, Savey A, et al. Attributable mortality of ventilator-associated pneumonia among patients with COVID-19. Am J Respir Crit Care Med 2022;206:161–9.

20. Pickens CO, Gao CA, Cuttica MJ, et al. NU COVID Investigators. Bacterial superinfection pneumonia in patients mechanically ventilated for COVID-19 pneumonia. Am J Respir Crit Care Med 2021;204:921–32.

21. Metersky ML, Wang Y, Klompas M, et al. Trend in Ventilator-Associated Pneumonia Rates between 2005 and 2013. JAMA 2016;316:2427–9.

22. Zilberberg MD, Nathanson BH, Puzniak LA, et al. Descriptive Epidemiology and Outcomes of Nonventilated Hospital-Acquired, Ventilated Hospital-Acquired, and Ventilator-Associated Bacterial Pneumonia in the United States, 2012-2019. Crit Care Med 2022;50:460–8.

23. Motowski H, Ilges D, Hampton N, et al. Determinants of Mortality for Ventilated Hospital-Acquired Pneumonia and Ventilator-Associated Pneumonia. Crit Care Explor 2023;5:e0867.

24. Bekaert M, Timsit JF, Vansteelandt S, et al. Attributable mortality of ventilator-associated pneumonia: a reappraisal using causal analysis. Am J Respir Crit Care Med 2011;184:1133–9.

25. Nguile-Makao M, Zahar J-R, Français A, et al. Attributable mortality of ventilator-associated pneumonia: respective impact of main characteristics at ICU admission and VAP onset using conditional logistic regression and multi-state models. Intensive Care Med 2010;36:781–9.

26. Kollef MH. Ventilator-associated Pneumonia Prevention. Is It Worth It? Am J Respir Crit Care Med 2015;192:5–7.

27. Botlet E, Yakusheva O, Costa DK. Nursing strategies to prevent ventilator-associated pneumonia. Am Nurse Today 2017;12:42–3.

28. Kollef MH, Sherman G, Ward S, et al. Inadequate antimicrobial treatment of infections: a risk factor for hospital mortality among critically ill patients. Chest 1999;115:462–74.

29. Iregi M, Ward S, Sherman G, et al. Clinical importance of delays in the initiation of appropriate antibiotic treatment for ventilator-associated pneumonia. Chest 2002;122:262–8.

30. Torres A, Serra-Batlles J, Ros E, et al. Pulmonary aspiration of gastric contents in patients receiving mechanical ventilation: the effect of body position. Ann Intern Med 1992;116:540–3.

31. Garrouste-Orgeas M, Chevret S, Arlet G, et al. Oropharyngeal or gastric colonization and nosocomial pneumonia in adult intensive care unit patients. A prospective study based on genomic DNA analysis. Am J Respir Crit Care Med 1997;156:1647–55.

32. Bonten MJ, Gaillard CA, van Tiel FH, et al. The stomach is not a source for colonization of the upper respiratory tract and pneumonia in ICU patients. Chest 1994;105:878–84.

33. Drakulovic MB, Torres A, Bauer TT, et al. Supine body position as a risk factor for nosocomial pneumonia in mechanically ventilated patients: a randomised trial. Lancet 1999;354:1851–8.

34. van Nieuwenhoven CA, Vandenbroucke-Grauls C, van Tiel FH, et al. Feasibility and effects of the semirecumbent position to prevent ventilator-associated pneumonia: a randomized study. Crit Care Med 2006;34:396–402.

35. Williams Z, Chan R, Kelly E. A simple device to increase rates of compliance in maintaining 30-degree head-of-bed elevation in ventilated patients. Crit Care Med 2008;36:1155–7.

36. Wolken RF, Woodruff RJ, Smith J, et al. Observational study of head of bed elevation adherence using a continuous monitoring system in a medical intensive care unit. Respir Care 2012;57:537–43.

37. Wang L, Li X, Yang Z, et al. Semi-recumbent position versus supine position for the prevention of ventilator-associated pneumonia in adults requiring mechanical ventilation. Cochrane Database Syst Rev 2016;CD009946.

38. Klompas M, Li L, Kleinman K, et al. Associations between Ventilator Bundle Components and Outcomes. JAMA Intern Med 2016;176:1277–83.

39. Li Bassi G, Panigada M, Ranzani OT, et al. Randomized, multicenter trial of lateral Trendelenburg versus semirecumbent body position for the prevention of ventilator-associated pneumonia. Intensive Care Med 2017;43:1572–84.

40. Zhu X, Lu Z, Xiao W, et al. The effect of prone position for ventilator-associated pneumonia in adult patients: a systematic review and meta-analysis. Emerg Crit Care Med 2021;1:37–44.

41. Head of bed elevation or semirecumbent positioning literature review. Content last reviewed January 2017. Agency for Healthcare Research and Quality, Rockville, MD. https://www.ahrq.gov/hai/tools/mvp/modules/technical/head-bed-elevation-lit-review.html. (Accessed 20 June 2023).

42. Kress JP, Pohlman AS, O'Connor MF, et al. Daily interruption of sedative infusions in critically ill patients undergoing mechanical ventilation. N Engl J Med 2000;342:1471–7.

43. Strøm T, Martinussen T, Toft P. A protocol of no sedation for critically ill patients receiving mechanical ventilation: a randomised trial. Lancet 2010;375:475–80.

44. Girard TD, Kress JP, Fuchs BD, et al. Efficacy and safety of a paired sedation and ventilator weaning protocol for mechanically ventilated patients in intensive care (Awakening and Breathing Controlled trial): a randomised controlled trial. Lancet 2008;371:126–34.

45. Mehta S, Burry L, Cook D, et al. Daily sedation interruption in mechanically ventilated critically ill patients cared for with a sedation protocol: a randomized controlled trial. JAMA 2012;308:1985–92.

46. Balas MC, Tan A, Mion LC, et al. Factors Associated With Spontaneous Awakening Trial and Spontaneous Breathing Trial Performance in Adults With Critical Illness: Analysis of a Multicenter, Nationwide, Cohort Study. Chest 2022;162:588–602.

47. Moraes FDS, Marengo LL, Moura MDG, et al. ABCDE and ABCDEF care bundles: A systematic review of the implementation process in intensive care units. Medicine (Baltim) 2022;101:e29499.

48. Ely EW, Baker AM, Dunagan DP, et al. Effect on the duration of mechanical ventilation of identifying patients capable of breathing spontaneously. N Engl J Med 1996;335:1864–9.

49. Kollef MH, Shapiro SD, Silver P, et al. A randomized, controlled trial of protocol-directed versus physician-directed weaning from mechanical ventilation. Crit Care Med 1997;25:567–74.

50. Lellouche F, Mancebo J, Jolliet P, et al. A multicenter randomized trial of computer-driven protocolized weaning from mechanical ventilation. Am J Respir Crit Care Med 2006;174:894–900.

51. Blackwood B, Burns KEA, Cardwell CR, et al. Protocolized versus non-protocolized weaning for reducing the duration of mechanical ventilation in critically ill adult patients. Cochrane Database Syst Rev 2014;CD006904.

52. Thille AW, Gacouin A, Coudroy R, et al. Spontaneous-Breathing Trials with Pressure-Support Ventilation or a T-Piece. N Engl J Med 2022;387. 1843-18.

53. Pohlman MC, Schweickert WD, Pohlman AS, et al. Feasibility of physical and occupational therapy beginning from initiation of mechanical ventilation. Crit Care Med 2010;38:2089–94.

54. Schweickert WD, Pohlman MC, Pohlman AS, et al. Early physical and occupational therapy in mechanically ventilated, critically ill patients: a randomised controlled trial. Lancet 2009;373:1874–82.

55. Patel BK, Wolfe KS, Patel SB, et al. Effect of early mobilisation on long-term cognitive impairment in critical illness in the USA: a randomised controlled trial. Lancet Respir Med 2023;11:563–72.

56. Su K-C, Kou YR, Lin F-C, et al. A simplified prevention bundle with dual hand hygiene audit reduces early-onset ventilator-associated pneumonia in cardiovascular surgery units: An interrupted time-series analysis. PLoS One 2017;12:e0182252.

57. Rello J, Afonso E, Lisboa T, et al. A care bundle approach for prevention of ventilator-associated pneumonia. Clin Microbiol Infect 2013;19:363–9.

58. Koff MD, Corwin HL, Beah ML, et al. Reduction in ventilator associated pneumonia in a mixed intensive care unit after initiation of a novel hand hygiene program. Crit Care 2011;26:489–95.

59. Ma S, Liu S, Huang L, et al. A meta-analysis of the effect of enhanced hand hygiene on the morbidity of ventilator-associated pneumonia. Zhonghua Wei Zhong Bing Ji Jiu Yi Xue 2014;26:304–8.

60. Kollef MH, Shapiro SD, Fraser VJ, et al. Mechanical ventilation with or without 7-day circuit changes. A randomized controlled trial. Ann Intern Med 1995;123:168–74.

61. Han J, Liu Y. Effect of ventilator circuit changes on ventilator-associated pneumonia: a systematic review and meta-analysis. Respir Care 2010;55:467–74.

62. Dezfulian C, Shojania K, Collard HR, et al. Subglottic secretion drainage for preventing ventilator-associated pneumonia: a meta-analysis. Am J Med 2005;118:11–8.

63. Muscedere J, Rewa O, McKechnie K, et al. Subglottic secretion drainage for the prevention of ventilator-associated pneumonia: a systematic review and meta-analysis. Crit Care Med 2011;39:1985–91.

64. Caroff DA, Li L, Muscedere J, et al. Subglottic Secretion Drainage and Objective Outcomes: A Systematic Review and Meta-Analysis. Crit Care Med 2016;44:830–40.

65. Zheng R-Q, Lin H, Shao J, et al. A clinical study of subglottic secretion drainage for prevention of ventilation associated pneumonia. Zhongguo Wei Zhong Bing Ji Jiu Yi Xue 2008;20:338–40.

66. Mastrogianni M, Katsoulas T, Galanis P, et al. The Impact of Care Bundles on Ventilator-Associated Pneumonia (VAP) Prevention in Adult ICUs: A Systematic Review. Antibiotics (Basel) 2023;12:227.
67. Sole ML, Penoyer DA, Su X, et al. Assessment of endotracheal cuff pressure by continuous monitoring: a pilot study. Am J Crit Care 2009;18:133–43.
68. Nseir S, Lorente L, Ferrer M, et al. Continuous control of tracheal cuff pressure for VAP prevention: a collaborative meta-analysis of individual participant data. Ann Intensive Care 2015;5:43.
69. Nseir S, Zerimech F, Fournier C, et al. Continuous control of tracheal cuff pressure and microaspiration of gastric contents in critically ill patients. Am J Respir Crit Care Med 2011;184:1041–7.
70. Letvin A, Kremer P, Silver PC, et al. Frequent Versus Infrequent Monitoring of Endotracheal Tube Cuff Pressures. Respir Care 2018;63:495–501.
71. Marjanovic N, Boisson M, Asehnoune K, et al. Continuous Pneumatic Regulation of Tracheal Cuff Pressure to Decrease Ventilator-associated Pneumonia in Trauma Patients Who Were Mechanically Ventilated: The AGATE Multicenter Randomized Controlled Study. Chest 2021;160:499–508.
72. Monsel A, Lu Q, Le Corre M, et al. Tapered-cuff Endotracheal Tube Does Not Prevent Early Postoperative Pneumonia Compared with Spherical-cuff Endotracheal Tube after Major Vascular Surgery: A Randomized Controlled Trial. Anesthesiology 2016;124:1041–52.
73. Philippart F, Gaudry S, Quinquis L, et al. Randomized intubation with polyurethane or conical cuffs to prevent pneumonia in ventilated patients. Am J Respir Crit Care Med 2015;191:637–45.
74. Jaillette E, Brunin G, Girault C, et al. Impact of tracheal cuff shape on microaspiration of gastric contents in intubated critically ill patients: study protocol for a randomized controlled trial. Trials 2015;16:429.
75. Dewavrin F, Zerimech F, Boyer A, et al. Accuracy of alpha amylase in diagnosing microaspiration in intubated critically-ill patients. PLoS One 2014;9:e90851.
76. Maertens B, Blot K, Blot S. Prevention of Ventilator-Associated and Early Postoperative Pneumonia through Tapered Endotracheal Tube Cuffs: A Systematic Review and Meta-Analysis of Randomized Controlled Trials. Crit Care Med 2018;46:316–23.
77. Kollef MH, Afessa B, Anzueto A, et al. Silver-coated endotracheal tubes and incidence of ventilator-associated pneumonia: the NASCENT randomized trial. JAMA 2008;300:805–13.
78. Branch-Elliman W, Wright SB, Howell MD. Determining the Ideal Strategy for Ventilator-associated Pneumonia Prevention. Cost-Benefit Analysis. Am J Respir Crit Care Med 2015;192:57–63.
79. Shorr AF, Zilberberg MD, Kollef M. Cost-effectiveness analysis of a silver-coated endotracheal tube to reduce the incidence of ventilator-associated pneumonia. Infect Control Hosp Epidemiol 2009;30:759–63.
80. Pirrone M, Imber DAE, Marrazzo F, et al. Silver-Coated Endotracheal Tubes Cleaned With a Mechanism for Secretion Removal. Respir Care 2019;64:1–9.
81. Reignier J, Mercier E, Le Gouge A, et al. Effect of not monitoring residual gastric volume on risk of ventilator-associated pneumonia in adults receiving mechanical ventilation and early enteral feeding: a randomized controlled trial. JAMA 2013;309:249–56.
82. Yasuda H, Kondo N, Yamamoto R, et al. Monitoring of gastric residual volume during enteral nutrition Cochrane. Database Syst Rev 2021;9:CD013335.

83. Leone M, Bouadma L, Bouhemad B, et al. Hospital-acquired pneumonia in ICU. Anaesth Crit Care Pain Med 2018;37:83–98.

84. de Smet AMGA, Kluytmans JW, Cooper BS, et al. Decontamination of the digestive tract and oropharynx in ICU patients. N Engl J Med 2009;360:20–31.

85. Oostdijk EAN, Kesecioglu J, Schultz MJ, et al. Notice of Retraction and Replacement: Oostdijk et al. Effects of Decontamination of the Oropharynx and Intestinal Tract on Antibiotic Resistance in ICUs: A Randomized Clinical Trial. JAMA. 2014;312(14):1429-1437. JAMA 2017;317:1583–4.

86. Roquilly A, Marret E, Abraham E, et al. Pneumonia prevention to decrease mortality in intensive care unit: a systematic review and meta-analysis. Clin Infect Dis 2015;60:64–75.

87. Hammond NE, Myburgh J, Seppelt I, et al. Association Between Selective Decontamination of the Digestive Tract and In-Hospital Mortality in Intensive Care Unit Patients Receiving Mechanical Ventilation. A Systematic Review and Meta-analysis. JAMA 2022;328:1922–34.

88. Myburgh JA, Seppelt IM, Goodman F, et al. Effect of Selective Decontamination of the Digestive Tract on Hospital Mortality in Critically Ill Patients Receiving Mechanical Ventilation. A Randomized Clinical Trial. JAMA 2022;328:1911–21.

89. Daneman N, Sarwar S, Fowler RA, et al. Effect of selective decontamination on antimicrobial resistance in intensive care units: a systematic review and meta-analysis. Lancet Infect Dis 2013;13:328–41.

90. Wittekamp BHJ, Oostdijk EAN, de Smet AMGA, et al. Colistin and tobramycin resistance during long- term use of selective decontamination strategies in the intensive care unit: a post hoc analysis. Crit Care 2015;19:113.

91. de Smet AMGA, Kluytmans JW, Blok HEM, et al. Selective digestive tract decontamination and selective oropharyngeal decontamination and antibiotic resistance in patients in intensive-care units: an open-label, clustered group-randomised, crossover study. Lancet Infect Dis 2011;11:372–80.

92. Houben AJM, Oostdijk EaN, van der Voort PHJ, et al. Selective decontamination of the oropharynx and the digestive tract, and antimicrobial resistance: a 4 year ecological study in 38 intensive care units in the Netherlands. J Antimicrob Chemother 2014;69:797–804.

93. van der Bij AK, Frentz D, Bonten MJM, ISIS-AR Study Group. Gram-positive cocci in Dutch ICUs with and without selective decontamination of the oropharyngeal and digestive tract: a retrospective database analysis. J Antimicrob Chemother 2016;71:816–20.

94. Oostdijk EAN, de Smet AMGA, Blok HEM, et al. Ecological effects of selective decontamination on resistant gram-negative bacterial colonization. Am J Respir Crit Care Med 2010;181:452–7.

95. Frencken JF, Wittekamp BHJ, Plantinga NL, et al. Associations between Enteral Colonization with Gram-Negative Bacteria and Intensive Care Unit-Acquired Infections and Colonization of the Respiratory Tract. Clin Infect Dis 2018;66: 497–503.

96. Torres A, Niederman MS, Chastre J, et al. Summary of the international clinical guidelines for the management of hospital-acquired and ventilator-acquired pneumonia. ERJ Open Res 2018;4:00028–2018.

97. Wittekamp BJH, Oostdijk EAN, Cuthbertson BH, et al. Selective decontamination of the digestive tract (SDD) in critically ill patients: a narrative review. Intensive Care Med 2020;46:343–9.

98. Gu W-J, Gong Y-Z, Pan L, et al. Impact of oral care with versus without tooth-brushing on the prevention of ventilator-associated pneumonia: a systematic review and meta-analysis of randomized controlled trials. Crit Care 2012;16:R190.

99. Silva PUJ, Paranhos LR, Meneses-Santos D, et al. Combination of toothbrushing and chlorhexidine compared with exclusive use of chlorhexidine to reduce the risk of ventilator-associated pneumonia: A systematic review with meta-analysis. Clinics 2021;76:e2659.

100. DeRiso AJ, Ladowski JS, Dillon TA, et al. Chlorhexidine gluconate 0.12% oral rinse reduces the incidence of total nosocomial respiratory infection and non-prophylactic systemic antibiotic use in patients undergoing heart surgery. Chest 1996;109:1556–61.

101. Labeau SO, Van de Vyver K, Brusselaers N, et al. Prevention of ventilator-associated pneumonia with oral antiseptics: a systematic review and meta-analysis. Lancet Infect Dis 2011;11:845–54.

102. Chan EY, Ruest A, Meade MO, et al. Oral decontamination for prevention of pneumonia in mechanically ventilated adults: systematic review and meta-analysis. BMJ 2007;334:889.

103. Hua F, Xie H, Worthington HV, et al. Oral hygiene care for critically ill patients to prevent ventilator-associated pneumonia. Cochrane Database Syst Rev 2016; 10:CD008367.

104. Price R, MacLennan G, Glen J, SuDDICU Collaboration. Selective digestive or oropharyngeal decontamination and topical oropharyngeal chlorhexidine for prevention of death in general intensive care: systematic review and network meta-analysis. BMJ 2014;348:g2197.

105. Klompas M, Speck K, Howell MD, et al. Reappraisal of routine oral care with chlorhexidine gluconate for patients receiving mechanical ventilation: systematic review and meta-analysis. JAMA Intern Med 2014;174:751–61.

106. Dai W, Yany X, Huang P, et al. Meta-Analysis of the Efficacy and Safety of Chlorhexidine for Ventilator-Associated Pneumonia Prevention in Mechanically Ventilated Patients. Evid Based Complement Alternat Med 2022;2022:5311034.

107. Cruz JC, Martins CK, Piassi JEV, et al. Does chlorhexidine reduce the incidence of ventilator-associated pneumonia in ICU patients? A systematic review and meta-analysis. Med Intensiva 2022. S2173-5727:00329-330.

108. Righy C, Brasil PEA, Vallés J, et al. Systemic antibiotics for preventing ventilator-associated pneumonia in comatose patients: a systematic review and meta-analysis. Ann Intensive Care 2017;7:67.

109. François B, Cariou A, Clere-Jehl R, et al. Prevention of Early Ventilator-Associated Pneumonia after Cardiac Arrest. N Engl J Med 2019;381:1831–42.

110. Bo L, Li J, Tao T, et al. Probiotics for preventing ventilator-associated pneumonia. Cochrane Database Syst Rev; 2014. p. CD009066.

111. Morrow LE, Kollef MH, Casale TB. Probiotic prophylaxis of ventilator-associated pneumonia: a blinded, randomized, controlled trial. Am J Respir Crit Care Med 2010;182:1058–64.

112. Johnstone J, Meade M, Lauzier F, et al. Effect of Probiotics on Incident Ventilator-Associated Pneumonia in Critically Ill Patients: A Randomized Clinical Trial. JAMA 2021;326:1024–33.

113. Darawad MW, Sa'aleek MA, Shawashi T. Evidence-based guidelines for prevention of ventilator-associated pneumonia: Evaluation of intensive care unit nurses' adherence. Am J Infect Control 2018;46:711–3.

114. Bouadma L, Mourvillier B, Deiler V, et al. A multifaceted program to prevent ventilator-associated pneumonia: impact on compliance with preventive measures. Crit Care Med 2010;38:789–96.

115. Rosenthal VD, Rodrigues C, Álvarez-Moreno C, et al. Effectiveness of a multidimensional approach for prevention of ventilator-associated pneumonia in adult intensive care units from 14 developing countries of four continents: findings of the International Nosocomial Infection Control Consortium. Crit Care Med 2012; 40:3121–8.

116. Harris BD, Thomas GA, Greene MH, et al. Ventilator Bundle Compliance and Risk of Ventilator-Associated Events. Infect Control Hosp Epidemiol 2018;39: 637–43.

117. Buterakos R, Jenkins PM, Cranford J, et al. An in-depth look at ventilator-associated pneumonia in trauma patients and efforts to increase bundle compliance, education and documentation in a surgical trauma critical care unit. Am J Infect Control 2022;50:1333–8.

118. Brownstein JS, Rader B, Astley CM, et al. Advances in Artificial Intelligence for Infectious-Disease Surveillance. N Engl J Med 2023;388:1597–607.

119. Fitzpatrick F, Doherty A, Lacey G. Using Artificial Intelligence in Infection Prevention. Curr Treat Options Infect Dis 2020;12:135–44.

120. Ladbrook E, Khaw D, Bouchoucha S, et al. A systematic scoping review of the cost-impact of ventilator-associated pneumonia (VAP) intervention bundles in intensive care. Am J Infect Control 2021;49:928–36.

121. Lee T, Tan QL, Sinuff T, et al. Outcomes of prolonged mechanical ventilation and tracheostomy in critically ill elderly patients: a historical cohort study. Can J Anaesth 2022;69:1107–16.

122. Mehta A, Walkey AJ, Curran-Everett, et al. One-Year Outcomes Following Tracheostomy for Acute Respiratory Failure. Crit Care Med 2019;47:1572–81.

123. Girou E, Brun-Buisson C, Taillé S, et al. Secular trends in nosocomial infections and mortality associated with noninvasive ventilation in patients with exacerbation of COPD and pulmonary edema. JAMA 2003;290:2985–91.

124. Burns KEA, Meade MO, Premji A, et al. Noninvasive positive-pressure ventilation as a weaning strategy for intubated adults with respiratory failure. Cochrane Database Syst Rev 2013;CD004127.

125. Harris AD, Pineles L, Belton B, et al. Universal glove and gown use and acquisition of antibiotic-resistant bacteria in the ICU: a randomized trial. JAMA 2013; 310:1571–80.

126. George DL, Falk PS, Umberto Meduri G, et al. Nosocomial sinusitis in patients in the medical intensive care unit: a prospective epidemiological study. Clin Infect Dis 1998;27:463–70.

Management of Ventilator-Associated Pneumonia
Guidelines

Mark L. Metersky, MD[a],*, Andre C. Kalil, MD, MPH[b]

KEYWORDS

- Guideline • Hospital-acquired pneumonia • Ventilator-associated pneumonia
- Nosocomial pneumonia

KEY POINTS

- Although the guidelines for the diagnosis and treatment of hospital-acquired pneumonia (HAP) and ventilator associated pneumonia (VAP) recently released by the Infectious Diseases Society of America with the American Thoracic Society, and the European Respiratory Society have some noteworthy differences, they are more similar than different.
- Appropriate initial empiric antibiotic treatment of HAP and VAP is important for optimum patient outcomes. Both excessive antibiotic treatment and ineffective initial treatment have the potential to cause patient harm.
- There is considerable patient-level and hospital-level variation in the prevalence of resistant pathogens causing HAP and VAP. Empiric antibiotic regimens should be based on local antibiogram data and knowledge of patient-level factors that predict antibiotic-resistant pathogens.
- Most patients with HAP and VAP can be treated with a 7-day course of antibiotics.
- Procalcitonin measurement is not useful for determining if a patient with suspected VAP should receive antibiotics, but is useful in decreasing the length of antibiotic treatment in centers that do not routinely use short-course therapy.

INTRODUCTION

Ventilator-associated pneumonia (VAP) remains a common problem among patients who require invasive mechanical ventilation in acute care hospitals. Despite widespread implementation of care processes thought to decrease VAP rates, including

This article was previously published in *Clinics in Chest Medicine* 39:4 December 2018.
No authors report financial conflict of interest related to the subject of this article.
[a] Division of Pulmonary, Critical Care and Sleep Medicine, University of Connecticut School of Medicine, UConn Health, 263 Farmington Avenue, Farmington, CT 06030-1321, USA;
[b] Department of Internal Medicine, Division of Infectious Diseases, University of Nebraska Medical Center, 985400 Nebraska Medical Center, Omaha, NE 68198, USA
* Corresponding author.
E-mail address: Metersky@uchc.edu

Infect Dis Clin N Am 38 (2024) 87–101
https://doi.org/10.1016/j.idc.2023.12.004
0891-5520/24/© 2023 Elsevier Inc. All rights reserved.

head of bed elevation, sedation vacations, and daily assessment of readiness to wean, approximately 10% of patients ventilated for more than 2 days still develop VAP, a rate that has remained stable for more than a decade.[1] The consequences of VAP are considerable. The attributable mortality is estimated at approximately 13%.[2] VAP also results in significant morbidity, evidenced by a markedly prolonged hospital length of stay[3] and increased ventilator days in patients[4] who develop VAP compared with those who do not, with associated increased costs estimated at $40,000.[3]

In 2005, the American Thoracic Society (ATS) and Infectious Diseases Society of America (IDSA) published guidelines for the prevention and management of VAP (and hospital-acquired pneumonia [HAP] and health care–associated pneumonia).[5] These guidelines were subsequently updated in 2016 by a panel convened jointly by the ATS and the IDSA.[6] The 2016 guideline did not address VAP prevention because a comprehensive VAP prevention guideline and subsequent update had been published shortly before.[7] Subsequently, in 2017, the European Respiratory Society (ERS) with involvement of the European Society of Intensive Care Medicine, the European Society of Clinical Microbiology and Infectious Diseases, and the Latin American Thoracic Association published their guidelines on the management of VAP.[8] Both guidelines used the Grading of Recommendations Assessment, Development and Evaluation (GRADE) methodology, which relies on framing specific clinical questions, systematic literature reviews, and a specified process for determining the direction and strength of recommendations that are based on the results of those systematic reviews.

This article summarizes the 2016 IDSA-ATS and 2017 ERS guideline recommendations, and in doing so highlights similarities and differences between the recommendations. We also comment on a few subsequent publications relevant to the recommendations we review.

DIAGNOSIS OF VENTILATOR-ASSOCIATED PNEUMONIA

The accurate diagnosis of VAP is difficult for numerous reasons, including the multitude of reasons why patients in the intensive care unit (ICU) can develop fever or elevated white blood cell count, difficulty in distinguishing between bacterial colonization of the airway and infection, and the limitations of portable chest imaging in the ICU. The IDSA/ATS guidelines suggest that blood cultures and respiratory cultures be obtained on all patients with suspected VAP, although they acknowledge that there is limited evidence to support either test.[6] The ERS guidelines also recommend respiratory tract cultures on all patients, but do not address blood cultures.[8] The rationale for blood cultures is that although bacteremic VAP is uncommon, the presence of bacteremia can provide definitive evidence of the infecting organism and consequently can improve the accuracy of using appropriate antibiotics. Also, if a pathogen not usually causing respiratory tract infection is isolated, it can point to a nonrespiratory source needing investigation.[9,10] Because of the high prevalence of multidrug resistant (MDR) pathogens causing VAP, there is no debate about the need to perform respiratory cultures to guide antibiotic therapy for VAP.

What has remained controversial since the publication of the 2005 ATS/IDSA guidelines[5] is the best way to obtain and process samples for respiratory culture. Two methods are most commonly used in clinical practice. One is the culture of suctioned endotracheal aspirates, in a semiquantitative fashion, which generates a report of bacterial growth as absent, or with one of three levels of growth (eg, no growth, small, moderate, large). The other method commonly used involves quantitative culturing of samples obtained in a manner that more preferentially samples the lower airways and alveoli (usually via protected bronchoalveolar lavage [BAL]), thereby minimizing collection of bacteria that may be colonizing the airways. Culture results are reported as colony-forming units (CFUs) per milliliter, with greater than 10^3 CFUs/mL considered as representing infection. The potential advantage of quantitative BAL culture is that it may decrease the frequency of false-positive diagnosis of VAP caused by airway colonization. The potential disadvantages include delays in antibiotic therapy while awaiting performance of the BAL, the potential for false-negative cultures in the setting of prior antibiotic therapy, and the cost and burden to the microbiology laboratory associated with quantitative cultures. The potential advantages of semiquantitative cultures of tracheal aspirates include the avoidance of the negative effects on gas exchange caused by BAL and the probable higher sensitivity in the setting of antibiotic treatment.

The 2005 ATS/IDSA guidelines described both methodologies and the competing rationales, but made no specific recommendation of one over the other.[5] The 2016 IDSA/ATS[6] and the 2017 ERS[8] guidelines both addressed this issue. A systematic review and meta-analysis of studies investigating outcomes of patients randomized to either invasive respiratory sampling with quantitative cultures versus noninvasive sampling and semiquantitative cultures demonstrated no improvement in patient outcomes including mortality, ventilator days or ICU days, or antibiotic changes.[11] Both guidelines concluded from the available data that invasive techniques with quantitative cultures are not likely to improve clinical outcomes, may decrease antibiotic exposure, may increase risk in the most severely ill patients, and that they increase laboratory cost. The ERS guidelines make the point that decreased antibiotic costs may mitigate the laboratory costs. Based on these findings, the IDSA/ATS guideline panel recommended not performing invasive modalities with quantitative cultures, whereas the ERS guideline recommended that one of the two modalities be used. In both guidelines, the recommendations were weak, indicating the limited and inconclusive evidence base. The IDSA/ATS panel recognized the degree of clinical equipoise associated with this issue, such that many institutions already performing invasive sampling and quantitative cultures are likely to continue to do so. The panel believed that if quantitative cultures were performed, the available evidence demonstrated that it was generally safe to discontinue antibiotics in patients with a quantitative culture below the accepted threshold.

It is noteworthy that despite using the same evidence base, and coming to a similar finding on the risks and benefits, the two guidelines panels arrived at different recommendations. This result demonstrates that despite the more structured methodology of the GRADE approach, when the magnitude of risks and benefits is unclear or is small, subjective expert opinion and experience can influence the ultimate recommendation.

BIOMARKERS FOR THE DIAGNOSIS OF VENTILATOR-ASSOCIATED PNEUMONIA

The IDSA/ATS guidelines also addressed the use of biomarkers to assist in the diagnosis of VAP.[6] Ideally, a recommendation to use one of these biomarkers would be based on evidence of improved outcomes with their use. However, there were no studies that reported patient outcomes related to the use of these biomarkers to diagnose the presence of VAP. Therefore, the recommendation was based solely on the performance characteristics of the test. Neither procalcitonin (PCT), C-reactive protein, nor soluble triggering receptor expressed on myeloid cells were found to have adequate sensitivity or specificity to inspire a recommendation for their use to assist in the diagnosis of VAP.

TREATMENT OF VENTILATOR-ASSOCIATED PNEUMONIA

Both the IDSA/ATS and ERS guidelines acknowledge the importance of appropriate initial antibiotic therapy,[6,8] because initial inappropriate therapy is associated with worsened patient outcomes.[12,13] Yet a major concern that has increased in magnitude is the danger posed by indiscriminant antibiotic usage, which results in increased resistance rates, Clostridium difficile colitis, and other antibiotic-associated side effects. Guidelines for VAP walk a tightrope trying to balance the risk of undertreatment versus the risks of overtreatment. It is an unfortunate reality that there are limited data that provide reliable estimates on the magnitude of morbidity and mortality associated with these competing risks. The IDSA/ATS guidelines accepted a somewhat arbitrary target of creating initial empiric antibiotic regimens that would provide appropriate therapy for 95% of patients. Even with triple antibiotics for all patients, it might not be possible to achieve 100% appropriate initial empiric therapy; there would be diminishing returns and increased antibiotic usage associated with attempting to achieve appropriate coverage rates greater than 95%.

The difficulty in crafting such regimens is that antibiotic resistance rates vary widely among ICUs in different hospitals and even among different ICUs in the same hospital. Furthermore, patient-related risk factors for MDR pathogens are not well understood; it remains difficult to predict at a patient level which case of VAP will be caused by resistant organisms.

Although there have been numerous randomized controlled trials (RCTs) of antibiotics for VAP, essentially all of them were for the purpose of obtaining regulatory approval of specific antibiotics and therefore were not always designed to answer the most clinically relevant questions. Consequently, most of these trials are limited in their ability to answer questions about initial empiric therapy for various reasons, including limiting enrollment of patients with risk factors for MDR pathogens, and allowing initial broader spectrum coverage for a period of time preceding enrollment or until culture results were obtained. For all of these reasons, recommendations for initial empiric antibiotic treatment of VAP must be considered as a "best effort," of knowledgeable and thoughtful guideline panelists, but based on an incomplete evidence base.

INITIAL EMPIRIC REGIMEN FOR "EARLY ONSET" VENTILATOR-ASSOCIATED PNEUMONIA

Several studies have suggested that patients with early onset VAP are less likely to develop VAP with MDR organisms, such as methicillin-resistant Staphylococcus aureus (MRSA) or Pseudomonas aeruginosa, than patients who develop VAP later in their hospital stay.[14–18] Importantly, early onset VAP should be defined as VAP occurring within 4 to 5 days of hospitalization, not within 4 to 5 days of the onset of mechanical ventilation. Hospitalized patients are at increased risk of infection with MDR pathogens even before being intubated. Based on these observations, the 2005 guidelines recommended that empiric therapy for early onset VAP need not include coverage for P aeruginosa or MRSA if the patient had no risk factors for infection with MDR pathogens.[5] The ERS guidelines specifically developed a recommendation for antibiotic treatment of early onset VAP,[8] whereas the IDSA/ATS guidelines considered late-onset VAP a risk for MDR pathogens.[6]

When one examines the rate of MDR pathogens as a cause of early onset VAP, there are considerable rates of MDR pathogens, including MRSA and potentially drug-resistant gram-negative bacilli, such as Pseudomonas (Table 1). Of course, many of these patients have risk factors for MDR pathogens independent of length of hospital

Table 1
Frequency of potentially MDR pathogens in early onset nosocomial pneumonia versus late-onset pneumonia in studies published since 2010

First Author, Year of Publication	Potential MDR Pathogens in Early Onset Nosocomial Pneumonia (%)	Potential MDR Pathogens in Late-Onset Nosocomial Pneumonia (%)
Ferrer et al,[14] 2010	26[a]	29[b]
Restrepo et al,[15] 2013	28	32
Martin-Loeches et al,[16] 2013	51[b]	60[b]
Arvanitis et al,[17] 2014	10	32
Khan et al,[18] 2016	32	41

[a] Includes only early onset nosocomial without risks for MDR pathogens.
[b] Includes early onset with risks for MDR pathogens.

stay. The important question, then, is whether a subpopulation of patients with early onset VAP can be identified who are at sufficiently low risk of MDR pathogens that narrow-spectrum antibiotic treatment can be safely used.

Patients with early onset VAP after traumatic or medical brain injury have been considered by some experts as especially likely to develop early onset VAP with community-type nonresistant organisms, given the significant risk for aspiration at the time of the brain injury. A study of 48 such patients by Ewig and colleagues[19] in 1999 found that at the time of ICU admission, no patients had MRSA in their tracheobronchial aspirate or protected specimen brush, at least 4 of 41 had gram-negative enterics, and at least four had P aeruginosa. Serial cultures demonstrated an increase rate of isolation of potentially MDR pathogens starting at around Day 5. A study published in 2010 found that among 45 patients with head trauma who developed early onset VAP, one (2%) was caused by MRSA, four (9%) were caused by P aeruginosa, and nine (20%) were caused by gram-negative enterics. Although these percentages were generally lower than among the patients with late-onset VAP, they still represent a considerable risk for initial inappropriate antibiotic therapy if coverage for MDR pathogens was not used.[20]

In an observational study from a single ICU including 124 patients with nosocomial pneumonia (83% VAP), analysis identified certain factors associated with a lower risk of MDR pathogens. The absence of prior antimicrobial treatment, the presence of prior antimicrobial treatment with neurologic disturbances on ICU admission and early onset pneumonia, and the presence of prior antimicrobial treatment without neurologic disturbances but with aspiration on ICU admission were always associated with antimicrobial-susceptible pneumonia. The combination of these factors in a validation cohort of 26 patients allowed the validation of an algorithm that identified all patients with antimicrobial-susceptible nosocomial pneumonia.[21]

A prospective cohort study carried out to assess the rate of appropriateness of empirical antimicrobial therapy in 115 VAP patients showed that the mortality rate was significantly higher in the patients with inappropriate empirical therapy than in those with appropriate treatment (47% and 20%, respectively). A limited-spectrum therapy was used in 79 patients (69%) according to the criteria of early onset VAP (<5 days) without recent prior hospitalization or prior antibiotic treatment. Among these patients, there was a requirement for treatment escalation in 21 out of 79 patients (27%). The mortality rate was significantly higher in the patients in whom empirical therapy was inappropriate than in those in whom treatment was appropriate (47 vs 20%; P = .04).[12]

The ERS guidelines suggest using narrow-spectrum antibiotics (ertapenem, ceftriaxone, cefotaxime, moxifloxacin, or levofloxacin) in patients with suspected low risk of resistance and early onset HAP/VAP.[8] This was a weak recommendation, based on a very low quality of evidence. Patients defined as being at low risk were those without septic shock, with no other risk factors for MDR pathogens and those who are not in hospitals with a high background rate of resistant pathogens. However, the presence of other clinical conditions may make individuals unsuitable for this recommendation. A prevalence of resistant pathogens in the ICU caring for the patient in question of greater than 25% was considered a high background rate. It is not clear if patients with septic shock were defined as higher risk because such patients are at higher risk of having MDR pathogens or because the danger to the patient resulting from inadequate initial therapy is greater. However, both issues are likely relevant.

The IDSA/ATS guidelines, in contrast, did not separate out early onset VAP for a less broad-spectrum initial empiric regimen.[6] The guideline panelists believed that there was not adequate data to safely use narrow-spectrum antibiotic therapy in this patient population. Rather, a hospital length of stay of 5 or more days was considered a risk factor for MDR pathogens. Patients with less than 5 days of hospitalization and no other risk factors for MDR pathogens were still suggested for MDR gram-negative coverage, but MRSA coverage could be omitted if there was a low prevalence of MRSA in the facility.

The available evidence suggests that there are some patients with early onset VAP who are at low risk of MDR pathogens. However, there is limited evidence to suggest that clinicians can accurately define such patients at this time, because a sizable proportion of these patients will be infected with potentially resistant gram negatives or MRSA. The ERS recommendation that either ertapenem, cefotaxime, or ceftriaxone alone (agents without activity against *Pseudomonas* or MRSA) can be used for early onset VAP in patients without other risk factors for MDR pathogens is arguably the most significant area of difference between the ERS and IDSA/ATS guidelines.

INITIAL EMPIRIC ANTIBIOTIC THERAPY FOR NON–EARLY ONSET VENTILATOR-ASSOCIATED PNEUMONIA

There are marked geographic variations in the prevalence of MRSA and MDR gram negatives, and what classes of antibiotics these gram negatives are susceptible to. This fact makes it imperative that the clinician be aware of antibiotic resistance patterns in their hospital, and if possible their ICU. Both the IDSA/ATS and the ERS guidelines stress the importance of knowledge of local antibiotic resistance patterns as being integral for the informed choice of empiric antibiotic for patients in a given ICU. The ERS stressed this in a "good practice," statement, whereas the IDSA/ATS performed a systematic review of the literature and provided a strong recommendation.

Both the IDSA/ATS and the ERS guidelines provide recommendations for initial empiric antibiotic regimens. However, the wording of the specific clinical question being addressed differs greatly between the two guidelines. The ERS recommendation addresses the question of whether monotherapy can be used, or whether dual antibiotic coverage is always necessary.[8] Practically speaking, because essentially all patients whose VAP is not early onset require coverage for MDR gram-negative pathogens, for most patients, this is thought of as a question of whether MRSA coverage is required. Based on the risk for MDR pathogens and the patient's estimated risk of mortality, the ERS guidelines provided a suggested algorithm for initial empiric antibiotics in patients with HAP and VAP, although this algorithm was not directly linked to a formal recommendation (**Fig. 1**). Patients at low risk for mortality and low risk for MDR pathogens were recommended for monotherapy that would not cover MRSA, with some of the antibiotic choices potentially covering some isolates of nonfermenting gram negatives, such as *Pseudomonas*, and some not covering *Pseudomonas*.

The IDSA/ATS guidelines structured their question differently, addressing in a more general fashion the question of which antibiotics are recommended for the empiric treatment of VAP.[6] Gram-negative and gram-positive antibiotic coverage were addressed separately; the resulting regimen would be derived from the recommendations for gram-negative and gram-positive coverage relevant to the individual patient and the specific institution. IDSA/ATS an included coverage for MRSA and double coverage for MDR gram-negative bacilli for patients at high risk for MDR pathogens (**Table 2**). However, single gram-negative coverage was recommended in ICUs where the hospital or ICU antibiogram suggested that at least 90% of gram negatives would be sensitive to a single antibiotic. In such situations, certain antibiotics would allow monotherapy in settings where there were no risk factors for MRSA, as long as the antibiotic used was active against MSSA. Appropriate antibiotics in such situations could include piperacillin-tazobactam, cefepime, levofloxacin, or carbapenems depending on the local resistance patterns.

Both the IDSA/ATS and ERS guidelines recommend initial empiric coverage for *Pseudomonas* and MRSA in patients with risk factors for antibiotic resistance, including recent antibiotic exposure and treatment in an ICU with a high prevalence of MDR pathogens.

Recently, Ekren and colleagues[22] assessed the performance of the IDSA/ATS recommendations for initial empiric therapy in several ICUs in a single hospital. They found that guideline-concordant therapy resulted in initial appropriate empiric therapy for 97% of patients. In contrast, only 80% of patients with nonconcordant therapy receive appropriate empiric therapy (rate calculated based on numbers reported in

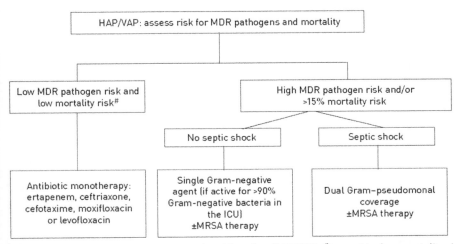

Fig. 1. Empiric antibiotic treatment algorithm for HAP/VAP. #Low risk for mortality is defined as a <15% chance of dying, a mortality rate that has been associated with better outcome using monotherapy than combination therapy when treating serious infection. (Reproduced with permission of the ERS 2023: European Respiratory Journal Sep 2017, 50 (3) 1700582; https://doi.org/10.1183/13993003.00582-2017.)

Table 2

Suggested empiric treatment options for clinically suspected ventilator-associated pneumonia in units where empiric methicillin-resistant *Staphylococcus aureus* coverage and double antipseudomonal/gram-negative coverage are appropriate

A. Gram-Positive Antibiotics with MRSA Activity	B. Gram-Negative Antibiotics with Antipseudomonal Activity: β-Lactam-Based Agents	C. Gram-Negative Antibiotics with Antipseudomonal Activity: Non-β-Lactam-Based Agents
Glycopeptides[a] Vancomycin, 15 mg/kg IV q 8–12 h (consider a loading dose of 25–30 mg/kg × 1 for severe illness)	Antipseudomonal penicillins[b] Piperacillin-tazobactam, 4.5 g IV q 6 h[b]	Fluoroquinolones Ciprofloxacin, 400 mg IV q 8 h Levofloxacin, 750 mg IV q 24 h
OR	OR	OR
Oxazolidinones Linezolid, 600 mg IV q 12 h	Cephalosporins[b] Cefepime, 2 g IV q 8 h Ceftazidime, 2 g IV q 8 h	Aminoglycosides[a,c] Amikacin, 15–20 mg/kg IV q 24 h Gentamicin, 5–7 mg/kg IV q 24 h Tobramycin, 5–7 mg/kg IV q 24 h
	OR	OR
	Carbapenems[b,d] Imipenem, 500 mg IV q 6 h[a] Meropenem, 1 g IV q 8 h	Polymyxins[a,e] Colistin, 5 mg/kg IV × 1 (loading dose) followed by 2.5 mg × (1.5 × CrCl + 30) IV daily, divided q 12 h (maintenance dose) Polymyxin B, 2.5–3.0 mg/kg/d divided in 2 daily IV doses
	OR	
	Monobactams[f] Aztreonam, 2 g IV q 8 h	

Abbreviations: CrCl, creatinine clearance; IV, Intravenous.

Choose one gram-positive option from column A, one gram-negative option from column B, and one gram-negative option from column C. Note that the initial doses suggested in this table may need to be modified for patients with hepatic or renal dysfunction.

[a] Drug levels and adjustment of doses and/or intervals required.

[b] Extended infusions may be appropriate. Please see the section on pharmacokinetic/pharmacodynamic optimization of antibiotic therapy.

[c] On meta-analysis, aminoglycoside regimens were associated with lower clinical response rates with no differences in mortality.

[d] The dose may need to be lowered in patients weighing less than 70 kg to prevent seizures.

[e] Polymyxins should be reserved for settings where there is a high prevalence of multidrug resistance and local expertise in using this medication. Dosing is based on colistin-base activity; for example, 1 million IU of colistin is equivalent to about 30 mg of colistin-base activity, which corresponds to about 80 mg of the prodrug colistimethate. Polymyxin B (1 mg = 10,000 units).

[f] In the absence of other options, it is acceptable to use aztreonam as an adjunctive agent with another β-lactam-based agent because it has different targets within the bacterial cell wall.

the research letter). This high appropriate therapy rate associated with guideline-concordant therapy might have come at a cost of antibiotic overuse; 60% of patients receiving guideline-concordant therapy received what was defined as overtreatment. However, the authors did not describe how they defined overtreatment; for example, it is unclear if double gram-negative coverage was defined as overtreatment if only one of the antibiotics would have covered the gram-negative pathogen ultimately isolated. Also, if antibiotic de-escalation and short-course treatment were appropriately performed as recommended in both guidelines, the initial empiric coverage should not have led to significant antibiotic overtreatment. The authors also noted that 25% of patients would have been adequately covered with community-acquired pneumonia-type antibiotics. It would have been interesting to know if these patients had characteristics that could have allowed then to be reliably identified. For example, were they mostly early onset? Despite the limitations represented by a single-center study and the unanswered questions, this study represents an interesting preliminary evaluation of a few aspects of the IDSA/ATS guidelines. It is hoped that further studies can help identify factors that would allow progress toward the "Holy Grail" of less broad-spectrum antibiotic coverage combined with a high rate of initial appropriate coverage. Unfortunately, we suspect that no single guideline will be able to achieve this goal, because of the marked variations in antibiotic resistance rates from ICU to ICU, hospital to hospital, and region to region. Ideally, hospitals will review their antibiograms in specific subpopulations, such as early onset VAP, to adapt antibiotic decisions to their local situation.

LENGTH OF ANTIBIOTIC THERAPY

The 2005 ATS/IDSA guidelines recommended 7 to 8 days of antibiotic therapy for most VAP patients who respond well to therapy, with the exception of patients infected by nonfermenting gram-negative bacilli (NF-GNB), including *Pseudomonas* spp, *Acinetobacter* spp, and *Stenotrophomonas maltophilia*.[5] This was based on a large multicenter trial demonstrating overall similar outcomes with the shorter course treatment, compared with a 15-day course of antibiotics.[23] However, the investigators noted a higher rate of recurrent VAP in the patients with NF-GNB who received short-course therapy. This finding was likely caused by the way in which the end point of recurrent VAP was calculated (at 28 days after the beginning of treatment). This meant that the short-course group had 21 days during which they were at risk for recurrence, whereas the longer course group had only 14 days at risk. When the recurrence rate was calculated per day at risk, there was no significant difference in recurrent VAP rate. Furthermore, the short course NF-GNB VAP patients had similar mortality, clinical cure, and ventilator days to patients receiving long-course therapy, suggesting that at least some of the recurrences may have been colonization, without clinical significance. The IDSA/ATS guideline panel further performed a systematic review with data provided by the authors of previous trials: the data analysis separated VAP caused by nonfermenting gram-negative rods, mostly *Pseudomonas* spp, *Acinetobacter* spp, and *Stenotrophomonas* spp, and found no significant differences between long and short courses for the following outcomes: mortality, clinical cure, pneumonia recurrence, and ventilation days. Two systematic reviews have concluded that short-course therapy (7–8 days) results in similar outcomes compared with longer course therapy (10–15 days).[24,25] Based on these data, the IDSA/ATS and the ERS guidelines recommended 7 to 8 days of therapy for most patients.[6,8] Although the ERS guideline does not exclude patients infected with NF-GNB from the recommendation for short-course therapy, they note that short-course therapy "may not be possible" for such patients and that therapy should be individualized. Of course, this is true for all patients; no matter what the infecting organism, if a patient is still febrile and producing copious amounts of purulent sputum on Day 5, a course of therapy greater than 7 days is likely appropriate. Furthermore, the ERS guidelines note that patients who received initially inappropriate therapy, might not be candidates for short-course therapy (perhaps the way to approach this issue is to consider the days of appropriate therapy when determining the length of therapy). The ERS guidelines also recommend that short-course therapy not be considered for patients with lung abscess or necrotizing pneumonia, although evidence is not provided to support this statement.[8] That being said, patients with lung abscess or necrotizing pneumonia are more likely to have prolonged symptomatology and/or slower clinical recovery, so they would likely fall within the IDSA/ATS recommendation to provide longer therapy based on individual patient response.

INHALED ANTIBIOTICS

The theoretic advantage of using inhaled antibiotics in VAP is the ability to deliver high concentrations of antibiotic directly to the airways. This might be especially relevant for such antibiotics as aminoglycosides, which penetrate poorly into the alveolar lining fluid when given intravenously. Several studies have evaluated the role of adjunctive inhaled antibiotics combined with intravenous antibiotics in patients with VAP. Most recruited patients were infected with organisms sensitive to only aminoglycosides or polymyxins (colistin or polymyxin B). A meta-analysis of these studies performed by the IDSA/ATS guidelines panelists demonstrated improved outcomes in patients who received adjunctive inhaled antibiotics.[6] The evidence was considered low quality because most were observational, unblinded studies, therefore subject to bias. Nonetheless, given the limited treatment options for these pathogens and lack of significant toxicity of adjunctive inhaled antibiotics in these studies, the IDSA/ATS guidelines suggested adjunctive inhaled antibiotics, but only for patients infected with MDR pathogens sensitive to only aminoglycosides or polymyxins. Fortunately, this remains a rare occurrence in the United States.

Recent studies of adjunctive inhaled amikacin[26] and amikacin-fosfamycin[27] with standard of care intravenous antibiotics failed to show benefit of adding inhaled antibiotics. However, the studies were not limited to pneumonia due to extremely drug resistant pathogens. At this point, evidence seems to be accumulating that adjunctive inhaled antibiotics should not be routinely used for VAP, but there is limited evidence suggesting that there may be benefit in the setting of pathogens that are only sensitive to aminoglycosides or polymyxins.

PHARMACOKINETIC/PHARMACODYNAMIC OPTIMIZED ANTIBIOTIC DOSING

A wealth of evidence in animal models has demonstrated that some antibiotics are more effective in killing bacteria when given in a manner not consistent with the parameters recommended by the manufacturers. For example, β-lactam antibiotics kill bacteria in a time-dependent fashion, such that killing is more effective the longer the serum antibiotic concentration remains higher than minimum inhibitory concentration. This finding suggests that continuous or prolonged infusion would be more effective than the traditional episodic bolus dosing. In contrast, such antibiotics as fluoroquinolones and aminoglycosides exhibit concentration-dependent killing, meaning that the higher the concentration achieved, the more effective the killing. This evidence, in addition to evidence suggesting lower toxicity with once-daily aminoglycoside dosing, has led to widespread adoption of this practice. The IDSA/ATS guideline panelists performed a systematic review of patient outcomes in patients who received pharmacokinetic/pharmacodynamic (PK/PD) optimized antibiotic dosing.[6] For the purposes of this recommendation, all antibiotics were considered in a single analysis, but most of the included studies were of prolonged infusion of β-lactam antibiotics. Two studies investigated serum concentration monitoring compared with manufacturer recommended dosing (eg, for vancomycin). Meta-analyses demonstrated a significant improvement in patient outcomes, including mortality, ICU length of stay, and clinical cure, associated with the use of PK/PD optimized dosing versus standard dosing. Based on these results, the IDSA/ATS guidelines gave a weak recommendation in favor of PK/PD optimized dosing. In doing so, the panel acknowledged the limitations of the data, because the amount of evidence for any specific antibiotic was limited. The Agency for Healthcare Research and Quality convened a panel to address this same question, and published their results in 2014.[28] In contrast to the IDSA/ATS recommendations, the Agency for Healthcare Research and Quality panel found insufficient evidence to either recommend or discourage PK/PD optimized dosing for VAP. The disparity between the findings of the two panels is likely because the Agency for Healthcare Research and Quality panel considered each antibiotic individually and excluded all observational studies, markedly limiting the amount of available evidence. Subsequent to the publication of the IDSA/ATS guidelines, a meta-analysis of RCTs investigating continuous infusion of β-lactams in severe sepsis was published. Approximately 55% of the patients had a pulmonary source of the sepsis. A significant improvement in mortality was noted; 19.6% versus 26.3% (relative risk, 0.74; 95% confidence interval, 0.56–1.00; $P = .045$).[29] A subsequent RCT in patients with severe sepsis also demonstrated improved clinical cure rates associated with continuous infusion of β-lactams.[30] Last, a newly updated systematic review and meta-analysis by a different research group also showed significant sepsis mortality reduction with prolonged antibiotic infusion compared with short-duration infusion.[31]

PROCALCITONIN FOR SHORTENING THE COURSE OF VENTILATOR-ASSOCIATED PNEUMONIA THERAPY

Three randomized trials,[32–34] including one published only in abstract form,[34] have assessed whether serial measurement of PCT can allow clinicians to safely shorten the length of antibiotic treatment of patients with VAP. Pooled analysis of these three trials demonstrated that the use of serial PCT measurement, when combined with clinical criteria, resulted in decreased antibiotic exposure (9.1 vs 12.1 days; $P<.00001$) with no difference in mortality. Other outcomes, such as ICU days and hospital length of stay, were assessed in some of these studies and also were not significantly different between groups. Based on these results, the IDSA/ATS guidelines gave a weak recommendation in favor of using serial PCT in combination with clinical criteria to shorten antibiotic exposure to patients with VAP.[6] However, the guideline noted that there is no evidence that doing so could decrease antibiotic exposure to less than 7 days, so this strategy is not likely to be of benefit in settings where clinicians accept the recommendation for 7 days as the standard length of antibiotic treatment of VAP. Subsequent to the publication of the IDSA/IDSA guidelines, a large multicenter RCT of ICU patients with suspected bacterial infection of any type demonstrated a significant decrease in antibiotic days with the use of serial PCT measurement.[35] In this study, the median length of antibiotic treatment in the PCT group was 5 days, whereas the standard of care treated group received antibiotics for a median of 7 days. Furthermore, the PCT-guided patients had a significantly higher survival (hazard ratio, 1.26; 95% confidence interval, 1.07–1.49). However, the applicability of this study to VAP is unclear. Although 65% of the patients included in the study had a suspected pulmonary source of infection, only about 49% of the patients had a hospital-acquired infection. A recent patient-level data meta-analysis by Schuetz and colleagues[36] also showed a significant mortality reduction and a significant decrease in antibiotic treatment duration specifically for acute respiratory infections from 8.1 days to 5.7 days.

The IDSA/ATS recommendation[6] differs somewhat from that made in the ERS guidelines, although the interpretation of the available literature and the intent of the two recommendations seem to be similar.[8] The European panel, similarly noting that an intended antibiotic course of 7 to 8 days was unlikely to be shortened by the use of PCT, recommended against routine PCT testing for this purpose when the anticipated length of antibiotic treatment was 7 to 8 days. However, they noted that in certain patient populations, a routine 7- to 8-day course of antibiotics might be unlikely. These include patients who had initially inappropriate antibiotic therapy, those with severe immunocompromise (neutropenia or stem cell transplant), patients with highly antibiotic-resistant pathogens (*P aeruginosa*, carbapenem-resistant *Acinetobacter* spp, carbapenem-resistant *Enterobacteriaceae*), and those being treated with second-line antibiotic therapy (eg, colistin, tigecycline). A good practice statement in the European guidelines suggested that the use of PCT in these settings, with the aim of decreasing the length of antibiotic therapy, represents good clinical practice. Of note, the use of PCT has not been studied specifically in any of these situations, either in original studies or as secondary/subgroup analyses of previously published studies.

OTHER RECOMMENDATIONS FOR HOSPITAL-ACQUIRED PNEUMONIA AND VENTILATOR-ASSOCIATED PNEUMONIA

Both the IDSA/ATS and the ERS guidelines included additional recommendations that are not discussed in this review. They are briefly listed in **Box 1** (IDSA/ATS guidelines) and **Box 2** (ERS guidelines).

Box 1
Recommendations from the 2016 IDSA/ATS HAP/VAP guidelines not discussed in this review

Recommendation against use of the clinical pulmonary infection score to assist with the decision of whether to start antibiotics in patients with suspected VAP

Recommendation against routine antibiotic treatment of ventilator-associated tracheobronchitis

Recommendations for initial empiric antibiotic regimens for HAP

Pathogen-specific therapy
   Recommendation for use of either vancomycin or linezolid for treatment of HAP/VAP caused by MRSA
   Recommendation against aminoglycoside monotherapy for treatment of *Pseudomonas* HAP/VAP
   Recommendation for combination therapy for *Pseudomonas* HAP/VAP for patients in septic shock or high risk of death at the time antibiotic susceptibility results become known
   No specific antibiotic class recommended for the treatment of extended-spectrum β-lactamase-producing gram-negative bacilli
   Recommendation for either ampicillin/sulbactam or a carbapenem for susceptible *Acinetobacter* species and against tigecycline

Recommendation in favor of antibiotic de-escalation

Recommendation against use of the clinical pulmonary infection score to assist with the decision of how long to continue antibiotics for VAP

Box 2
Recommendations from the 2017 European Respiratory Society Guidelines not discussed in this review

Recommendation against the routine use of biomarkers in patients being treated for nosocomial pneumonia to predict clinical response or likelihood of adverse outcomes

Recommendation against routine use of antibiotics for more than 3 days in patients with low probability of hospital-acquired pneumonia and no clinical deterioration within 3 days of symptom onset

Recommendation for the use of selective oral decontamination with nonabsorbable antibiotics to prevent VAP, in settings with low use of antibiotics (ICU with <1000 daily doses per patient days) and less than 5% prevalence of antibiotic-resistant bacteria

No recommendation on use of selective oral decontamination with chlorhexidine caused by unclear balance between potential reduction of pneumonia and increase in mortality

---

SUMMARY

During the past 2 years, two guidelines for the diagnosis and treatment of patients with HAP and VAP were released. Although these guidelines have some notable differences in their recommendations, they share more similarities than differences. A common theme among both guidelines is that high-quality evidence is lacking for many of the most commonly encountered diagnostic and treatment decisions. It is hoped that the publication of these guidelines will serve to define the areas of greatest need for clinical and basic research in HAP/VAP.

REFERENCES

1. Metersky ML, Wang Y, Klompas M, et al. Trend in ventilator-associated pneumonia rates between 2005 and 2013. JAMA 2016;316:2427–9.

2. Melsen WG, Rovers MM, Groenwold RH, et al. Attributable mortality of ventilator-associated pneumonia: a meta-analysis of individual patient data from randomised prevention studies. Lancet Infect Dis 2013;13:665–71.

3. Kollef MH, Hamilton CW, Ernst FR. Economic impact of ventilator-associated pneumonia in a large matched cohort. Infect Control Hosp Epidemiol 2012;33: 250–6.

4. Muscedere JG, Day A, Heyland DK. Mortality, attributable mortality, and clinical events as end points for clinical trials of ventilator-associated pneumonia and hospital-acquired pneumonia. Clin Infect Dis 2010;51(Suppl 1):S120–5.

5. American Thoracic Society; Infectious Diseases Society of America. Guidelines for the management of adults with hospital-acquired, ventilator-associated, and healthcare-associated pneumonia. Am J Respir Crit Care Med 2005;171: 388–416.

6. Kalil AC, Metersky ML, Klompas M, et al. Management of adults with hospital-acquired and ventilator-associated pneumonia: 2016 clinical practice guidelines by the infectious diseases society of America and the American Thoracic society. Clin Infect Dis 2016;63:e61–111.

7. Klompas M, Branson R, Eichenwald EC, et al. Strategies to prevent ventilator-associated pneumonia in acute care hospitals: 2014 update. Infect Control Hosp Epidemiol 2014;35(Suppl 2):S133–54.

8. Torres A, Niederman MS, Chastre J, et al. International ERS/ESICM/ESCMID/ALAT guidelines for the management of hospital-acquired pneumonia and ventilator-associated pneumonia: guidelines for the management of hospital-acquired pneumonia (HAP)/ventilator-associated pneumonia (VAP) of the European Respiratory Society (ERS), European Society of Intensive Care Medicine (ESICM), European Society of Clinical Microbiology and Infectious Diseases (ESCMID) and Asociacion Latinoamericana del Tórax (ALAT). Eur Respir J 2017;50 [pii:1700582].

9. Kunac A, Sifri ZC, Mohr AM, et al. Bacteremia and ventilator-associated pneumonia: a marker for contemporaneous extra-pulmonic infection. Surg Infect (Larchmt) 2014;15:77–83.

10. Luna CM, Videla A, Mattera J, et al. Blood cultures have limited value in predicting severity of illness and as a diagnostic tool in ventilator-associated pneumonia. Chest 1999;116(4):1075–84.

11. Berton DC, Kalil AC, Teixeira PJ. Quantitative versus qualitative cultures of respiratory secretions for clinical outcomes in patients with ventilator-associated pneumonia. Cochrane Database Syst Rev 2014;(10):CD006482.

12. Leone M, Garcin F, Bouvenot J, et al. Ventilator-associated pneumonia: breaking the vicious circle of antibiotic overuse. Crit Care Med 2007;35:379–85 [quizz: 386].

13. Luna CM, Vujacich P, Niederman MS, et al. Impact of BAL data on the therapy and outcome of ventilator-associated pneumonia. Chest 1997;111:676–85.

14. Ferrer M, Liapikou A, Valencia M, et al. Validation of the American Thoracic Society-Infectious Diseases Society of America guidelines for hospital-acquired pneumonia in the intensive care unit. Clin Infect Dis 2010;50:945–52.

15. Restrepo MI, Peterson J, Fernandez JF, et al. Comparison of the bacterial etiology of early-onset and late-onset ventilator-associated pneumonia in subjects enrolled in 2 large clinical studies. Respir Care 2013;58:1220–5.

16. Martin-Loeches I, Deja M, Koulenti D, et al. Potentially resistant microorganisms in intubated patients with hospital-acquired pneumonia: the interaction of ecology, shock and risk factors. Intensive Care Med 2013;39:672–81.

17. Arvanitis M, Anagnostou T, Kourkoumpetis TK, et al. The impact of antimicrobial resistance and aging in VAP outcomes: experience from a large tertiary care center. PLoS One 2014;9:e89984.

18. Khan R, Al-Dorzi HM, Tamim HM, et al. The impact of onset time on the isolated pathogens and outcomes in ventilator associated pneumonia. J Infect Public Health 2016;9:161–71.

19. Ewig S, Torres A, El-Ebiary M, et al. Bacterial colonization patterns in mechanically ventilated patients with traumatic and medical head injury. Incidence, risk factors, and association with ventilator-associated pneumonia. Am J Respir Crit Care Med 1999;159:188–98.

20. Lepelletier D, Roquilly A, Demeure dit latte D, et al. Retrospective analysis of the risk factors and pathogens associated with early-onset ventilator-associated pneumonia in surgical-ICU head-trauma patients. J Neurosurg Anesthesiol 2010;22:32–7.

21. Leroy O, Jaffre S, D'Escrivan T, et al. Hospital-acquired pneumonia: risk factors for antimicrobial-resistant causative pathogens in critically ill patients. Chest 2003;123:2034–42.

22. Ekren PK, Ranzani OT, Ceccato A, et al. Evaluation of the 2016 Infectious Diseases Society of America/American Thoracic Society guideline criteria for risk

of multidrug-resistant pathogens in patients with hospital-acquired and ventilator-associated pneumonia in the ICU. Am J Respir Crit Care Med 2018;197:826–30.

23. Chastre J, Wolff M, Fagon JY, et al. Comparison of 8 vs 15 days of antibiotic therapy for ventilator-associated pneumonia in adults: a randomized trial. JAMA 2003;290:2588–98.

24. Pugh R, Grant C, Cooke RP, et al. Short-course versus prolonged-course antibiotic therapy for hospital-acquired pneumonia in critically ill adults. Cochrane Database Syst Rev 2015;(8):CD007577.

25. Dimopoulos G, Poulakou G, Pneumatikos IA, et al. Short- vs long-duration antibiotic regimens for ventilator-associated pneumonia: a systematic review and meta-analysis. Chest 2013;144:1759–67.

26. Phase III study with Amikacin Inhale in intubated and mechanically ventilated patients with gram-negative pneumonia does not meet primary endpoint of superiority. 2017. https://www.prnewswire.com/news-releases/phase-iii-study-with-amikacin-inhale-in-intubated-and-mechanically-ventilated-patients-with-gram-negative-pneumonia-does-not-meet-primary-endpoint-of-superiority-300561095.html. Accessed April 10, 2018.

27. Kollef MH, Ricard JD, Roux D, et al. A randomized trial of the Amikacin Fosfomycin inhalation system for the adjunctive therapy of gram-negative ventilator-associated pneumonia: IASIS trial. Chest 2017;151:1239–46.

28. Lux LJ, Posey RE, Daniels LS, et al. Pharmacokinetic/pharmacodynamic measures for guiding antibiotic treatment for hospital-acquired pneumonia. Rockville (MD): Agency for Healthcare Research and Quality; 2014.

29. Abdul-Aziz MH, Dulhunty JM, Bellomo R, et al. Continuous beta-lactam infusion in critically ill patients: the clinical evidence. Ann Intensive Care 2012; 2:37.

30. Abdul-Aziz MH, Sulaiman H, Mat-Nor MB, et al. Beta-Lactam Infusion in Severe Sepsis (BLISS): a prospective, two-centre, open-labelled randomised controlled trial of continuous versus intermittent beta-lactam infusion in critically ill patients with severe sepsis. Intensive Care Med 2016;42:1535–45.

31. Vardakas KZ, Voulgaris GL, Maliaros A, et al. Prolonged versus short-term intravenous infusion of antipseudomonal beta-lactams for patients with sepsis: a systematic review and meta-analysis of randomised trials. Lancet Infect Dis 2018;18: 108–20.

32. Stolz D, Smyrnios N, Eggimann P, et al. Procalcitonin for reduced antibiotic exposure in ventilator-associated pneumonia: a randomised study. Eur Respir J 2009; 34:1364–75.

33. Bouadma L, Luyt CE, Tubach F, et al. Use of procalcitonin to reduce patients' exposure to antibiotics in intensive care units (PRORATA trial): a multicentre randomised controlled trial. Lancet 2010;375:463–74.

34. Pontet J, Paciel D, Olivera W, et al. Procalcitonin (PCT) guided antibiotic treatment in ventilator associated pneumonia (VAP). Multi-centre, clinical prospective, randomized-controlled study. Am J Respir Crit Care Med 2007;175: A212.

35. de Jong E, van Oers JA, Beishuizen A, et al. Efficacy and safety of procalcitonin guidance in reducing the duration of antibiotic treatment in critically ill patients: a randomised, controlled, open-label trial. Lancet Infect Dis 2016; 16:819–27.

36. Schuetz P, Wirz Y, Sager R, et al. Effect of procalcitonin-guided antibiotic treatment on mortality in acute respiratory infections: a patient level meta-analysis. Lancet Infect Dis 2018;18:95–107.

Infections in Heart and Lung Transplant Recipients

Mohammed Alsaeed, MD[a,b], Shahid Husain, MD, MS, FECMM, FRCP[a,*]

KEYWORDS

- Infections • Lung transplant • Heart transplant • Critical care

KEY POINTS

- Sepsis is the leading cause of admission to intensive care unit in heart/lung transplant recipients.
- Heart/lung transplant recipients with infection are less likely to present with fever and leukocytosis, but rather with organ dysfunction.
- Bloodstream infections are more common in the first 3 months posttransplant and are associated with high mortality.
- Pneumonia is the leading cause of infection in heart/lung transplant recipients especially in the first year posttransplant.
- Bacteria are the leading cause of infection in heart/lung transplant patients but always look for viral and fungal causes.

INTRODUCTION

Heart and lung transplantation has become the treatment modality of choice for end-stage cardiac and pulmonary disease. The critical care unit is the first step toward recovery and normal life afterward. According to the International Society for Heart and Lung transplantation in 2017, there were more than 60,000 lung transplants and 4000 heart-lung transplants performed worldwide that were reported to their registry.[1] With the rapidly increasing number of transplants, critical care physicians are more likely to be involved in the specialized care of these types of patients. The morbidity and mortality following heart and/or lung transplantation is largely due to infection and

This article was previously published in *Critical Care Clinics* 35:1 January 2019.

Disclosure Statement: S. Husain has received grant funding from Merck (Canada) and Astellas (Canada) and consultancy fees from Cidara. M. Alsaeed has nothing to disclose.

[a] Division of Infectious Diseases, Multi-Organ Transplant Program, Department of Medicine, University of Toronto, University Health Network, 585 University Avenue, 11 PMB 138, Toronto, Ontario M5G 2N2, Canada; [b] Division of Infectious Diseases, Department of Medicine, Prince Sultan Military Medical City, Makkah Al Mukarramah Road, As Sulimaniyah, Riyadh 12233, Saudi Arabia

* Corresponding author.

E-mail address: shahid.husain@uhn.ca

Infect Dis Clin N Am 38 (2024) 103–120

https://doi.org/10.1016/j.idc.2023.11.003

0891-5520/24/© 2023 Elsevier Inc. All rights reserved.

id.theclinics.com

rejection-related complications.[2,3] Critical care physicians should be aware of the common infections that develop in this population. In this article, the authors review the epidemiology, risk factors, specific clinical syndromes, and most frequent opportunistic infections in heart and/or lung transplant recipients and provide a practical approach of empirical management.

EPIDEMIOLOGY

Since the first lung and heart transplantations performed in the 1960s, there has been significant advancement in organ preservation, surgical techniques, immunosuppression, and postoperative care that has made long-term survival a reality. Despite these advancements, posttransplant infectious complications remain a significant contributor to overall morbidity and mortality.[4]

The epidemiology of infections has changed over time, which is primarily due to widespread use of different prophylactic strategies. Classically, infections in solid organ transplant patients have been divided into 3 periods[5]:

- Early period posttransplant (first month) has been attributed mostly to nosocomial pathogens.
- Intermediate period (2 to 6 months) has been attributed mostly to opportunistic pathogens.
- Late period (more than 6 months) has been attributed mostly to community pathogens.

This approach is simple but is rigid and has its limitations. It fails to take into account several factors such as type of transplant, antimicrobial prophylaxis, induction immunosuppression, and nosocomial exposure of the patient.

RISK FACTORS

The risk factors for heart and/or lung transplant recipients continue to change overtime but are broadly classified into recipient, donor, and graft (transplanted organ) factors. These factors are listed in **Box 1**. The evaluation of these risk factors is important when a critically ill heart and/or lung transplant recipient is seen in the intensive care unit (ICU).

SPECIFIC CLINICAL SYNDROMES
Sepsis

Sepsis has been studied extensively in the past 3 decades, but despite the growing number of solid organ transplant (SOT) patients worldwide the definition of sepsis has never been validated in these patients.[6,7] Solid organ transplant patients may lack classical signs and symptoms probably due to their immunosuppressed state, which blunts the inflammatory response.

They are less likely to present with fever and leukocytosis, but rather with organ dysfunction. Another important issue is that many other noninfectious transplant-related complications can mimic the clinical presentation of sepsis such as primary graft dysfunction and rejection.[8–11]

Sepsis is the leading cause of admission to hospital and critical care unit in solid organ transplant recipients. Trzeciak and colleagues[12] looked retrospectively into 325 emergency room visits by SOT patients; 6% were lung and heart transplant patients. The leading cause of admission was infections (35%); around 12% had severe sepsis

---

Box 1
Risk factors for heart and/or lung transplant recipients

Recipient Factors

- Age
- Diabetes
- Hypogammaglobulinemia
- Renal failure
- No immunity against CMV, toxoplasmosis, EBV, VZV
- Latent infection TB, CMV, HSV, VZV, EBV, endemic mycosis
- Colonization with MDR.
- Immunosuppressive therapy
- Rejection
- Environmental exposure (gardener, animals, caves, travel)
- Native lung colonization

Donor Factors

- Bacterial or fungal allograft colonization
- Allograft latent infection (toxoplasma, CMV, other viruses, endemic mycosis, TB)

Transplantation

- Allograft injury (ischemia, preservation)
- Complexity and length of surgery
- Postsurgical care (mechanical ventilation, intravenous catheters, drains, bladder catheters, extracorporeal membrane oxygenation)
- Transfusion
- Intensive care stay

Abbreviations: CMV, cytomegalovirus; EBV, Epstein-Barr virus; HSV, herpes simplex virus; MDR, multidrug resistance; TB, tuberculosis; VZV, varicella zoster virus.

---

and required ICU care. In comparison with nontransplant, SOT patients are 3 times more likely to be admitted with sepsis.

Sepsis is also a predominant cause of intensive care readmission and death. Pietrantoni and colleagues[13] looked into 210 lung transplant recipients for ICU readmission after initial 30-day posttransplant period over a 4-year period and found 46% admission due to sepsis with a mortality rate approaching 52%.

Kalil and colleagues[14] compared mortality in blood culture–proven sepsis in SOT patients and non-SOT patients. They surprisingly found that SOT patients had better survival at 28 days and 90 days in comparison to non-SOT patients. This could be explained by the fact that the transplant group was more likely to receive appropriate initial antibiotic therapy. They also found SOT recipients had 20 times more nosocomial infections than non-SOT recipients.

Inadequate empirical antibiotic therapy is associated with poor outcome in SOT patients. Hamandi and colleagues[15] looked into 312 SOT patients admitted with culture-proven sepsis. Fifty-four percent of patients received inadequate therapy with a mortality approaching 25% while a mortality of only 7% in those who received appropriate empirical antibiotic therapy.

The choice of appropriate antibiotic therapy depends on many factors, including the knowledge of colonization with multidrug-resistant organisms, recent antibiotic exposure, source of infection, local epidemiology, and any recent procedures or surgeries.[10]

Bloodstream Infections

Bloodstream infections is a well-recognized problem among heart/and or lung transplant patients. It is associated with graft loss and increased mortality. The incidence of bloodstream infections in heart transplant approaches 16%, whereas in lung transplants this goes up to 25%.[16,17]

Rodríguez and colleagues[16] looked into 309 consecutive heart transplant patients for bloodstream infections and found an incidence of 15.8% with direct mortality of 12.2% related to bloodstream infection. Over the 15-year study period they noted a decline in the incidence of bloodstream infections, which they attributed to a change in immunosuppression regimens, antimicrobial protocols, and better improvement in infection control measures. They also observed that most of the bloodstream infections occurred within the first 2 months after transplantation and around 65% were nosocomial. The most common source of infection was pulmonary. Almost half (55.3%) were gram-negative, followed closely by gram-positive (44.6%), whereas only one case of candidemia was noted.

Palmer and colleagues[17] looked into 176 consecutive lung transplant recipients for bloodstream infections and found an incidence of 25%. Risk factors associated with bacteremia are as follows: younger age, have cystic fibrosis, have undergone bilateral lung transplant, or have undergone pretransplant mechanical ventilation. In comparison to lung transplant patients without bloodstream infection, patients who had a first bloodstream infection had higher mortality. The most common source of infection was pneumonia. During the transplant period, gram-negative bacteria (46%) and candida (23%) were the most common cause of bloodstream infections, whereas after transplant discharge gram-positive organisms (38%) were more prevalent.

Husain and colleagues[18] have also looked prospectively into bacteremia among lung transplant recipients: they found that 50% of bacteremias in the first posttransplant year were pulmonary in origin. After 1 year, the proportion of bacteremias that were due to pulmonary infection declined to 26.7% and vascular catheters emerged as a leading source of bacteremia (53.3%). Mortality rate at 28 days after the onset of bacteremia was 25%. Multiple antibiotic–resistant (multidrug-resistant [MDR]) organisms were isolated in 48% of the bacteremia episodes. Patients with cystic fibrosis were more likely to have MDR (35% vs 8%). The approach to gram-negative and positive bacteremia in heart and/or lung transplant recipients is summarized in **Figs. 1** and **2**.

Vascular catheters should always be considered as a source of bloodstream infection in the ICU. Most exit site infections can be treated with antiinfective therapy without line removal. However, vascular catheters should be immediately removed in patients with septic shock, septic phlebitis, and tunnel or port pocket infections. Catheter infections with certain organisms such as *Staphylococcus aureus*, *Pseudomonas aeruginosa*, nontuberculous mycobacteria, yeast, and molds should also be removed. Treating catheter-related bloodstream infection in heart and/or lung transplant patients is similar to treating other patients according to published guidelines.[19,20]

Candida bloodstream infection in critically ill patients is usually severe and life threatening. Although uncommon in heart and lung transplant recipients, it is nevertheless associated with significant mortality and morbidity. Gadre and colleagues[21] have

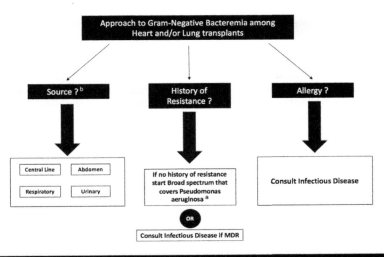

Fig. 1. The approach to gram-negative bacteremia in heart and/or lung transplant recipients. [a] Based on hospital susceptibility pattern. [b] By proper imaging and cultures.

looked into 1053 lung transplant patients for candida bloodstream infections. Only 11 patients (1.04%) developed candidemia. Most patients were hospitalized pretransplant and exposed to high-dose steroids, antibiotics, and immunomodulators in the 3 months before transplant. Posttransplant, extra-corporeal life support was also associated with increased risk for candidemia, with the most common source being surgical site infection and the most common species being *Candida albicans*. Mortality was more than 50%.

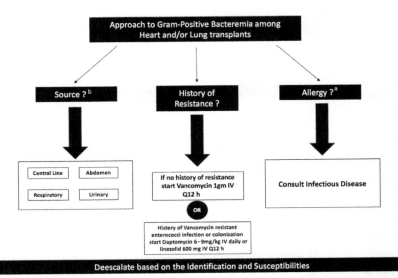

Fig. 2. The approach to gram-positive bacteremia in heart and/or lung transplant recipients. [a] If allergic to first-line drugs consult an Infectious Disease Specialist. [b] By proper imaging and culture.

Treatment for candida bloodstream infection in heart and/or lung transplant patients is similar to other patient population based on 2016 Infectious Disease Society of America guidelines. There is no randomized study for the treatment of candidemia in this heart and/or lung transplant recipients.[22] Delaying empirical treatment of candida bloodstream infection until positive blood cultures may pretend to worse outcome in this patient population.[23] However, empirical management with an echinocandin did not increase the survival in 2 randomized controlled trails in nonneutropenic candidemic individuals.[24,25] In patients with septic shock attributed to candida infection, delaying appropriate antifungal treatment and proper source control is associated with worse outcome.[26] The approaches to suspected and confirmed candidemia are summarized in **Figs. 3** and **4**.

Pneumonia

Pneumonia is the leading cause of infection in both heart and lung transplant patients. Two separate studies from Spain looked into pneumonia among heart and lung transplant patients. The first study was a multicenter retrospective study that evaluated 307 heart transplant recipients for pneumonia and found that 20% of patients developed pneumonia; 75% of episodes of pneumonia were in the first 3 months after transplant and 60% of the organisms were opportunistic.[27] The second study was a multicenter prospective study that observed 236 lung transplant patients for 180 days; 85 episodes of pneumonia were documented with an incidence of 72 episodes/100 lung transplant years; around 44% developed pneumonia in the first month; 82% were bacterial and 72% were due to gram-negative organisms most commonly *Pseudomonas*. The study also showed reduced survival at 1 year in patients who had

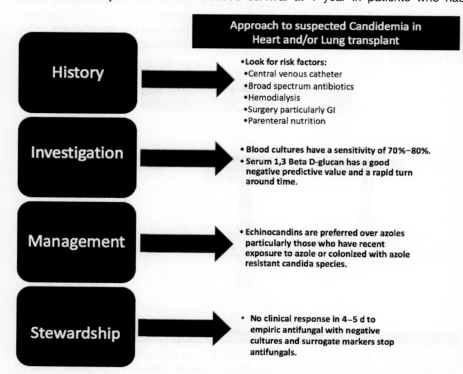

Fig. 3. The approach to suspected candidemia in heart and/or lung transplant recipients.

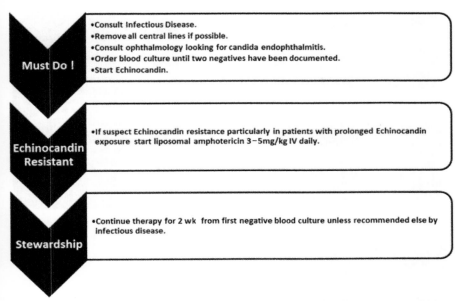

Fig. 4. The approach to confirmed candidemia in heart and/or lung transplant recipients.

developed an episode of pneumonia (74%) as compared with those who did not develop pneumonia (99%).[28]

Lung transplant recipients have the greatest risk of developing pneumonia for several reasons, including continuous and direct exposure of the allograft to microbes, denervation of the allograft with subsequent impairment of cough reflex and mucociliary clearance; impaired lymphatic drainage; complications associated with anastomosis[29]; transmission of infection from donor lungs[30]; infection from native lung in single lung transplantation; and need for prolonged mechanical ventilatory support.[31]

Understanding the epidemiologic characteristics is of paramount importance in predicting the suspected cause of pneumonia; for example, local ecology of MDR organisms,[32] recent exposure to sick contacts particularly viral infections in children, history of travel to endemic areas for fungal and mycobacterial infections,[33] recent exposure to construction sites or environmental source for *Aspergillus* or *Nocardia*[34] and water sources such as *Legionella* or nontuberculous mycobacteria.[35]

Clinical presentation can differ according to the pathogen. Typical presentation with fever may be absent due to immunosuppression. Dry cough is present with cytomegalovirus (CMV) and *Pneumocystis jiroveci* pneumonias (PJP).[36,37] Hemoptysis is more frequent with *Aspergillus* pneumonia.[38] Nosocomial pneumonias usually have an acute presentation, whereas *Mycobacterium tuberculosis* has a subacute presentation.[39]

Diagnosis of pneumonia particularly in lung transplantation may be difficult, because the presence of organisms in the airway may reflect airway colonization. Moreover, other noninfectious cause, especially acute cellular rejection or primary graft dysfunction, may mimic pneumonia. **Fig. 5** summarizes the diagnostic criteria for proven pneumonia in heart and lung recipients.[40]

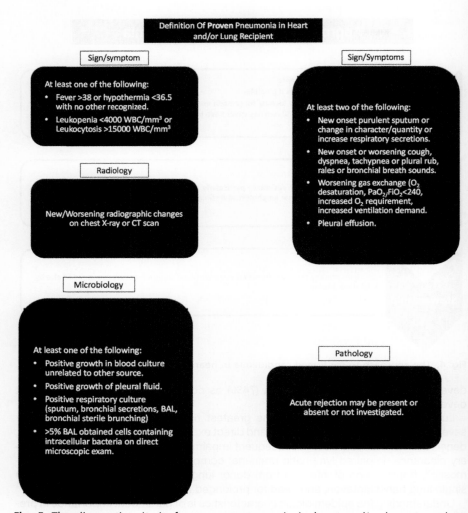

Fig. 5. The diagnostic criteria for proven pneumonia in heart and/or lung transplant recipients.

Respiratory viruses, CMV, and fungi should be worked up as potential cause of pneumonia.[41] Computed tomography is more sensitive than regular X-rays in detecting pulmonary complications in immunosuppressed individuals. Although being nonspecific, certain characteristics on radiograph images can favor certain causes such as bilateral interstitial infiltrates go with PJP, whereas the presence of cavitation indicates an *Aspergillus* infection.[42] Bronchoscopy and bronchoalveolar lavage are crucial tools for evaluating respiratory symptoms in heart and/or lung transplant recipients. A transbronchial biopsy provides an excellent route for excluding allograft rejection.[43] **Fig. 6** summarizes the diagnostic tests for the evaluation of pneumonia.

Empirical treatment of pneumonia depends on prior colonization or infection, especially in lung transplant recipients. In general, empirical antibiotics should cover gram-negative bacteria including *Pseudomonas*. In addition, if the patient has specific risk factors of methicillin-resistant *Stephylococcus aureus* (MRSA) (eg, MRSA

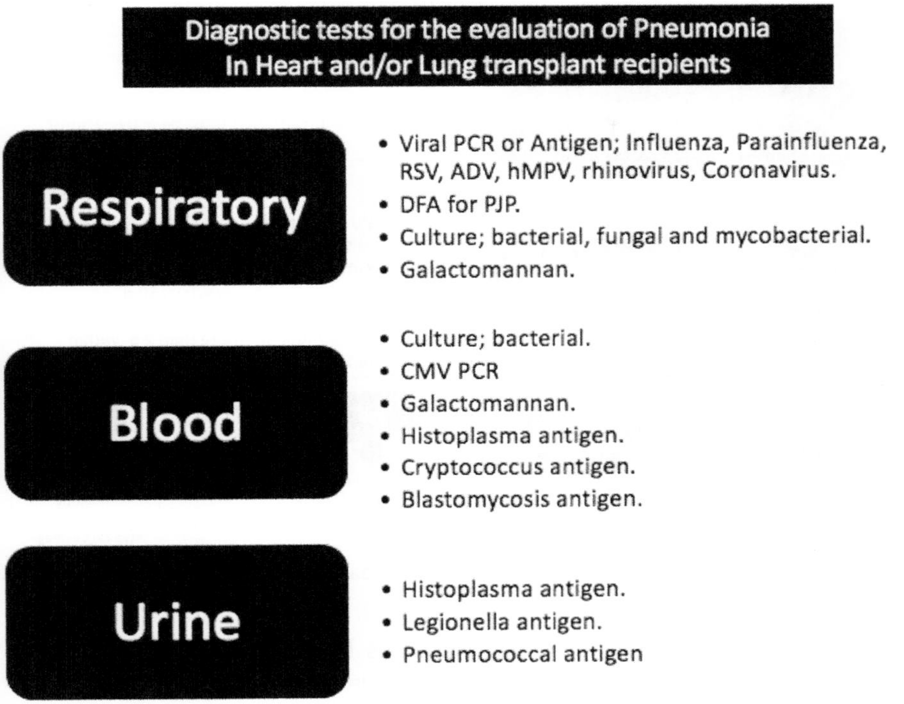

Fig. 6. The diagnostic tests for the evaluation of pneumonia in heart and/or lung transplant recipients.

colonization) S aureus coverage should be included. Patients should be treated according to the results of microbiological studies performed.

Guided by clinical response and the specific infectious organism, an 8- to 14-day course is recommended for bacterial infections.[44] The approach to pneumonia management in heart and/or lung transplant recipients is summarized in **Fig. 7**.

Mediastinitis

Postsurgical mediastinitis is a rare but a life-threatening complication occurring after heart and lung transplantation. In most series, the reported incidence is between 1% and 2%.[45] The associated mortality is high and varies between 14% and 47%.[46] In comparison to lung transplant, heart transplant patients have a higher risk of developing mediastinitis. Abid and colleagues[47] have reported their 15 years of experience on mediastinitis in heart and lung transplant recipients. Between 1985 and 2000, 776 patients underwent heart and/or lung transplant; 21 (2.7%) developed mediastinitis: 14 hearts, 3 heart-lung, and 4 lungs. There were 6 (28.6%) deaths. In heart transplant patients, the most common organism was S aureus, whereas in lung transplant gram-negative rods were the predominant organisms.

Major risk factors associated with mediastinitis include obesity, diabetes mellitus, length of postoperative hospitalization, ventricular assistance device before surgery, and duration of mechanical ventilation after transplantation.

Clinical presentation is frequently not typical. A high index of suspicion is required. The most frequent symptom is pain, disproportionate to sternotomy. Elevated white

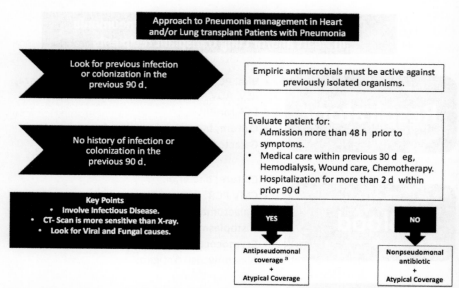

Fig. 7. The approach to pneumonia management in heart and/or lung transplant recipients with pneumonia.

blood cells, temperature, and erythema are less frequent. Diagnosis is made by computed tomography with sampling mediastinal tissue or fluid collection for culture.[48–50]

Empirical treatment should include coverage for *S aureus*, *Staphylococcus epidermis*, and gram-negative rods after blood cultures have been obtained. Duration of treatment depends on surgical resection of the sternum. If the sternum is resected, a 2- to 3-week course is sufficient, whereas if only debridement is done then a minimum of 4 to 6 weeks is required.[51]

OPPORTUNISTIC INFECTIONS
Cytomegalovirus Infection

CMV infection is the most prevalent opportunistic infection in both heart and lung transplant recipients.[52] It comes second only to bacterial infections as an overall cause of infections in heart and lung recipients.[53,54] CMV is one of the herpesviruses and can stay latent within the body for life with possible reactivation.[55] Among the multitude of risk factors associated with CMV disease, the serostatus of the donor and recipient is the most important (donor seropositive and recipient seronegative) followed by use of antithymocyte globulins for rejection.[56]

CMV is known to augment the net state of immunosuppression and may result in facilitating the occurrence of other opportunistic bacterial and fungal infections.[57] It may also predispose to acute allograft rejection in both heart and lung transplant recipients. Similarly, it has been reported to be associated with cardiac allograft vasculopathy and bronchiolitis obliterans in lung transplant recipients.[58]

Before the era of universal prophylaxis administration, 30% to 90% of CMV-seropositive patients would have evidence of the virus in their blood and most would progress to disease. The incidence and timing of CMV infection and disease has changed over the last decade. Median time to the onset of CMV disease or infection has significantly increased after the widespread use of universal prophylaxis.[59–61]

The virus is commonly detected in patients admitted to the ICU.[62,63] The presence of CMV in the blood warrants treatment.[64,65] However, the authors do not recommend treatment of CMV if the test is only positive in bronchoalveolar lavage with concomitantly negative CMV in the blood.[66,67]

Patients on CMV treatment should have their viral load assay repeated on a weekly basis using quantitative polymerase chain reaction to monitor response to treatment.[68,69] In CMV pneumonitis, administering intravenous immunoglobulin or CMV-specific immunoglobulin is controversial.[70,71]

Aspergillosis

Invasive aspergillosis is a major cause of morbidity and mortality in patients who had undergone heart and/or lung transplants.[72,73] It is estimated that 9% of deaths after lung transplant is attributed to invasive aspergillosis.[74] In the solid organ population, it mainly affects lung transplant patients. Pappas and colleagues[75] looked into the incidence of invasive fungal infections among 1063 organ transplant recipients in 23 US transplant centers. They found invasive aspergillosis to be the second most common cause in 19% of patients. Almost half (48%) of these cases occurred in lung transplant recipients and 10% in heart transplant recipients. Most of the cases happened in the first 6 months after transplant.

Risks factors for invasive aspergillosis in lung transplant recipients include colonization with *Aspergillus*, CMV disease, airway ischemia, and single lung transplantation, whereas in heart transplant recipients risk factors include CMV disease and posttransplant hemodialysis.[76–80]

Invasive pulmonary aspergillosis should be suspected in heart and/or lung transplant recipients who present with fever and/or respiratory symptoms in the first 3 months after transplantation, have a positive culture result of *Aspergillus* species, and have abnormal radiological findings in particular nodules.[81]

Lung and sinuses are involved in more than 90% of cases of aspergillosis. Singh and colleagues[82] reviewed 159 cases of aspergillosis after lung transplant published in the literature. The most common presentation was tracheobronchitis or bronchial anastomotic infection in 58% of cases, whereas 32% had invasive pulmonary and 22% had disseminated infection.

The diagnosis of invasive aspergillosis in transplant patients is hampered by the lack of specific clinical and radiological signs and low sensitivity of culture-based diagnostic methods.[40,83] Galactomannan has been proposed as surrogate marker for invasive aspergillosis. However, with limited sensitivity of serum galactomannan in transplant patients, bronchoalveolar lavage has been proved to be highly sensitive (approaching 98%). Hence, in pneumonia workup BAL galactomannan should be assessed.[84] Conversely $(1,3)$-β-D-glucan is very nonspecific in the setting of lung transplant recipients.[85]

Voriconazole is the recommended first-line therapy.[86,87] Liposomal amphotericin B or caspofungin could be considered as an alternative.[88] Duration of therapy depends on extent of disease, clinical response, and immunologic status of the patients.[89,90] To ensure proper exposure of voriconazole treatment, monitoring of serum trough levels should be performed. Regular monitoring of liver enzymes and serum concentration calcineurin inhibitors is required to avoid hepatotoxicity and nephrotoxicity.[91]

Pneumocystis Jirovecii Pneumonia

Pneumocystis jirovecii is an opportunistic fungus that causes life-threatening pulmonary infection in SOT recipients.[92] Before the era of universal prophylaxis, the incidence in heart and/or lung transplant recipients was 10% to 40%.[93] PJP is associated with graft loss, and mortality remains high (up to 60%) despite treatment with trimethoprim-sulfamethoxazole (TMP-SMX).[94] Heart and lung transplant recipients should stay on PJP prophylaxis for life.[95,96]

Critical care physicians should consider PJP as one differential in heart and/or lung transplant recipients admitted with pneumonia to the critical care unit, especially if not on PJP prophylaxis. Lehto and colleagues[97] reviewed 609 bronchoscopies on 40 lung or heart/lung transplant recipients, and they found that 23 (4.9%) of bronchoscopy specimens had PJP. Of these 15 (65%) were on prophylaxis.

Signs and symptoms are nonspecific, mostly presenting with dry cough, fever, and shortness of breath. Imaging is also nonspecific and can show bilateral interstitial infiltrates.[98] Diagnosis is based on direct identification of the organism in respiratory tract or secretions.[99] Serum (1,3)-D-glucan has high sensitivity (up to 95%) and if negative can exclude PJP.[100]

TMP-SMX is the drug of choice for PJP given 15 to 20 mg/kg/d intravenously divided every 6 to 8 hours.[101] Corticosteroids are commonly administered; yet their use is not well substantiated in transplantation.[102] Patients on TMP-SMX should have their cell count, creatinine, and potassium monitored at regular intervals. Intravenous TMP-SMX can be switched to oral once patient is improving to complete 21 days. In patients with sulfa drug allergy and suspected PJP an infectious disease consult should be sought for appropriate management.

Mycoplasma Hominis and Ureaplasma Urealyticum Infection

In lung transplant recipients, hyperammonemia is a rare but fatal condition in the early posttransplant period.[103] Chen and colleagues[104] evaluated 807 lung transplant patients for developing hyperammonemia syndrome and found that only 8 (1%) had developed it, of which 6 (75%) died.

Systemic infection with M hominis and U Urealyticum is a unique cause of hyperammonemia in lung transplant recipients.[105] Any recent lung transplant recipients with lethargy, seizure, or coma should have their ammonia levels checked and if high a macrolide, fluoroquinolone, or a tetracycline should be started. Combination therapy could be considered, especially with high resistance. Diagnosis is based on special cultures and polymerase chain reaction. Recently there has been a suggestion that this may be a donor-derived infection.[106]

REFERENCES

1. Chambers DC, Yusen RD, Cherikh WS, et al. The Registry of the International Society for Heart and Lung Transplantation: thirty-fourth adult lung and heart-lung transplantation report-2017; focus theme: allograft ischemic time. J Heart Lung Transplant 2017;36(10):1047-59.

2. Yusen RD, Edwards LB, Kucheryavaya AY, et al. The Registry of the International Society for Heart and Lung Transplantation: thirty-second official adult lung and heart-lung transplantation report-2015; focus theme: early graft failure. J Heart Lung Transplant 2015;34(10):1264-77.

3. Fishman JA. Infection in organ transplantation. Am J Transplant 2017;17(4): 856-79.

4. Green M. Introduction: infections in solid organ transplantation. Am J Transplant 2013;13(Suppl 4):3-8.

5. Fishman JA. Infection in solid-organ transplant recipients. N Engl J Med 2007; 357:2601-14.

6. Singer M, Deutschman CS, Seymour CW, et al. The third international consensus definitions for sepsis and septic shock (Sepsis-3). JAMA 2016; 315:801–10.

7. Seymour CW, Liu VX, Iwashyna TJ, et al. Assessment of clinical criteria for sepsis: for the third international consensus definitions for sepsis and septic shock (sepsis-3). JAMA 2016;315(8):762–74.

8. Kalil AC, Dakroub H, Freifeld AG. Sepsis and solid organ transplantation. Curr Drug Targets 2007;8(4):533–41.

9. Donnelly JP, Locke JE, MacLennan PA, et al. Inpatient mortality among solid organ transplant recipients hospitalized for sepsis and severe sepsis. Clin Infect Dis 2016;63(2):186–94.

10. Kalil AC, Sandkovsky U, Florescu DF. Severe infections in critically ill solid organ transplant patients. Clin Microbiol Infect 2018 [pii:S1198-743X(18)30362-8]. [Epub ahead of print].

11. Florescu DF, Sandkovsky U, Kalil AC. Sepsis and challenging infections in the immunosuppressed patient in the intensive care unit. Infect Dis Clin North Am 2017;31(3):415–34.

12. Trzeciak S1, Sharer R, Piper D, et al. Infections and severe sepsis in solid-organ transplant patients admitted from a university-based ED. Am J Emerg Med 2004;22(7):530–3.

13. Pietrantoni C, Minai OA, Yu NC, et al. Respiratory failure and sepsis are the major causes of ICU admissions and mortality in survivors of lung transplants. Chest 2003;123(2):504–9.

14. Kalil AC, Syed A, Rupp ME, et al. Is bacteremic sepsis associated with higher mortality in transplant recipients than in nontransplant patients? A matched case-control propensity-adjusted study. Clin Infect Dis 2015;60(2):216–22.

15. Hamandi B, Holbrook AM, Humar A, et al. Delay of adequate empiric antibiotic therapy is associated with increased mortality among solid-organ transplant patients. Am J Transplant 2009;9(7):1657–65.

16. Rodríguez C, Muñoz P, Rodríguez-Créixems M, et al. Bloodstream infections among heart transplant recipients. Transplantation 2006;81(3):384–91.

17. Palmer SM, Alexander BD, Sanders LL, et al. Significance of blood stream infection after lung transplantation: analysis in 176 consecutive patients. Transplantation 2000;69(11):2360–6.

18. Husain S, Chan KM, Palmer SM, et al. Bacteremia in lung transplant recipients in the current era. Am J Transplant 2006;6(12):3000–7.

19. Baden LR, Swaminathan S, Angarone M, et al. Prevention and treatment of cancer-related infections, version 2.2016, NCCN clinical practice guidelines in oncology. J Natl Compr Canc Netw 2016;14(7):882–913.

20. Mermel LA, Allon M, Bouza E, et al. Clinical practice guidelines for the diagnosis and management of intravascular catheter-related infection: 2009 Update by the Infectious Diseases Society of America. Clin Infect Dis 2009;49(1):1–45.

21. Gadre SK, Koval C, Budev M. Candida blood stream infections post lung transplant. J Heart Lung Transplant 2017;36(4):S241.

22. Pappas PG, Kauffman CA, Andes DR, et al. Clinical practice guideline for the management of candidiasis: 2016 update by the infectious diseases society of America. Clin Infect Dis 2016;62(4):e1–50.

23. Morrell M, Fraser VJ, Kollef MH. Delaying the empiric treatment of candida bloodstream infection until positive blood culture results are obtained: a potential risk factor for hospital mortality. Antimicrob Agents Chemother 2005;49(9): 3640–5.

24. Ostrosky-Zeichner L, Shoham S, Vazquez J, et al. MSG-01: a randomized, double-blind, placebo-controlled trial of caspofungin prophylaxis followed by preemptive therapy for invasive candidiasis in high-risk adults in the critical care setting. Clin Infect Dis 2014;58(9):1219–26.
25. Knitsch W, Vincent JL, Utzolino S, et al. A randomized, placebo-controlled trial of preemptive antifungal therapy for the prevention of invasive candidiasis following gastrointestinal surgery for intra-abdominal infections. Clin Infect Dis 2015;61(11):1671–8.
26. Kollef M, Micek S, Hampton N, et al. Septic shock attributed to Candida infection: importance of empiric therapy and source control. Clin Infect Dis 2012; 54(12):1739–46.
27. Cisneros JM1, Muñoz P, Torre-Cisneros J, et al. Pneumonia after heart transplantation: a multi-institutional study. Spanish transplantation infection study group. Clin Infect Dis 1998;27(2):324–31.
28. Aguilar-Guisado M1, Givaldá J, Ussetti P, et al, RESITRA cohort. Pneumonia after lung transplantation in the RESITRA Cohort: a multicenter prospective study. Am J Transplant 2007;7(8):1989–96.
29. Olland A, Reeb J, Puyraveau M, et al. Bronchial complications after lung transplantation are associated with primary lung graft dysfunction and surgical technique. J Heart Lung Transplant 2017;36(2):157–65.
30. Ruiz I, Gavaldà J, Monforte V, et al. Donor-to-host transmission of bacterial and fungal infections in lung transplantation. Am J Transplant 2006;6(1):178–82.
31. Maurer JR, Tullis DE, Grossman RF, et al. Infectious complications following isolated lung transplantation. Chest 1992;101(4):1056–9.
32. Mattner F, Fischer S, Weissbrodt H, et al. Post-operative nosocomial infections after lung and heart transplantation. J Heart Lung Transplant 2007;26(3):241–9.
33. Gasink LB, Blumberg EA. Bacterial and mycobacterial pneumonia in transplant recipients. Clin Chest Med 2005;26(4):647–59.
34. Clark NM, Reid GE, AST Infectious Diseases Community of Practice. Nocardia infections in solid organ transplantation. Am J Transplant 2013;13(Suppl 4): 83–92.
35. Avery RK, Michaels MG, AST Infectious Diseases Community of Practice. Strategies for safe living after solid organ transplantation. Am J Transplant 2013; 13(Suppl 4):304–10.
36. Ison MG1, Fishman JA. Cytomegalovirus pneumonia in transplant recipients. Clin Chest Med 2005;26(4):691–705.
37. Kovacs JA, Hiemenz JW, Macher AM, et al. Pneumocystis carinii pneumonia: a comparison between patients with the acquired immunodeficiency syndrome and patients with other immunodeficiencies. Ann Intern Med 1984;100(5): 663–71.
38. Singh N1, Paterson DL. Aspergillus infections in transplant recipients. Clin Microbiol Rev 2005;18(1):44–69.
39. Meije Y, Piersimoni C, Torre-Cisneros J, et al, ESCMID Study Group of Infection in Compromised Hosts. Mycobacterial infections in solid organ transplant recipients. Clin Microbiol Infect 2014;20(Suppl 7):89–101.
40. Husain S, Mooney ML, Danziger-Isakov L, et al, ISHLT Infectious Diseases Council Working Group on Definitions. A 2010 working formulation for the standardization of definitions of infections in cardiothoracic transplant recipients. J Heart Lung Transplant 2011;30(4):361–74.
41. Chakinala MM, Trulock EP. Pneumonia in the solid organ transplant patient. Clin Chest Med 2005;26(1):113–21.

42. Fujii T, Nakamura T, Iwamoto A. Pneumocystis pneumonia in patients with HIV infection: clinical manifestations, laboratory findings, and radiological features. J Infect Chemother 2007;13(1):1–7.

43. Guilinger RA, Paradis IL, Dauber JH, et al. The importance of bronchoscopy with transbronchial biopsy and bronchoalveolar lavage in the management of lung transplant recipients. Am J Respir Crit Care Med 1995;152(6 Pt 1): 2037–43.

44. Kalil AC, Metersky ML, Klompas M, et al. Executive summary: management of adults with hospital-acquired and ventilator-associated pneumonia: 2016 clinical practice guidelines by the infectious diseases society of America and the American Thoracic Society. Clin Infect Dis 2016;63(5):575–82.

45. Karwande SV, Renlund DG, Olsen SL, et al. Mediastinitis in heart transplantation. Ann Thorac Surg 1992;54(6):1039–45.

46. Gummert JF, Barten MJ, Hans C, et al. Mediastinitis and cardiac surgery–an updated risk factor analysis in 10,373 consecutive adult patients. Thorac Cardiovasc Surg 2002;50(2):87–91.

47. Abid Q, Nkere UU, Hasan A, et al. Mediastinitis in heart and lung transplantation: 15 years' experience. Ann Thorac Surg 2003;75(5):1565–71.

48. Sénéchal M, LePrince P, Tezenas du Montcel S, et al. Bacterial mediastinitis after heart transplantation: clinical presentation, risk factors and treatment. J Heart Lung Transplant 2004;23(2):165–70.

49. Misawa Y, Fuse K, Hasegawa T. Infectious mediastinitis after cardiac operations: computed tomographic findings. Ann Thorac Surg 1998;65(3):622–4.

50. Yamaguchi H, Yamauchi H, Yamada T, et al. Diagnostic validity of computed tomography for mediastinitis after cardiac surgery. Ann Thorac Cardiovasc Surg 2001;7(2):94–8.

51. El Oakley RM, Wright JE. Postoperative mediastinitis: classification and management. Ann Thorac Surg 1996;61(3):1030–6.

52. Fisher RA. Cytomegalovirus infection and disease in the new era of immunosuppression following solid organ transplantation. Transpl Infect Dis 2009;11(3): 195–202.

53. Vaska PL. Common infections in heart transplant patients. Am J Crit Care 1993; 2(2):145–54.

54. Zamora MR. Cytomegalovirus and lung transplantation. Am J Transplant 2004; 4(8):1219–26.

55. Fishman JA. Overview: cytomegalovirus and the herpesviruses in transplantation. Am J Transplant 2013;13(Suppl 3):1–8.

56. Harvala H, Stewart C, Muller K, et al. High risk of cytomegalovirus infection following solid organ transplantation despite prophylactic therapy. J Med Virol 2013;85(5):893–8.

57. Snyder LD, Finlen-Copeland CA, Turbyfill WJ, et al. Cytomegalovirus pneumonitis is a risk for bronchiolitis obliterans syndrome in lung transplantation. Am J Respir Crit Care Med 2010;181(12):1391–6.

58. Delgado JF, Reyne AG, de Dios S, et al. Influence of cytomegalovirus infection in the development of cardiac allograft vasculopathy after heart transplantation. J Heart Lung Transplant 2015;34(8):1112–9.

59. Hodson EM, Ladhani M, Webster AC, et al. Antiviral medications for preventing cytomegalovirus disease in solid organ transplant recipients. Cochrane Database Syst Rev 2013;(2):CD003774.

60. Schoeppler KE1, Lyu DM, Grazia TJ, et al. Late-onset cytomegalovirus (CMV) in lung transplant recipients: can CMV serostatus guide the duration of prophylaxis? Am J Transplant 2013;13(2):376–82.

61. Potena L, Solidoro P, Patrucco F, et al. Treatment and prevention of cytomegalovirus infection in heart and lung transplantation: an update. Expert Opin Pharmacother 2016;17(12):1611–22.

62. Papazian L, Hraiech S, Lehingue S, et al. Cytomegalovirus reactivation in ICU patients. Intensive Care Med 2016;42(1):28–37.

63. Lachance P, Chen J, Featherstone R, et al. Impact of cytomegalovirus reactivation on clinical outcomes in immunocompetent critically ill patients: protocol for a systematic review and meta-analysis. Syst Rev 2016;5(1):127.

64. Asberg A, Humar A, Rollag H, et al, VICTOR Study Group. Oral valganciclovir is noninferior to intravenous ganciclovir for the treatment of cytomegalovirus disease in solid organ transplant recipients. Am J Transplant 2007;7(9):2106–13.

65. Kotton CN1, Kumar D, Caliendo AM, et al, Transplantation Society International CMV Consensus Group. Updated international consensus guidelines on the management of cytomegalovirus in solid-organ transplantation. Transplantation 2013;96(4):333–60.

66. Lodding IP, Schultz HH, Jensen JU, et al. Cytomegalovirus viral load in bronchoalveolar lavage to diagnose lung transplant associated CMV pneumonia. Transplantation 2018;102(2):326–32.

67. Coussement J, Steensels D, Nollevaux MC, et al. When polymerase chain reaction does not help: cytomegalovirus pneumonitis associated with very low or undetectable viral load in both blood and bronchoalveolar lavage samples after lung transplantation. Transpl Infect Dis 2016;18(2):284–7.

68. Caliendo AM, St George K, Allega J, et al. Distinguishing cytomegalovirus (CMV) infection and disease with CMV nucleic acid assays. J Clin Microbiol 2002;40(5):1581–6.

69. Humar A, Kumar D, Boivin G, et al. Cytomegalovirus (CMV) virus load kinetics to predict recurrent disease in solid-organ transplant patients with CMV disease. J Infect Dis 2002;186(6):829–33.

70. Snydman DR. Cytomegalovirus immunoglobulins in the prevention and treatment of cytomegalovirus disease. Rev Infect Dis 1990;12(Suppl 7):S839–48.

71. Haidar G, Singh N. Viral infections in solid organ transplant recipients: novel updates and a review of the classics. Curr Opin Infect Dis 2017;30(6):579–88.

72. Singh N, Husain S, AST Infectious Diseases Community of Practice. Aspergillosis in solid organ transplantation. Am J Transplant 2013;13(Suppl 4):228–41.

73. Neofytos D, Fishman JA, Horn D, et al. Epidemiology and outcome of invasive fungal infections in solid organ transplant recipients. Transpl Infect Dis 2010; 12(3):220–9.

74. Paterson DL, Singh N. Invasive aspergillosis in transplant recipients. Medicine (Baltimore) 1999;78(2):123–38.

75. Pappas PG, Alexander BD, Andes DR, et al. Invasive fungal infections among organ transplant recipients: results of the Transplant-Associated Infection Surveillance Network (TRANSNET). Clin Infect Dis 2010;50(8):1101–11.

76. Montoya JG, Chaparro SV, Celis D, et al. Invasive aspergillosis in the setting of cardiac transplantation. Clin Infect Dis 2003;37(Suppl 3):S281–92.

77. Montoya JG, Giraldo LF, Efron B, et al. Infectious complications among 620 consecutive heart transplant patients at Stanford University Medical Center. Clin Infect Dis 2001;33(5):629–40.

78. Munoz P, Rodriguez C, Bouza E, et al. Risk factors of invasive aspergillosis after heart transplantation: protective role of oral itraconazole prophylaxis. Am J Transplant 2004;4:636–43.

79. Speziali G, McDougall JC, Midthun DE, et al. Native lung complications after single lung transplantation for emphysema. Transpl Int 1997;10:113–5.

80. Husni RN, Gordon SM, Longworth DL, et al. Cytomegalovirus infection is a risk factor for invasive aspergillosis in lung transplant recipients. Clin Infect Dis 1998;26(3):753–5.

81. Muñoz P1, Alcalá L, Sánchez Conde M, et al. The isolation of Aspergillus fumigatus from respiratory tract specimens in heart transplant recipients is highly predictive of invasive aspergillosis. Transplantation 2003;75(3):326–9.

82. Singh N, Husain S. Aspergillus infections after lung transplantation: clinical differences in type of transplant and implications for management. J Heart Lung Transplant 2003;22(3):258–66.

83. Park YS, Seo JB, Lee YK, et al. Radiological and clinical findings of pulmonary aspergillosis following solid organ transplant. Clin Radiol 2008;63(6):673–80.

84. Pasqualotto AC, Xavier MO, Sánchez LB, et al. Diagnosis of invasive aspergillosis in lung transplant recipients by detection of galactomannan in the bronchoalveolar lavage fluid. Transplantation 2010;90(3):306–11.

85. Mutschlechner W, Risslegger B, Willinger B, et al. Bronchoalveolar lavage fluid (1,3)β-D-glucan for the diagnosis of invasive fungal infections in solid organ transplantation: a prospective multicenter study. Transplantation 2015;99(9): e140–4.

86. Fortún J, Martín-Dávila P, Sánchez MA, et al. Voriconazole in the treatment of invasive mold infections in transplant recipients. Eur J Clin Microbiol Infect Dis 2003;22(7):408–13.

87. Denning DW, Ribaud P, Milpied N, et al. Efficacy and safety of voriconazole in the treatment of acute invasive aspergillosis. Clin Infect Dis 2002;34(5):563–71.

88. Wieland T, Liebold A, Jagiello M, et al. Superiority of voriconazole over amphotericin B in the treatment of invasive aspergillosis after heart transplantation. J Heart Lung Transplant 2005;24(1):102–4.

89. Herbrecht R, Denning DW, Patterson TF, et al. Invasive Fungal Infections Group of the European Organisation for Research and Treatment of Cancer and the Global Aspergillus Study Group. Voriconazole versus amphotericin B for primary therapy of invasive aspergillosis. N Engl J Med 2002;347(6):408–15.

90. Patterson TF, Thompson GR, Denning DW, et al. Practice guidelines for the diagnosis and management of aspergillosis: 2016 update by the infectious diseases society of America. Clin Infect Dis 2016;63(4):e1–60.

91. Kulkarni HS, Witt CA. Voriconazole in lung transplant recipients - how worried should we be? Am J Transplant 2018;18(1):5–6.

92. Martin SI, Fishman JA, AST Infectious Diseases Community of Practice. Pneumocystis pneumonia in solid organ transplantation. Am J Transplant 2013; 13(Suppl 4):272–9.

93. Kramer MR, Stoehr C, Lewiston NJ, et al. Trimethoprim-sulfamethoxazole prophylaxis for Pneumocystis carinii infections in heart-lung and lung transplantation–how effective and for how long? Transplantation 1992;53(3): 586–9.

94. Rodriguez M, Fishman JA. Prevention of infection due to Pneumocystis spp. in human immunodeficiency virus-negative immunocompromised patients. Clin Microbiol Rev 2004;17(4):770–82.

95. Gordon SM, LaRosa SP, Kalmadi S, et al. Should prophylaxis for Pneumocystis carinii pneumonia in solid organ transplant recipients ever be discontinued? Clin Infect Dis 1999;28(2):240–6.

96. Perez-Ordoño L, Hoyo I, Sanclemente G, et al. Late-onset Pneumocystis jirovecii pneumonia in solid organ transplant recipients. Transpl Infect Dis 2014;16(2): 324–8.

97. Lehto JT, Koskinen PK, Anttila VJ, et al. Bronchoscopy in the diagnosis and surveillance of respiratory infections in lung and heart-lung transplant recipients. Transpl Int 2005;18(5):562–71.

98. Kanne JP, Yandow DR, Meyer CA. Pneumocystis jiroveci pneumonia: high-resolution CT findings in patients with and without HIV infection. AJR Am J Roentgenol 2012;198(6):W555–61.

99. LaRocque RC, Katz JT, Perruzzi P, et al. The utility of sputum induction for diagnosis of Pneumocystis pneumonia in immunocompromised patients without human immunodeficiency virus. Clin Infect Dis 2003;37(10):1380–3.

100. Karageorgopoulos DE, Qu JM, Korbila IP, et al. Accuracy of β-D-glucan for the diagnosis of Pneumocystis jirovecii pneumonia: a meta-analysis. Clin Microbiol Infect 2013;19(1):39–49.

101. Garnacho-Montero J, Olaechea P, Alvarez-Lerma F, et al. Epidemiology, diagnosis and treatment of fungal respiratory infections in the critically ill patient. Rev Esp Quimioter 2013;26(2):173–88.

102. McKinnell JA, Cannella AP, Injean P, et al. Adjunctive glucocorticoid therapy for non-HIV-related pneumocystis carinii pneumonia (NH-PCP). Am J Transplant 2014;14(4):982–3.

103. Lichtenstein GR, Yang YX, Nunes FA, et al. Fatal hyperammonemia after orthotopic lung transplantation. Ann Intern Med 2000;132(4):283–7.

104. Chen C, Bain KB, Iuppa JA, et al. Hyperammonemia syndrome after lung transplantation: a single center experience. Transplantation 2016;100(3):678–84.

105. Bharat A, Cunningham SA, Scott Budinger GR, et al. Disseminated Ureaplasma infection as a cause of fatal hyperammonemia in humans. Sci Transl Med 2015; 7(284):284re3.

106. Fernandez R, Ratliff A, Crabb D, et al. Ureaplasma transmitted from donor lungs is pathogenic after lung transplantation. Ann Thorac Surg 2017;103(2):670–1.

Opportunistic Infections Post-Lung Transplantation: Viral, Fungal, and Mycobacterial

Gabriela Magda, MD

KEYWORDS

• Lung transplant • Opportunistic infection • Immunocompromised hosts

KEY POINTS

- Comprehensive donor and recipient screening for infection risk pre-transplant can reduce infection incidence post-transplant and guide prophylaxis.
- Certain infections (eg, cytomegalovirus, *Aspergillus*, community-acquired respiratory viruses affecting the lower respiratory tract) are more strongly associated with the development of chronic lung allograft dysfunction; prevention, early diagnosis, and aggressive treatment are critical to preserving long-term allograft function.
- Antifungal prophylaxis strategies are variable across transplant centers; there are supportive data for universal prophylaxis, but available evidence has not proven it to be a clearly superior strategy to preemptive approaches.

INTRODUCTION

Lung transplant recipient (LTR) outcomes have improved significantly but remain inferior to other solid organ transplant (SOT) outcomes despite advances in surgical techniques and immunosuppressive strategies, partly because of infection-related complications.[1] Between the first 30 days and 1-year post-transplant, infections are the leading cause of LTR mortality. Certain infections are associated with the development of acute rejection and chronic lung allograft dysfunction (CLAD).[2] Gram-negative bacterial infections are most common, but viruses, fungi, and mycobacteria are also important contributors to LTR outcomes. Risk factors for infection include continuous exposure of the lung allograft to the external environment, high immunosuppression levels, disruptions to allograft bronchial blood supply, lymphatic drainage, and vagal nerve paths causing impaired mucociliary clearance from airway epithelium changes and decreased cough reflex, and impact of the native lung microbiome in single

This article was previously published in *Clinics in Chest Medicine* 44:1 March 2023.
Columbia University Lung Transplant Program, Division of Pulmonary, Allergy, and Critical Care Medicine, Columbia University Irving Medical Center, Columbia University Vagelos College of Physicians and Surgeons, 622 West 168th Street PH-14, New York, NY 10032, USA
E-mail address: gm2339@cumc.columbia.edu

Infect Dis Clin N Am 38 (2024) 121–147
https://doi.org/10.1016/j.idc.2023.12.001
id.theclinics.com

LTRs.[3,4] Infection risk is mitigated through careful pre-transplant screening of recipients and donors, implementation of antimicrobial prophylaxis strategies, and routine post-transplant surveillance.[5] This review describes common viral, fungal, and mycobacterial infectious after lung transplant and provides prevention and treatment recommendations.

INFECTION SCREENING AND PREVENTION

LTR infections can be derived from the donor, reactivated latent infections in the recipient, or newly acquired (**Fig. 1**). Donors and recipients should undergo thorough pre-

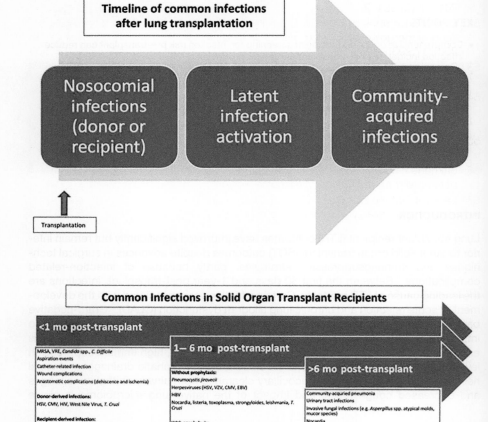

Fig. 1. Types and timing of infections after lung transplantation. (*Modified from* Fishman JA. Infection in solid-organ transplant recipients. N Engl J Med. 2007;357(25):2606.)

transplant evaluation of infection risk. Prior infectious exposures can be ascertained through taking comprehensive medical, social, travel, and immunization histories. Serostatus, sputum, and nucleic acid tests should be confirmed pre-transplant to risk stratify donor to recipient transmission and guide post-transplant infectious prophylaxis (**Table 1**). LTRs with suppurative underlying lung diseases, who have been frequently hospitalized, or who have received broad-spectrum antimicrobials may be colonized with fungi or bacteria. Antimicrobial susceptibilities of colonizing organisms should be known pre-transplant for appropriate perioperative and postoperative antimicrobial selection.[6,7]

Effort should be made to vaccinate potential LTRs when absence of immunity to specific pathogens is identified (**Table 2**). Vaccination timing may be impacted by degree of immunosuppression pre-transplant and post-transplant and transplant urgency. Vaccination may be deferred until immunosuppression levels are significantly reduced post-transplant to better ensure protective immune response. Live attenuated vaccines are contraindicated after SOT.[8–10] Household members and close contacts of LTRs also should adhere to routine immunization schedules.

Infection risk depends on time since transplant surgery. In the first month posttransplant, infections are generally due to donor allograft transmission, reactivation of recipient infections, or acquired from the hospitalization or surgical procedures. Infection risk may be increased in LTRs with comorbid immunodeficiencies or who received immunosuppression pre-transplant. Bacterial infections are most common. Pleural effusions within the first 3 months posttransplant should not be presumed to benign without infection evaluation.[11] Up to 6 months post-transplant, opportunistic infections predominate, though donor-derived infections may still occur. After the first 6 months, infections from broader range bacteria become more common.[12,13]

VIRUSES

Viral infections in LTRs can be grouped into pathogens primarily affecting extrapulmonary tissues (eg, the herpesviruses) and pathogens primarily affecting the respiratory tract (eg, the community-acquired respiratory viruses [CARVs]).

Cytomegalovirus

Cytomegalovirus (CMV) is a ubiquitous herpesvirus that can reactivate from latent infection in SOT recipients; transmission also occurs through allografts or blood product transfusions from CMV-infected donors or close contact with CMV-infected people. Over half of United States adults have serologic evidence of prior CMV infection.[14,15] Owing to relatively increased immunosuppression levels in LTRs and higher viral load transmission from seropositive lung allografts, CMV infection occurs more frequently in LTRs than other SOTs.[16,17] Immunomodulatory effects of CMV increase risks of infection from other opportunistic pathogens, Epstein–Barr virus (EBV)-related post-transplant lymphoproliferative disease, and allograft dysfunction.[18–20] CMV infection is variably associated with acute rejection and CLAD.[21–23] Without antiviral prophylaxis, 54% to 92% of LTRs develop CMV infection or disease.[24,25] Negative serostatus recipients with positive serostatus donors (CMV D+/R-) are at highest risk. CMV D+/R+ recipients have higher rate of infection than CMV D-/R+ recipients (69% and 58%, respectively) due to potential for CMV reactivation or infection with new strains.[26–29] CMV prophylaxis significantly decreases rates of CLAD.[30,31]

CMV disease requires evidence of viral replication in the presence of attributable symptoms or tissue invasion, whereas CMV infection is defined by viral replication regardless of symptom presence.[32] CMV disease most frequently occurs in the early

Table 1
Infection risk screening of lung transplant donors and recipients

Pathogen	Donor and Recipient Screening Test	Special Considerations
Cytomegalovirus (CMV)	CMV Immunoglobulin G (IgG)	
Epstein–Barr virus (EBV)	EBV nuclear antigen, viral capsid IgG	
Varicella-Zoster virus (VZV)	VZV IgG	
Herpes simplex 1 and 2 (HSV-1/HSV-2)	HSV-1 IgG HSV-2 IgG	
Hepatitis B virus (HBV)	HBV nucleic acid test (NAT), anti-HBc antibody, HBsAG	
Hepatitis C virus (HCV)	HCV NAT anti-HCV antibody	Perform testing in LTR immediately before transplant and 4–6 wk post-transplant
HIV	NAT and anti-HIV antibody	Repeat testing in LTR 4–6 wk post-transplant
SARS-CoV-2	Nasopharyngeal PCR	BAL can be considered in donor lung
Measles, mumps, rubella	Measles IgG, mumps IgG, rubella IgG	
Tuberculosis	Tuberculin skin testing (TST) or interferon gamma release assay (IGRA)	TST and IGRA are not validated in donors BAL and sputum can be obtained from donor for AFB smear, culture, and molecular testing Repeat testing in LTR 4–6 wk post-transplant
Treponema pallidum (syphilis)	Venereal Disease Research Laboratory or Rapid Plasma Reagin	
Toxoplasma gondii	Toxoplasma IgG	Toxoplasma IgG
Strongyloides stercoralis	Strongyloides IgG	Can limit screening to endemic areas

	Region Specific Screening	
Pathogen	Endemic Regions	Special Considerations
Schistosoma spp	Africa, South America, Caribbean, Middle East, southern China, southeast Asia	Cystoscopy may be indicated in renal transplant patients
Trypanosoma cruzi (Chagas disease)	Mexico, Central America, South America	
Leishmania spp	Africa, Asia, Middle East, southern Europe, Mexico, Central America, South America	May cross-react with T Cruzi

Coccidioides spp	Southeastern United States, California Central Valley, Mexico, part of Central and South America	
Histoplasma spp	Central and Eastern North America, Central America, South America, Africa, Asia, Australia	
Blastomyces spp.	Midwestern/South-Central/Southeastern United States, Eastern Canada, Africa, South Asia	
HTLV1 and HTLV2	Southern Japan, South America, Caribbean, Middle East, Sub-Saharan Africa, Central Australia, Papua New Guinea	Screening tests may be suboptimal in low prevalence areas
Hepatitis A	Areas with contaminated food and water supply, inadequate sanitation	Consider consultation with infectious diseases experts to determine if testing is indicated

Table 2
Vaccination recommendations for lung transplant recipients

Pathogen Target	Vaccine Type	Current Recommendation	Special Considerations
Influenza	Nonlive	Before and after transplant	Only inactivated, nonlive vaccine should be administered Annual administration to account for changing seasonal strains
Hepatitis B	Nonlive	Before and after transplant if not previously immunized of inadequate immunity	Monitor serostatus to confirm immunity
Hepatitis A	Nonlive	Before and after transplant	
Streptococcus pneumoniae	Nonlive	Before and after transplant if not previously immunized	
Neisseria meningitidis	Nonlive	Before and after transplant for high-risk patients not previously immunized	Risk factors include impaired splenic function and treatment with eculizumab
Haemophilus influenzae	Nonlive	Before and after transplant for high-risk patients not previously immunized	Risk factors include impaired splenic function
Human papillomavirus	Nonlive	Before and after transplant	
Tetanus, diphtheria, pertussis (Tdap)	Nonlive	Before and after transplant	
SARS-CoV-2	Nonlive	Before and after transplant	Boosters should be administrated at recommended intervals
Zoster	Nonlive (recombinant zoster vaccine)	Before and after transplant in LTRs > 19 year old	
Zoster	Live, attenuated zoster vaccine	Before transplant in candidates > 50 year old; contraindicated posttransplant and in immunosuppressed patients	
Varicella	Live, attenuated	Before transplant; contraindicated posttransplant and in immunosuppressed patients	
Measles, mumps, rubella	Live, attenuated	Before transplant; contraindicated posttransplant and in immunosuppressed patients	
Rotavirus	Live, attenuated	Before transplant; contraindicated posttransplant and in immunosuppressed patients	

post-transplant period and times of augmented immunosuppression. CMV pneumonitis is the most common presentation in LTRs; characteristics include fever, dyspnea, dry cough, lung function decline on spirometry, and radiographic findings such as ground-glass opacities and patchy consolidations.[33] Some tissue-invasive disease (CMV enteritis) presents with negative serum viral loads. Tissue biopsy with histopathologic findings of CMV inclusion bodies and/or viral antigens confirms diagnosis. Viral shedding in bronchoalveolar lavage (BAL) or bronchial washings cannot be distinguished from tissue-invasive disease and must be interpreted in clinical context.[34–39]

Although no trials have compared the approaches, universal antiviral prophylaxis in the first 6 to 12 months post-transplant with either oral valganciclovir or intravenous ganciclovir is recommended over preemptive serial monitoring of CMV viral loads with initiation of antivirals on viral replication detection.[31,40–42] A recently developed CMV T-Cell immunity panel, measuring CMV-specific CD4+ and CD8+ T-cell immunity by flow cytometry and intracellular cytokine staining has potential to personalize prophylaxis choice and duration and to predict clinically significant CMV events or inability to clear viremia. A measure of 0.2% of CMV reactive CD4+ and CD8+ T cells indicates existing immunity to CMV in a healthy population. The utilization of this test in combination with CMV polymerase chain reaction (PCR) testing is currently being studied in LTRs and could guide treating physicians in deciding continuation of CMV prophylaxis beyond 3 months post-transplant.[43–46]

Ongoing prophylaxis may be considered in CMV D+/R+ or CMV D-/R+ recipients receiving augmented immunosuppression with high-dose glucocorticoids or antilymphocyte antibodies. Myelosuppression is a common treatment toxicity. Oral letermovir lacks the myelosuppressive effects of valganciclovir and has been approved for CMV prophylaxis in hematopoietic stem cell transplant recipients.[47] Successful letermovir use in LTRs has been described in small studies, but there reports of breakthrough viremia and letermovir resistance exist.[48–50]

CMV treatment consists of valganciclovir or ganciclovir and concomitant immunosuppression reduction (particularly in moderate to severe disease). Treatment of asymptomatic viremia to prevent the development of invasive disease is advised. Valganciclovir is equivalent to ganciclovir for mild to moderate disease.[51,52] Ganciclovir is recommended for CMV pneumonitis, with transition to oral medication on clinical and virologic resolution. Treatment duration depends on clinical response and virologic clearance. Antiviral drug dosing should not be reduced if leukopenia emerges because of risk of drug resistance. Treatment with CMV immune globulin (CytoGam) might be considered in severe disease, though data are limited. If no virologic or clinical improvement is observed after 2 weeks of therapy, genotypic resistance testing should be performed.[53–56] The most common mutation conferring resistance is UL97 phosphotransferase. Resistant CMV treatment includes immunosuppression reduction and changing antivirals to foscarnet or cidofovir.[26] Oral maribavir is an alternative salvage treatment of resistant CMV disease approved for use in SOTs, with limited data in LTRs.[56–58] Letermovir can also be considered.

Non-Cytomegalovirus Herpesviruses

Herpes simplex 1 (HSV-1) and HSV-2 disease in LTRs is usually due to reactivation of latent virus in the dorsal root ganglia when herpesvirus prophylaxis is not used.[59] Acyclovir, valacyclovir, or famciclovir should be used in patients not receiving CMV prophylaxis.[60] Patients with limited mucocutaneous infection should be treated with oral medications until lesions are fully healed.[61] LTRs with severe or disseminated infection should be treated with intravenous acyclovir.

Varicella-zoster virus (VZV) infection occurs by airborne acquisition or reactivation from primary infection and presents as herpes zoster in up to 20% of LTRs in the first 5 years post-transplant.[62,63] Prophylaxis is similar in HSV; treatment is with valacyclovir or famciclovir. If lesions progress or new lesions develop despite therapy, treatment should be changed to intravenous acyclovir. Intravenous acyclovir is recommended for primary VZV infection, disseminated disease, or VZV affecting the trigeminal nerve.

Community-Acquired Respiratory Viruses

CARVs are associated with significant morbidity and mortality in LTRs.[64–66] Infection incidence in LTRs may be underestimated because historically studies have been retrospective and only of inpatient populations, whereas severity may be overestimated because studies used culture-based diagnostics in patients with severe respiratory symptoms.[66–68] Seasonal and geographic patterns of CARV infection in LTRs and immunocompetent individuals are similar.[69] Infection prevention strategies generally focus on contact avoidance and isolation and vaccination when available.

Immunosuppression can mute systemic inflammatory responses to CARV infection, and lung function declines from baseline on spirometry might be the sole infection indicators. Radiographic parenchymal abnormalities include ground-glass opacities, tree-in-bud opacities, nodules, and/or airspace consolidations.[70] Progression to lower respiratory tract disease or severe illness increases in LTRs who have had early post-transplant infections and who are receiving augmented immunosuppression or rejection treatment.[64,71]

Definitive diagnosis is achieved through testing respiratory tract samples. Initial testing should be through nasopharyngeal swab or washing and include a wide range of viruses to account for high likelihood of coinfection. Available tests and techniques vary by institution. Washings are more sensitive than swabs.[72] Molecular diagnostic tests are more sensitive than viral culture, direct fluorescent antibody, or rapid antigen detection in symptomatic and asymptomatic immunocompromised patients in outpatient and inpatient settings.[73–78] If initial testing is negative but clinical suspicion remains high, repeat confirmatory testing is advised, particularly if effective antiviral therapeutics are available. BAL may be indicated. When prolonged viral shedding is detected, serial quantitative molecular testing can guide treatment responsiveness.[79]

CARV infection stimulates cytokine and chemokine production that attracts damaging inflammatory cells, thereby changing mucosal epithelium integrity and composition.[80–83] Risk of secondary infection with locally invading bacterial or fungal airway colonizers is increased. Local alloantigen production can incite immune-mediated injury leading to episodes of acute rejection and CLAD development.[84,85] High BAL chemokine concentration prognosticates significant forced expiratory volume in the first second (FEV1) decline 6 months after initial infection.[86] CARV infections (particularly in the lower respiratory tract) are independent risk factors for CLAD, but contemporary studies have failed to demonstrate a strong relationship to acute rejection, possibly because most studies are retrospective single center analyses with variable definitions of acute rejection.[87–96] As expected host response to viral infection is perivascular lymphocytic infiltrate, the presence of lymphocytes on allograft biopsy can signify appropriate response to infection or rejection.

Influenza

LTRs have the highest incidence of influenza among SOTs. Unlike in immunocompetent patients, antiviral therapies are advised for all LTRs with suspected or confirmed influenza infection, regardless of illness severity or interval between symptom onset and diagnosis, due to secondary infections and rejection risks.[79,97] Confirmatory testing to guide antiviral therapy should be obtained when drug resistance is a concern. Neuraminidase inhibitors (oseltamivir, zanamivir, peramivir) are typical first-line treatments; M2 inhibitors (amantadine, rimantadine) are no longer recommended because of resistance and inactivity.[74,98] Therapy should continue until viral shedding is undetectable. Resistance testing should be performed in patients with prolonged symptom duration or clinical deterioration with ongoing viral shedding; empiric treatment with alternative antivirals should be considered while awaiting testing results. Antiviral prophylaxis is generally avoided to minimize development of resistance, except in LTRs likely to have inadequate immunity due to augmented immunosuppression or recent transplantation.[79]

Adenovirus
Adenovirus infection can be acquired throughout the year or reactivate from latent childhood infection to cause pneumonia or disseminated disease.[99] Mild disease is generally managed through immunosuppression reduction. Disseminated disease carries 50% mortality. Cidofovir is recommended for severe pneumonia or disseminated disease. Treatment can cause nephrotoxicity, neutropenia, and Fanconi-type anemia. Weekly quantitative serum viral load is recommended in addition to serial monitoring of renal function, serum electrolytes, and urine protein content.[100]

Respiratory syncytial virus
Respiratory syncytial virus (RSV) is a common cause of childhood bronchiolitis that carries 10% to 20% mortality in LTRs. Infection ranges from mild upper respiratory to severe lower respiratory tract disease associated with allograft dysfunction.[101,102] Prophylaxis with palivizumab can be considered. Ribavirin has in vitro activity against RSV; limited data in LTRs suggest ribavirin, with or without concomitant glucocorticoids or intravenous immunoglobulin (IVIG), successfully prevents progression to lower respiratory infection.[103,104]

Human metapneumovirus
Human metapneumovirus has similar presentation to RSV infection in LTRs and has been associated with allograft dysfunction. The main therapy is supportive care; ribavirin with or without IVIG has been used in few severe cases with successful outcome.[102,105]

Parainfluenza
Parainfluenza infects up to 10% of LTRs, with peak seasonal distribution in spring and summer. Infection is usually mild but can progress to severe lower respiratory tract illness and be associated with CLAD.[106,107] Ribavirin has been used in few reported cases with successful outcome.[108] Antivirals, adjunctive steroids, and IVIG generally have not proven beneficial.[71]

FUNGAL INFECTIONS

Invasive fungal infections (IFIs) have an 8% to 10% yearly cumulative incidence in LTRs. *Aspergillus* and *Candida* spp are the most common causative organisms; other culprits include the geographically endemic mycoses (*Histoplasma, Blastomyces,* and *Coccidioides* spp), *Pneumocystis, Cryptococcus* spp, mucormycosis agents, and non-*Aspergillus* molds (*Scedosporium* and *Fusarium* spp).[109] Incidence and type of IFI are influenced by immunosuppression intensity, pre-transplant airway colonization and ischemia, microbiome alterations from antimicrobial usage, timing since transplant, and antifungal prophylaxis. Invasive *Candida* spp (IC) infections typically occur in the early post-transplant period as complications associated with surgery, hospitalization, and ICU length of stay. Most non-*Candida* IFIs are acquired through inhalation or develop from recipient airway colonization. *Aspergillus* infections occur most frequently within the first 6 to 12 months posttransplant.[109] Non-*Aspergillus* mold infections occur later post-transplant and are associated with significantly higher mortality than *Aspergillus* (60.5% vs 39.5%, respectively).[110] IFIs are notably associated with allograft dysfunction. *Aspergillus* colonization is an independent risk factor for CLAD.[111] IFI testing and treatment is summarized in **Table 3**.

For all suspected IFIs, early bronchoscopy is recommended to evaluate anastomotic integrity, inspect airways for tracheobronchial abnormalities (pseudomembranes, erythema, ulcerations, or necrosis), and obtain BAL. Anastomotic dehiscence can be confirmed by chest imaging. Cavitary and nodular lesions are characteristic radiographic features. Cultures and fungal stains are positive in 50% to 70% of cases.[112] *Aspergillus* BAL PCR sensitivity is over 90% but testing cannot distinguish between infection and colonization.[113] Definitive IFI diagnosis necessitates tissue biopsy for visualization of fungal presence or tissue invasion at the suspected infection site.

Galactomannan antigen and 1,3-beta-D-glucan serum assays have variable utility in diagnosing IFIs in LTRs. Galactomannan is a cell wall component of *Aspergillus* sp released during fungal replication that can be detected in serum using enzyme immunoassay (EIA).[114] Serum galactomannan sensitivity is greatest in severely neutropenic patients because preserved immune systems consume circulating galactomannan; sensitivity in LTRs is 30%, versus over 70% in hematopoietic stem cell transplants.[115,116] In BALs of nonneutropenic SOT recipients, sensitivity increases to 88%.[114] Serum and BAL specificity are over 90% in all patients.[115,117,118] Galactomannan EIA cross-reactivity can occur with non-*Aspergillus* molds (*Fusarium* and *Penicillium*) and penicillin antibiotics (less so recently due to improved antibiotic purification).[109] The 1,3-beta-D-glucan is present in most fungal cell walls and particularly abundant in *Candida* spp; 1,3-beta-D-glucan sensitivity and specificity for IC is 80% and 60%, respectively. Patients with *Pneumocystis* pneumonia also have characteristically high levels; 1,3-beta-D-glucan is notably absent in cell walls of *Blastomyces*, *Cryptococcus*, and *Mucorales*. Falsely elevated levels of 1,3-beta-D-glucan can occur in patients on hemodialysis or who have received blood transfusions and intravenous immunoglobulin.[119,120] There is paucity of evidence on 1,3-beta-D-glucan testing in LTRs, and it is best used as a diagnostic adjunct in clinical context.

Prophylaxis strategies targeting both *Candida* spp and molds vary among transplant centers.[116] Questions remain regarding universal versus preemptive prophylaxis, choice of drug, need for monotherapy versus combination therapy, and prophylaxis duration. Studies of IFI prophylaxis have been limited by retrospective, single-center, and nonrandomized designs.[121] Some transplant centers begin universal antifungal prophylaxis immediately post-transplant, whereas others limit prophylaxis to recipients with high risk for IFIs (underlying cystic fibrosis or bronchiectatic lung diseases, evidence of airway colonization, primary graft dysfunction, and history of CMV infection).[122–126] Data on superiority of either strategy are mixed.[127–129] Most centers use monotherapy with aerosolized amphotericin B, or systemic voriconazole or itraconazole; the remainder use combination therapy with inhaled and systemic antifungals. Isavuconazole has been demonstrated to be a safe and effective alternative agent.[130] Duration of prophylaxis varies from 3 to over 12 months post-transplant. In one large retrospective study, incidences of IC and mold IFI were greater than previously reported despite micafungin and amphotericin B prophylaxis, suggesting breakthrough infection because of inadequate tissue penetration of echinocandins, reduced systemic drug concentration in the presence of ECMO circuits, and resistance to

Table 3
Diagnosis and treatment of invasive fungal infections in lung transplant recipients

Pathogen	Diagnostic Tests	Treatment	Special Considerations
Aspergillus sp	• Cultures • Histopathology • Serum galactomannan • BAL galactomannan • Serum PCR: single negative test rules out IA; two positive tests help rule in IA • BAL PCR: Identifies the presence of mold but cannot distinguish infection from colonization without appropriate clinical context • 1,3-beta-D-glucan variably helpful	First-line for IA: voriconazole Alternative agents: • Azoles: posaconazole, isavuconazole • Echinocandins: caspofungin, anidulafungin • Combination therapy can be considered Tracheobronchitis: inhaled amphotericin B in combination with systemic therapy	Treatment considerations: • Azoles: monitoring of hepatic function and calcineurin/mTOR inhibitor levels is advised • Liposomal amphotericin: monitoring of electrolytes, renal and hepatic function is advised • Caspofungin and micafungin: monitoring of hepatic function is advised • Anidulafungin and caspofungin: role as single agent therapy is controversial • Trimethoprim-sulfamethoxazole (TMP-SMX): correct for renal function and maintain adequate hydration • Pentamidine side effects include pancreatitis, hypo- and hyperglycemia, myelosuppression, renal failure, electrolyte disturbances • Avoid primaquine and dapsone in G6PD deficiency
Candida spp.	• Cultures • Histopathology • 1,3-beta-D-glucan can be helpful in clinical context T2 Candida assay (detects whole blood Candida cells of the 5 most common species with high sensitivity and specificity) • PCR testing not clinically available	IC and candidemia: • Echinocandins (micafungin, anidulafungin) are initial empiric therapy • Fluconazole as empiric therapy when azole resistance is not a concern • Liposomal amphotericin B Mild oropharyngeal disease: • Clotrimazole, fluconazole • Nystatin Endovascular infection/implantable Device infection: • Liposomal amphotericin B as initial therapy	

(continued on next page)

Table 3
(continued)

Pathogen	Diagnostic Tests	Treatment	Special Considerations
Mucormycosis	• Mucorales PCR is not clinically available • Cultures grow within 24–48 h • Cultures might be negative despite positive tissue staining • Galactomannan notably not useful	• High-dose echinocandin as alternative therapy Invasive mucormycosis: • Induction therapy with high dose liposomal amphotericin B • Combination of liposomal amphotericin B with echinocandin or posaconazole can be considered for refractory cases but data are weak • Posaconazole or isavuconazole can be used in patients not tolerating amphotericin but data are weak • Surgical excision and debridement for all extrapulmonary manifestations	
Cryptococcus	• Cryptococcus antigen testing of CSF and serum • CSF culture and stain • BAL culture and stain • Biopsy whenever possible	CNS disease: • Induction with liposomal amphotericin B and flucytosine for 2–4 wk • Consolidation with high-dose fluconazole for 8 wk • Maintenance with lower dose fluconazole for a year • Lumbar puncture as needed to relieve elevated intracranial pressure Pulmonary disease: • Asymptomatic or mild to moderate disease: Fluconazole for 6–12 mo • Severe pulmonary disease: same as CNS treatment	

Organism	Diagnostics	Treatment
Fusarium	• Cultures • Histopathology	Invasive fusariosis: • No treatment is clearly superior; voriconazole is typically first line • Amphotericin B in combination with voriconazole for resistant cases • Posaconazole as alternative • Surgical excision and debridement where indicated
Scedosporium	• Cultures • Histopathology	Invasive scedosporiosis • Voriconazole is first line • Amphotericin B, voriconazole, posaconazole, isavuconazole are all options and can be considered in combination • Surgical excision and debridement
Pneumocystis jirovecii	• BAL or tissue biopsy • Immunofluroscent assays are the most sensitive diagnostics • Nucleic acid testing in BAL cannot distinguish colonization from disease without clinical context • Silver stain on BAL excludes *Pneumocystis* pneumonia (PCP) if negative • LDH is nonspecific • 1,3-beta-D-glucan can be a helpful adjunct but is not specific for PCP	*Pneumocystis* Pneumonia: • Trimethoprim–sulfamethoxazole is first-line treatment • Alternatives: inhaled pentamidine: dapsone and trimethoprim • For mild to moderate disease only: atovaquone; combination primaquine and clindamycin • Combination echinocandins and TMP-SMX have shown benefit in animal models but clinical benefit is unknown • Adjunctive steroids are not clearly beneficial in non-HIV populations

inhaled amphotericin B. A recent meta-analysis of 12 antifungal prophylactic strategies among 13 studies did not establish a strong recommendation for a particular regimen.[131,132]

Aspergillus

Aspergillus spp is the most common cause of IFIs after lung transplantation. Owing to higher immunosuppression levels, invasive aspergillosis (IA) occurs more frequently in LTRs than other SOTs. Other risk factors include airway ischemia and prior airway colonization. *Aspergillus fumigatus* most commonly causes IA; other causative species include *Aspergillus terreus* (notable for in vitro resistance to amphotericin B), *Aspergillus flavus*, and *Aspergillus niger*. *Aspergillus* infection can present as tracheobronchitis, anastomotic dehiscence, pneumonia, aspergilloma, and disseminated disease to the sinuses, central nervous system (CNS), spine, pleural or pericardial spaces, or skin. Tracheobronchial aspergillosis typically occurs within 3 months posttransplant with fever, cough, wheezing, hemoptysis, or can be asymptomatic. Pulmonary aspergillosis generally presents 6 months post-transplant.[133,134] Single LTRs are at an increased risk of developing IA posttransplant and consequently experience higher mortality than bilateral or combined heart-LTRs. Among bilateral LTRs cystic fibrosis patients are at higher risk of aspergillosis.[133,135,136]

Voriconazole is the preferred initial treatment for IA; alternative agents include caspofungin and isavuconazole.[137] Azoles increase levels of tacrolimus, cyclosporine, and sirolimus; therefore, immunosuppression reduction and close serum drug concentration monitoring is required during treatment. Nebulized amphotericin B can be an adjunct therapy at the devascularized anastomotic site in tracheobronchial aspergillosis. Anastomotic debridement of necrotic tissue or debris is necessary when there is a threat of airway obstruction. Severe pulmonary and disseminated aspergillosis is typically treated in combination with echinocandins. Treatment duration is not well established but at least 3 months is advised with therapy extension if there is no clinical improvement.

Candida

Candida spp is the second most common cause of IFIs in LTRs. Infections typically occur within the first 3 months post-transplant and are associated with prolonged hospital exposure or critical illness, indwelling catheters, prolonged antibacterial therapy, and neutropenia.[138] Presentation ranges from candidemia to deep tissue infection in the pleural space and at the incision or anastomoses. Although *Candida* is frequently isolated from sputum and BAL specimens, invasive pulmonary disease is rare. Species identification is crucial for guiding treatment because of variable antifungal therapy resistance (fluconazole resistance in *C krusei*; dose-dependent susceptibility to fluconazole and amphotericin, respectively *C glabrata* and *C lusitaniae*). Echinocandins (micafungin, caspofungin) are suggested initial empiric therapy; high-dose fluconazole can alternatively be used in mild to moderate IC with low risk for *glabrata*, pending organism identification. Prompt source control including removal of infected catheters improves outcomes.

Mucormycosis

Mucormycosis is the third most common IFI in LTRs in the first-year post-transplant (2% incidence) and carries high morbidity and mortality (76% in pneumonia, 95% in disseminated disease). *Rhizopus*, *Mucor*, and *Rhizomucor* are the most implicated organisms.[139] Disease can be pulmonary, rhinocerebral, gastrointestinal, cutaneous, anastomotic, or disseminated. Fungal cell wall biomarkers are classically negative, making diagnosis challenging. Successful treatment depends on early diagnosis and resection of involved tissue when there is evidence of vascular invasion and tissue necrosis.

Cryptococcus

Yearly cumulative incidence of Cryptococcus in LTRs is under 1%, but infection risk is higher than other SOTs. Disease onsets within the first 6 to 12 months posttransplant; presentation can be pulmonary or disseminated. Concomitant immunosuppression reduction at the initiation of antifungal therapy is associated with the development of immune reconstitution inflammatory syndrome (IRIS).[140,141]

Non-Aspergillus Molds

Fusarium spp are environmentally ubiquitous but uncommonly pathogenic in LTRs; when they cause IFIs, mortality is high (65% in disseminated disease). Infection occurs through inhalation or mucosal or cutaneous invasion with potential for hematogenous spread.[142] LTRs, especially those with underlying cystic fibrosis (CF), are at increased risk for focal or disseminated IFI with Scedosporium. Treatment involves voriconazole, immunosuppression reduction, and surgical debridement.

Pneumocystis Jirovecii

Immunocompromised hosts with depleted T-cell immunity are at increased risk for Pneumocystis infection. LTRs are at higher risk than other SOTs. Before universal prophylaxis with trimethoprim–sulfamethoxazole, incidence of Pneumocystis pneumonia in LTRs ranged from 10% to 40%; lifelong prophylaxis reduces incidence to 5%.[143,144] Diagnostic testing sensitivity is decreased in LTRs because of reduced organismal burden in non-HIV patients with severe infection.[145]

Endemic Fungi

Infection with Histoplasma, Coccidioides, and Blastomyces may be reactivation of latent recipient infection, transmitted from donors from endemic areas, or acquired de novo from the environment. LTRs are more likely to present with severe pneumonia and disseminated disease.[146]

MYCOBACTERIAL INFECTIONS

Over 200 species of genus Mycobacterium exist with wide heterogeneity in prevalence, pathogenicity, and management. Mycobacteria are further divided into species complexes, the most notable being Mycobacterium tuberculosis complex which causes tuberculosis (TB). Active pulmonary TB affects more than 10 million people worldwide, and number of latent infections exceeds that. Nontuberculous mycobacteria (NTM) are ubiquitously found in soil and water and more frequently encountered in areas with low TB prevalence. Most NTM infections arise from environmental exposure, though nosocomial infections have also been described.[147,148]

Tuberculosis

Incidence of active TB in LTRs is less than 2% but mortality is highest among SOTs; mortality in all SOT is between 10% and 20%.[149,150] All donors and LTRs should be screened with tuberculin skin test (TST) or interferon gamma release assay (IGRA) and preferably treated for latent TB infection (LTBI) pre-transplant. Transplant urgency may preclude full treatment pre-transplant; if active TB is excluded, LTBI is not a contraindication for transplant and treatment should continue post-transplant.[151,152]

Negative recipients should undergo repeat IGRA testing at an interval post-transplant to verify donor transmission (noting that IGRA sensitivity is decreased with immunosuppression). LTBI treatment options are isoniazid for 9 months, rifampin for 4 months, or combination therapy with isoniazid and rifapentine for 3 months; rifampin and rifapentine are generally avoided post-transplant because of immunosuppressant drug interactions.

Active TB is an absolute contraindication for transplant because of dissemination risk and poor outcomes post-transplant.[153,154] It is not clear when a patient who has been successfully treated for active TB can safely undergo transplant. Diagnosing active TB after SOT can be difficult because of muted immune response, atypical radiographic presentation, and difficulty isolating organisms in culture; late diagnosis increases disseminated disease risk. First-line treatment of susceptible active TB is combination therapy with isoniazid, rifampin, pyrazinamide, and ethambutol for 2 months followed by at least an additional 4 months of rifampin and isoniazid.[155] Prolonged treatment is challenging because of drug toxicities and immunosuppressant interactions.

Nontuberculous Mycobacteria

NTM infection incidence in LTRs may be underestimated due to asymptomatic colonization and lack of reporting to public health agencies. Difficulty in diagnosis and treatment leads to significant morbidity and mortality. There is no clear association between NTM infection and CLAD. LTRs colonized or infected with NTM pretransplant should receive multidrug treatment to reduce disease burden; delay of transplant to complete at least 6 months of therapy can be considered.[156] Infection generally occurs 12 months posttransplant.[157,158] *Mycobacterium avium* complex species are the most common causative organisms. *Mycobacterium abscessus*, *Mycobacterium chelonae*, and *Mycobacterium kansasii* are most frequently associated with disseminated infection.[159] *M abscessus* is a virulent, fast growing NTM notable for human-to-human transmission among CF patients and high mortality without significant allograft dysfunction.[160,161] CF patients are at higher risk for NTM infection; risk increases with chronic macrolide therapy or airway colonization with *Pseudomonas aeruginosa* or *Burkholderia cepacia*.[162–164] CF patients with pretransplant *M abscessus* colonization have higher rates of disseminated infection.[165]

Symptoms depend on organism and infection site. In all SOTs, pleuropulmonary disease is the most common presentation with features including chronic productive cough, occasional hemoptysis, and nodular, bronchiectatic, or cavitary parenchymal abnormalities on imaging.[166] Cutaneous, musculoskeletal, and disseminated infection can occur. Immunosuppression might mute expected constitutional symptoms. Treatment is based on distinguishing NTM colonization from disease. Positive BAL acid-fast bacilli (AFB) culture can represent infection or contaminant from the laboratory or environment.[164] Molecular testing is available for some NTM species. Suspicious dermatologic lesions should be evaluated by skin biopsy with AFB staining and culture. The presence of virulent NTM such as *M abscessus* is highly suspicious for infection.

There are limited data and no randomized trials on NTM treatment in LTRs. Initial management involves combination therapy with multiple antimycobacterial drugs and surgical resection for complicated skin or soft tissue involvement. Typical combination therapies can include macrolides, rifamycins, ethambutol, isoniazid, fluoroquinolones, linezolid, tetracyclines, or aminoglycosides for duration of months to years depending on infection site and severity. Treatment is generally longer in LTRs than immunocompetent patients to prevent relapse.[156,167] Bacteriophages are being investigated as potential therapeutic options for management of drug resistant NTM.[168] Immunosuppression reduction should be considered with caution because of risk of IRIS. A minimum 12 months of treatment following negative sputum cultures is recommended for pulmonary disease. At least 4 to 6 months of therapy is recommended for focal soft tissue or bone infections. The rifamycins, particularly rifampin, reduce serum concentration of tacrolimus, cyclosporine, sirolimus, and everolimus through cytochrome p450 induction. Careful immunosuppressive drug monitoring and adjustment must be made to prevent rejection. Macrolides such as clarithromycin can increase serum concentrations of calcineurin inhibitors and sirolimus through cytochrome p450 inhibition; azithromycin is less likely to cause this effect. Outcomes of treatment are not well established due to relatively low incidence of infection.

SUMMARY

LTR outcomes are compromised by the wide range of infections to which the allograft is exposed. Comprehensive pre-transplant screening and careful post-transplant prophylaxis can mitigate infection risk and prevent infectious complications including development of allograft dysfunction. Future research in infection prevention, diagnostics, and therapeutics can further reduce LTR morbidity and mortality from infection.

CLINICS CARE POINTS

- Risk factors for infection in lung transplant recipients (LTRs) include continuous exposure of the lung allograft to the external environment, high levels of immunosuppression, impaired mucociliary clearance from airway epithelium changes due to disruptions in allograft blood supply and lymphatic drainage, and impact of the native lung microbiome in single LTRs.

- In the first month post-transplant, infections are generally due to donor allograft transmission, reactivation of recipient infections, or acquired from the hospitalization or surgical procedures; bacterial infections are the most common.

- Up to 6 months post-transplant, opportunistic infections predominate, though donor-derived infections may still occur; after the first 6 months, infections from broader range bacteria become more common.

- Comprehensive donor and recipient screening for infection risk pre-transplant, and vaccination of potential LTRs when absence of immunity to specific pathogens is identified, can reduce infection incidence post-transplant and guide prophylaxis choice and duration.

- Cytomegalovirus, *Aspergillus*, and community-acquired respiratory viruses affecting the lower respiratory tract are among the infections more strongly associated with the development of chronic lung allograft dysfunction; prevention, early diagnosis, and aggressive treatment are critical to preserving long-term allograft function.

- There are supportive data for the use of universal antifungal prophylaxis in lung transplant recipients, but available evidence has not proven it to be a clearly superior strategy to preemptive approaches in preventing invasive fungal infections, and antifungal prophylaxis strategies are variable across transplant centers

DISCLOSURE

The author has nothing to disclose.

REFERENCES

1. Chambers DC, Perch M, Zuckerman A, et al. The international thoracic organ transplant Registry of the international Society for heart and lung transplantation: Thirty-eighth adult lung transplantation report- 2021; focus on recipient characteristics. J Heart Lung Transpl 2021;40(10):1060–72.
2. Martin-Gandul C, Mueller NJ, Pascual M, et al. The impact of infection on chronic allograft dysfunction and allograft survival after solid organ transplantation. Am J Transpl 2015;15(12):3024–40.
3. Adegunsoye A, Strek ME, Garrity E, et al. Comprehensive care of the lung transplant patient. Chest 2017;152(1):150–64.
4. Bos S, Vos R, Van Raemdonck DR, et al. Survival in adult lung transplantation: where are we in 2020? Curr Opin Organ Transpl 2020;25(3):268–73.
5. Costa J, Benvenuto LJ, Sonett JR. Long-term outcomes and management of lung transplant recipients. Best Pract Res Clin Anaesthesiol 2017;31(2):285–97.
6. Avery RK. Recipient screening prior to solid-organ transplantation. Clin Infect Dis 2002;35(12):1513–9.
7. Trachuk P, Bartash R, Abbasi M, et al. Infectious complications in lung transplant Recipients. Lung 2020;198(6):879–87.
8. Malinas M, Boucher HW. Screening of donor and candidate prior to solid organ transplantation- guidelines from the American Society of transplantation infectious diseases community of practice. Clin Transpl 2019;33(9):e13548.
9. Danziger-Isakov L, Kumar D. Vaccination of solid organ transplant candidates and recipients: guidelines from the American Society of transplantation infectious diseases community of practice. Clin Transpl 2019;33(9):e13563.
10. Wolfe CR, Ison MG. Donor-derived infections: guidelines from the American Society of transplantation infectious diseases community of practice. Clin Transpl 2019;33(9):e13547.
11. Fishman JA. Infection in organ transplantation. Am J Transpl 2017;17(4):856–79.
12. Wahidi MM, Willner DA, Snyder LD, et al. Diagnosis and outcome of early pleural space infection following lung transplantation. Chest 2009;135(2):484–91.
13. Fishman JA. Infections in solid organ transplant recipients. N Engl J Med 2007; 357(25):2606–14.
14. Munting A, Manuel O. Viral infections in lung transplantation. J Thorac Dis 2021; 13(11):6673–94.
15. Bate SL, Dollard SC, Cannon MJ. Cytomegalovirus seroprevalence in the United States: the national health and nutrition examination surveys, 1988-2004. Clin Infect Dis 2010;50(11):1439–47.
16. Humar A, Snydman D. Cytomegalovirus in solid organ transplant recipients. Am J Transpl 2009;9(Suppl 4):S78–86.
17. Zamora MR. Cytomegalovirus and lung transplantation. Am J Transpl 2004;4(8): 1219–26.
18. Rubin RH. The indirect effects of cytomegalovirus infection on the outcome of organ transplantation. JAMA 1989;261:3607–9.
19. Hakimi Z, Aballea S, Ferchichi S, et al. Burden of cytomegalovirus disease in solid organ transplant recipients: a national matched cohort study in an inpatient setting. Transpl Infect Dis 2017;19(5):1–11.
20. Reinke P, Prosch S, Kern F, et al. Mechanisms of human cytomegalovirus (HCMV) (re)activation and its impact on organ transplant pateints. Transpl Infect Dis 1999;1(3):157–64.

21. Snyder LD, Finlen-Copeland CA, Turbyfill WJ, et al. Cytomegalovirus pneumonitis is a risk for bronchiolitis obliterans syndrome in lung transplantation. Am J Respir Crit Care Med 2010;181(12):1391–6.
22. Paraskeva M, Bailey M, Levvey NJ, et al. Cytomegalovirus replication within the lung allograft is associated with bronchiolitis obliterans syndrome. Am J Transpl 2011;11(10):2190–6.
23. Stern M, Hirsch H, Cusini A, et al. Cytomegalovirus serology and replication remain associated with solid organ graft rejection and graft loss in the era of prophylactic treatment. Transplantation 2014;98(9):1013–8.
24. Duncan AJ, Dummer JS, Paradis IL, et al. Cytomegalovirus infection and survival in lung transplant recipients. J Heart Lung Trnasplant 1991;10(5 Pt 1):638.
25. Zamora MR, Davis RD, Leonard C, CMV Adviso4y Board Expert Committee. Management of cytomegalovirus infection in lung transplant recipients: evidence-based recommendations. Transplantation 2005;80(2):157.
26. Razonable RR, Humar A. Cytomegalovirus in solid organ transplant recipients-guidelines of the American Society of transplantation infectious diseases community of practice. Clin Transpl 2019;33:e13512.
27. Manuel O, Husain S, Kumar D, et al. Assessment of cytomegalovirus-specific cell-mediated immunity for the prediction of cytomegalovirus disease in high-risk solid organ transplant recipients: a multicenter cohort study. Clin Infec Dis 2013;56(6):817–24.
28. Hammond SP, Martin ST, Roberts K, et al. Cytomegalovirus disease in lung transplantation: impact of recipient seropositivity and duration of antiviral prophylaxis. Transpl Infect Dis 2013;15(2):163–70.
29. Zamora MR. Controversies in lung transplantation: management of cytomegalovirus infections. J Heart Lung Transpl 2002;21(8):841.
30. Chmiel C, Speich R, Hofer M, et al. Ganciclovir/valganciclovir prophylaxis decreases cytomegalovirus-related events and bronchiolitis obliterans syndrome after lung transplantation. Clin Infect Dis 2008;46(6):831–9.
31. Jaamei N, Koutsoker A, Pasquier J, et al. Clinical significance of post-prophylaxis cytomegalovirus infection in lung transplant recipients. Transpl Infect Dis 2018;20(4):e12893.
32. Ljungman P, Boeckh M, Hirsch HH, et al. Definitions of cytomegalovirus infection and disease in transplant patients for Use in clinical trials. Clin Infect Dis 2017; 64(1):87–91.
33. Kang EY, Patz EF Jr, Muller NL. Cytomegalovirus pneumonia in transplant patients: CT findings. J Comput Assist Tomogr 1996;20(2):295–9.
34. Kotton CN, Kumar D, Caliendo AM, et al. The third international Consensus guidelines on the management of cytomegalovirus in solid-organ transplantation. Transplantation 2018;102(6):900–31.
35. Nakhleh RE, Bolman RM 3rd, Henke CA, et al. Lung transplant pathology. A comparative study of pulmonary acute rejection and cytomegalovirus infection. Am J Surg Pathol 1991;15(12):1197–201.
36. Chemaly RF, Yen-Lieberman B, Castilla EA, et al. Correlation between viral loads of cytomegalovirus in blood and bronchoalveolar lavage specimens from lung transplant recipients determined by histology and immunohistochemistry. J Clin Microbiol 2004 May;42(5):2168–72.
37. Riise GC, Andersson R, Bergstrom T, et al. Quantification of cytomegalovirus DNA in BAL fluid: a longitudinal study in lung transplant recipients. Chest 2000;118(6):1653–60.

38. Westall GP, Michaelidies A, Williams TJ, et al. Human cytomegalovirus load in plasma and bronchoalveolar lavage fluid: a longitudinal study of lung transplant recipeints. J Infect Dis 2004;190(6):1076–83.

39. Lodding IP, Schultz HH, Jensen JU, et al. Cytomegalovirus viral load in bronchoalveolar lavage to diagnose lung transplant associated CMV pneumonia. Transplantation 2018;102(2):326–32.

40. Manuel O, Kralidis G, Mueller NJ, et al. Impact of antiviral preventive strategies on the incidence and outcomes of cytomegalovirus disease in solid organ transplant recipients. Am J Transpl 2013;13(9):2402–10.

41. Palmer SM, Limaye AP, Banks M, et al. Extended valganciclovir prophylaxis to prevent cytomegalovirus after lung transplantation: a randomized, controlled trial. Ann Intern Med 2010;152(12):761–9.

42. Paya C, Humar A, Dominguez E, et al. Efficacy and safety of valganciclovir vs. oral ganciclovir for prevention of cytomegalovirus disease in solid organ transplant recipients. Am J Transpl 2004;4(4):611–20.

43. Veit T, Pan M, Munker D, et al. Association of CMV-specific T-cell immunity and risk of CMV infection in lung transplant recipients. Clin Transpl Jun 2021;35(6): e14294.

44. Sester U, Gärtner BC, Wilkens H, et al. Differences in CMV-specific T-cell levels and long-term susceptibility to CMV infection after kidney, heart and lung transplantation. Am J Transpl Jun 2005;5(6):1483–9.

45. Paez-Vega A, Cantisan S, Vaquero JM, et al. Efficacy and safety of the combination of reduced duration prophylaxis followed by immuno-guided prophylaxis to prevent cytomegalovirus disease in lung transplant recipients (CYTOCOR STUDY): an open-label, randomised, non-inferiority clinical trial. BMJ Open 2019;9(8):e030648.

46. Rogers R, Saharia K, Chandorkar A, et al. Clinical experience with a novel assay measuring cytomegalovirus (CMV)-specific CD4+ and CD8+ T-cell immunity by flow cytometry and intracellular cytokine staining to predict clinically significant CMV events. BMC Infect Dis 2020;20(1):58.

47. Frange P, Leruez-Ville M. Maribavir, brincidofovir, and letermovir: efficacy and safety of new antiviral drugs for treating cytomegalovirus infections. Med Mal Infect 2018;48(8):495–502.

48. Cherrier L, Nasar A, Goodlet KJ, et al. Emergence of letermovir resistance in a lung transplant recipient with ganciclovir-resistant cytomegalovirus infection. Am J Transpl 2018;18(12):3060–4.

49. Aryal S, Katugaha SB, Cochrane A, et al. Single-center experience with use of letermovir for CMV prophylaxis or treatment in thoracic organ transplant recipients. Transpl Infect Dis 2019;21(6):e13166.

50. Veit T, Munker D, Kauke T, et al. Letermovir for difficult to treat cytomegalovirus infection in lung transplant recipeints. Transplantation 2020;104(2):410–4.

51. Asberg A, Humar A, Rollag H, et al. Oral valganciclovir is noninferior to intravenous ganciclovir for the treatment of cytomegalovirus disease in solid organ transplant recipients. Am J Transpl 2007;7(9):2106–13.

52. Asberg A, Humar A, Jardine AG, et al. Long-term outcomes of CMV disease treatment with valganciclovir versus IV ganciclovir in solid organ transplant recipients. Am J Transpl 2009;9(5):1205–13.

53. Fisher CE, Knudsen JL, Lease ED, et al. Risk factors and outcomes of ganciclovir-resistant cytomegalovirus infection in solid organ transplant recipients. Clin Infect Dis 2017;65(1):57–63.

54. Khurana MP, Lodding IP, Mocroft A, et al. Risk factors for failure of primary val-ganciclovir prophylaxis against cytomegalovirus infection and disease in solid organ transplant recipients. Open Forum Infect Dis 2019;6(6):ofz215.
55. Le Page AK, Jager MM, Iwasenko JM, et al. Clinical aspects of cytomegalovirus antiviral resistance in solid organ transplant recipients. Clin Infect Dis 2013; 56(7):1018.
56. Pierce B, Richaedson CL, Lacloche L, et al. Safety and efficacy of foscarnet for the management of ganciclovir-resistant or refractory cytomegalovirus infections: a single-center study. Transpl Infect Dis 2018;20(2):e12852.
57. Chou S. Cytomegalovirus UL97 mutations in the era of ganciclovir and maribavir. Rev Med Virol 2008;18(4):233–46.
58. Papanicoloau GA, Silveira FP, Langston AA, et al. Maribavir for refractory or resistant cytomegalovirus infections in hematopoietic-cell or solid-organ trans-plant recipients: a randomized, dose-ranging, double-blind phase 2 study. Clin Infect Dis 2019;68(8):1255–64.
59. Fishman JA. Overview: cytomegalovirus and the herpesviruses in transplanta-tion. Am J Transpl 2013;13(Suppl 3):1–8, quiz 8.
60. Martin-Gandul C, Stampf S, Hequet D, et al. Preventive strategies against cyto-megalovirus and incidence of alpha-herpesvirus infections in solid organ trans-plant recipients: a nationwide cohort study. Am J Transpl 2017;17(7):1813–22.
61. Zuckerman RA, Limaye AP. Varicella zoster virus and herpes simplex virus in solid organ transplant patients. AM J Transpl 2013;13(Suppl 3):55–66, quiz 66.
62. Gourishankar S, McDermid JC, Jhangri GS, et al. Herpes zoster infection following solid organ transplantation: incidence, risk factors and outcomes in the current immunosuppressive era. Am J Transpl 2004;4(1):108–15.
63. Manuel O, Kumar D, Singer LG, et al. Incidence and clinical characteristics of herpes zoster after lung transplantation. J Jeart Lung Transpl 2008;27(1):11–6.
64. Kumar D, Husain S, Chen MH, et al. A prospective molecular surveillance study evaluating the clinical impact of community-acquired respiratory viruses in lung transplant recipients. Transplantation 2010;89(8):1028–33.
65. Vu DL, Bridevaux PO, Aubert JD, et al. Respiratory viruses in lung transplant re-cipients: a critical review and pooled analysis of clinical studies. Am J Transpl 2011;11(5):1071–8.
66. Palmer SM Jr, Henshaw NG, Howell DN, et al. Community acquired respiratory viral infection in adult lung transplant recipients. Chest 1998;113(4):944–50.
67. Milstone AP, Brumble LM, Barnes J, et al. A single-season prospective study of respiratory viral infections in lung transplant recipients. Eur Respir J 2006;28(1): 131–7.
68. Garbino J, Soccal PM, Aubert JD, et al. Respiratory virus in bronchoalveolar lavage: a hospital based cohort study in adults. Thorax 2009;64(5):399–404.
69. Couch RB, Englund JA, Whimbey E. Respiratory viral infections in immunocom-petent and immunocompromised persons. Am J Med 1997;102(3A):2–9, dis-cussion 25-6.
70. Franquet T. Imaging of pulmonary viral pneumonia. Radiology 2011;260(1): 18–39.
71. Ison MG. Respiratory viral infections in transplant recipients. Antivir Ther 2007; 12(4 Pt B):627–38.
72. Lieberman D, Lieberman D, Shimoni A, et al. Identification of respiratory viruses in adults: nasopharyngeal versus oropharyngeal sampling. J Clin Microbiol 2009;47(11):3439–43.

73. Kumar D, Michaels MG, Morris MI, et al. Outcomes from pandemic influenza A H1N1 infection in recipients of solid organ transplants: a multicenter cohort study. Lancet Infect Dis 2010;10:521–6.

74. Kumar D, Ferreira VH, Blumberg E, et al. A 5-year prospective multicenter evaluation of influenza infection in transplant recipients. Clin Infect Dis 2018;67(9): 1322–9.

75. Bridevaux PO, Aubert JD, Soccal PM, et al. Incidence and outcomes of respiratory viral infections in lung transplant recipients: a prospective study. Thorax 2014;69(1):32–8.

76. Mahony JB. Nucleic acid amplification-based diagnosis of respiratory virus infections. Expert Rev Anti Infect Ther 2010 Nov;8(11):1273–92.

77. Weinberg A, Zamora MR, Li S, et al. The value of polymerase chain reaction for the diagnosis of viral respiratory tract infections in lung transplant recipients. J Clin Virol 2002;25:171–5.

78. Englund JA, Piedra PA, Jewell A, et al. Rapid diagnosis of respiratory syncytial virus infections in immunocompromised adults. J Clin Microbiol 1996 Jul;34(7): 1649–53.

79. Manuel O, Estabrook M, AST Infectious Diseases Community of Practice. RNA respiratory viruses in solid organ transplantation. Am J Transpl 2013;13(Suppl 4):212–9.

80. Colvin BL, Thomson AW. Chemokines, their receptors, and transplant outcome. Transplantation 2002;74(2):149–55.

81. Skoner DP, Gentile DA, Patel A, et al. Evidence for cytokine mediation of disease expression in adults experimentally infected with influenza A virus. J Infect Dis 1999;180(1):10–4.

82. Arnold R, Humbert B, Werchau H, et al. Interleukin-8, interleukin-6, and soluble tumor necrosis factor receptor type 1 release from a human pulmonary epithelial cell line (A549) exposed to respiratory syncytial virus. Immunology 1994;82(1): 126–33.

83. Matsukura S, Kokobu F, Noda H, et al. Expression of IL-6, IL-8, and RANTES on human bronchial epithelial cells, NCI-H292, induced by influenza virus A. J Allergy Clin Immunol 1996;98(6, Pt 1):1080–7.

84. Belperio JA, Keane MP, Burdick MD, et al. Critical role for CXCR3 chemokine biology in the pathogenesis of bronchiolitis obliterans syndrome. J Immunol 2002;169(2):1037–49.

85. Belperio JA, Keane MP, Burdick MD, et al. Role of CXCL9/CXCR3 chemokine biology during pathogenesis of acute lung allograft rejection. J Immunol 2003; 171(9):4844–52.

86. Weigt SS, Derhovanessian A, Liao E, et al. CXCR3 chemokine ligands during respiratory viral infections predict lung allograft dysfunction. Am J Transpl 2012 Feb;12(2):477–84.

87. Soccal PM, Aubert JD, Bridevaux PO, et al. Upper and lower respiratory tract viral infections and acute graft rejection in lung transplant recipients. Clin Infect Dis 2010;51:163–70.

88. Peghin M, Hirsch HH, Len O, et al. Epidemiology and immediate indirect effects of respiratory viruses in lung transplant recipients: a 5-year prospective study. Am J Trnasplant 2017;17(5):1304–12.

89. Peghin M, Los-Arcos I, Hirsch HH, et al. Community-acquired respiratory viruses are a risk factor for chronic lung allograft dysfunction. Clin Infect Dis 2019;69(7):1192–7.

90. Allyn PR, Duffy EL, Humphires RM, et al. Graft loss and CLAD-onset is hastened by viral pneumonia after lung transplantation. Transplantation 2016;100(11): 2424–31.

91. Magnussen J, Westin J, Andersson LM, et al. Viral respiratory tract infection during the first postoperative year is a risk factor for chronic rejection after lung transplantation. Transpl Direct 2018;4(8):e370.

92. Khalifah AP, Hachem RR, Chakinala MM, et al. Respiratory viral infections are a distinct risk for bronchiolitis obliterans syndrome and death. Am J Respir Crit Care Med 2004;170(02):181–7.

93. Fisher CE, Preiksaitis CM, Lease ED, et al. Symptomatic respiratory virus infection and chronic lung allograft dysfunction. Clin Infect Dis 2016;62(3):313–9.

94. Billings JL, Hertz MI, Savik K, et al. Respiratory viruses and chronic rejection in lung transplant recipeints. J Heart Lung Transpl 2002;21(5):559–66.

95. Vilchez RA, Dauber J, Kusne S. Infectious etiology of bronchiolitis obliterans: the respiratory viruses connection- myth or reality? Am J Transpl 2003;3:245–9.

96. Sweet SC. Community-acquired respiratory viruses post-lung transplant. Semin Respir Crit Care Med 2021;42(3):449–59.

97. Vilchez RA, McCurry K, Dauber J, et al. Influenza virus infection in adult solid organ transplant recipients. Am J Transpl 2002 Mar;2(3):287–91.

98. Ison MG. Anti-influenza therapy: the emerging challenge of resistance. Therapy 2009;6:883.

99. Ison MG. Adenovirus infections in transplant recipients. Clin Infect Dis 2006; 43(3):331–9.

100. Florescu DF, Schaenman JM. AST infectious diseases community of practice. Adenovirus in solid organ transplant recipients. Guidelines from the American Society of transplantation infectious diseases community of practice. Clin Transpl 2019;33(9):e13527.

101. McCurdy LH, Milstone A, Dummer S. Clinical features and outcomes of paramyxoviral infection in lung transplant recipients treated with ribavirin. J Heart Lung Transpl 2003;22(7):745–53.

102. Hopkins P, McNeil K, Kermeen F, et al. Human metapneumovirus in lung transplant recipients and comparison to respiratory syncytial virus. Am J Respir Crit Care Med 2008;178(8):876–81.

103. Peleaz A, Lyon GM, Force SD, et al. Efficacy of oral ribavirin in lung transplant patients with respiratory syncytial virus lower respiratory tract infection. J Heart Lung Trasnplant 2009;28(1):67–71.

104. Burrows FS, Carlos LM, Benzimra M, et al. Oral ribavirin for respiratory syncytial virus infection after lung transplantation: efficacy and cost-efficiency. J Heart Lung Transpl 2015;34(7):958–62.

105. Raza K, Ismailjee SB, Crespo M, et al. Successful outcome of human metapneumovirus (hMPV) pneumonia in a lung transplant recipient treated with intravenous ribavirin. J Heart Lung Transpl 2007;26(8):862–4.

106. Vilchez R, McCurry K, Dauber J, et al. Influenza and parainfluenza respiratory viral infection requiring admission in adult lung transplant recipients. Transplantation 2002;73(7):1075–8.

107. Hall CB. Respiratory syncytial virus and parainfluenza virus. N Engl J Med 2001; 344(25):1917–28.

108. Liu V, Dhillon GS, Weill D. A multi-drug regimen for respiratory syncytial virus and parainfluenza virus infections in adult lung and heart-lung transplant recipients. Transpl Infect Dis 2010;12(1):38–44.

109. Kennedy CC, Pennington KM, Beam E, et al. Fungal infection in lung transplantation. Semin Respir Crit Care Med 2021;42(3):471–82.
110. Vasquez R, Vasquez-Guillamet MC, Suarez J, et al. Invasive mold infections in lung and heart-lung transplant recipients: Stanford University Experience. Transpl Infect Dis 2015;17(2):259–66.
111. Weigt SS, Elashoff RM, Huang C, et al. Aspergillus colonization of the lung allograft is a risk factor for bronchiolitis obliterans syndrome. Am J Transpl 2009; 9(8):1903–11.
112. Geltner C, Lass-Florl C. Invasive pulmonary Aspergillosis in organ transplants-Focus on lung transplants. Respir Investig 2016;54(2):76–84.
113. Lass-Florl C, Aigner M, Nachbaur D, et al. Diagnosing filamentous fungal infections in immunocompromised patients applying computed tomography-guided percutaneous lung biopsies: as 12-year experience. Infection 2017;45(6): 867–75.
114. Pfeiffer CD, Fine JP, Safdar N. Diagnosis of invasive aspergillosis using a galactomannan assay: a meta-analysis. Clin Infect Dis 2006;42(10):1417–27.
115. Husain S, Carmago JF. Invasive aspergillosis in solid-organ transplant recipients: guidelines from the American Society of transplantation infectious disease community of practice. Clin Transpl 2019;33(9):e13544.
116. Bergeron A, Belle A, Sulahian A, et al. Contribution of galactomannan antigen detection in BAL to the diagnosis of invasive pulmonary asspergillosis in patients with hematologic malignancies. Chest 2010;137(2):410–5.
117. Guo YL, Chen YQ, Wang K, et al. Accuracy of BAL galactomannan in diagnosing invasive aspergillosis: a bivariate metaanlysis and systematic review. Chest 2010;138(4):817–24.
118. Racil Z, Kocmanova I, Toskova M, et al. Galactomannan detection in bronchoalveolar lavage fluid for the diagnosis of invasive aspergillosis in patients with hematological diseases- the role of factors affecting assay performance. Int J Infect Dis 2011;15(12):e874–81.
119. Tran T, Beal SG. Application of the 1,3-B-D-Glucan (Fungitell) assay in the diagnosis of invasive fungal infections. Arch Pathol Lab Med 2016;140(2):181–5.
120. Patel TS, Eschenauer GA, Stuckey LJ, et al. Antifungal prophylaxis in lung transplant recipients. Transplantation 2016 Sep;100(9):1815–26.
121. Baker AW, Maziarz EK, Arnold CJ, et al. Invasive fungal infection after lung transplantation: epidemiology in the setting of antigunfal prophylaxis. Clin Infect Dis 2020;70(1):30–9.
122. Husain S, Zaldonis D, Kusne S, et al. Variation in antifungal prophylaxis strategies in lung transplantation. Transpl Infect Dis 2006;8(4):213–8.
123. He SY, Makhzoumi ZH, Singer JP, et al. Practice variation in Aspergillus prophylaxis and treatment among lung transplant centers: a national survey. Transpl Infect Dis 2015;17(1):14–20.
124. Hsu JL, Khan MA, Sobel RA, et al. Aspergillus fumigatus invasion increases with progressive airway ischemia. PLOS One 2013;8(10):e77136.
125. Verleden GM, Vos R, van Raemodonck D, et al. Pulmonary infection defense after lung transplantation: does airway ischemia play a role? Curr Opin Organ Transpl 2010;15(5):568–71.
126. Phoompoung P, Villalobos AP-C, Jain S, et al. Risk factors of invasive fungal infections in lung transplant recipients: a systematic review and meta-analysis. J Heart Lung Transpl 2022;41(2):255–62.
127. Bitterman R, Marinelli T, Husain S. Strategies for the prevention of invasive fungal infections after lung transplant. J Fungi (Basel) 2021;7(2):122.

128. Villalobos AP-C, Husain S. Infection prophylaxis and management of fungal infections in lung transplant. Ann Transl Med 2020;8(6):414.
129. Linder KA, Kauffman CA, Patel TS, et al. Evaluation of targeted versus universal prophylaxis for the prevention of invasive fungal infection following lung transplantation. Transpl Infect Dis 2021;23(1):e13448.
130. Samanta P, Clancy CJ, Marini RV, et al. Isavuconazole is as effective as and better Tolerated than voriconazole for antifungal prophylaxis in lung transplant recipients. Clin Infect Dis 2021;73(3):416–26.
131. Marinelli T, Rotstein C. Comment: invasive fungal infections in lung transplant recipients. Clin Infect Dis 2021;72(2):365–6.
132. Marinelli T, Davoudi S, Foroutan F, et al. Antifungal prophylaxis in adult lung transplant recipients: Uncertainty despite 30 years of experience. A systematic review of the literature and network meta-analysis. Transpl Infect Dis 2022;24(3): e13832.
133. Singh N, Husain S. Aspergillus infections after lung transplantation: clinical differences in type of transplant and implications for management. J Heart Lung Transpl 2003;22(3):258–66.
134. Gordon SM, Avery RK. Aspergillosis in lung transplantation: incidence, risk factors, and prophylactic strategies. Transpl Infect Dis 2001;3(3):161–7.
135. Aguilar CA, Hamandi B, Fegbeutel C, et al. Clinical risk factors for invasive aspergillosis in lung transplant recipients: results of an international cohort study. J Heart Lung Transpl 2018;37(10):1226–34.
136. Helmi M, Love RB, Welter D, et al. Aspergillus infection in lung transplant recipients with cystic fibrosis: risk factors and outcomes comparison to other types of transplant recipients. Chest 2003;123(3):800–8.
137. Paterson TF, Thompson GR 3rd, Denning DW, et al. Practice guidelines for the diagnosis and management of aspergillosis: 2016 update by the infectious diseases Society of America. Clin Infect Dis 2016;63(4):e1–60.
138. Marinelli T, Pennington KM, Hamandi B, et al. Epidemiology of candidemia in lung transplant recipeints and risk factors for candidemia in the early posttransplant period in the absence of universal antifungal prophylaxis. Transpl Infect Dis 2022;24(2):e13812.
139. Roden MM, Zaoutis TE, Buchanan WL, et al. Epidemiology and Outcome of Zygomycosis: a review of 929 reported cases. Clin Infect Dis 2005;41(5):634–53.
140. George IA, Santos CAQ, Olsen MA, et al. Epidemiology of Cryptococcosis and Cryptococcal meningitis in a large retrospective cohort of patients after solid organ transplantation. Open Forum Infect Dis 2017;4(1):ofx004.
141. Singh N, Lortholary Q, Alexander BD, et al. An immune reconstitution syndrome-like illness associated with Cryptococcus neoformans infection in organ transplant recipients. Clin Infect Dis 2005;40(12):1756–61.
142. Carneiro HA, Coleman JJ, Restrep A, et al. Fusarium infection in lung ttransplant patients: report of 6 cases and review of the literature. Medicine (Baltimore) 2011;90(01):69–80.
143. Sepkowitz KA. Opportunistic infections in patients with and patients without acquired immunodeficiency syndrome. Clin Infect Dis 2002;34:1098–107.
144. Gordon SM, LaRose SP, Kalmadi S, et al. Should prophylaxis for Pneuocystis carinii pneumonia in solid organ transplant recipients ever be discontinued? Clin Infect Dis 1999;28(2):240–6.
145. Thomas CF Jr, Limper AH. Pneumocystis pneumonia. N Engl J Med 2004; 350(24):2487–98.

146. Miller R, Assi M. AST infectious diseases community of practice. Endemic fungal infections in solid organ transplant recipients- guidelines from the American Society of transplantation infectious diseases community of practice. Clin Transpl 2019;33(9):e13553.

147. Friedman DZP, Doucette K. Mycobacteria: selection of transplant candidates and post-lung transplant outcomes. Semin Respir Crit Care Med 2021 Jun; 42(3):460–70.

148. Forbes BA, Hall GS, Miller MB, et al. Practical guidance for clinical microbiology laboratories: mycobacteria. Clin Microbiol Rev 2018;31(02):e00038.

149. Abad CLR, Razonable RR. Donor derived Mycobacterial tuberculosis infection after solid-organ transplantation: a comprehensive review. Transpl Infect Dis 2018;20(05):e12971.

150. Abad CLR, Razonable RR. Mycobacterium tuberculosis after solid organ transplantation: a review of more than 2000 cases. Clin Transpl 2018;32(06):e13259.

151. Subramanian AK, Theodoropoulos NM. Infectious Diseases Community of Practice of the American Society of Transplantation. Mycobacterium tuberculosis infections in solid organ transplantation: guidelines from the infectious diseases community of practice of the American Society of Transplantation. Clin Transpl 2019;33(09):e13513.

152. Subramanian AK. Tuberculosis in solid organ transplant candidates and recipients: current and future challenges. Curr Opin Infect Dis 2014 Aug;27(04): 316–21.

153. Leard LE, Holm AM, Valapour M, et al. Consensus document for the selection of lung transplant candidates: an update from the International Society for Heart and Lung Transplantation. J Heart Lung Transpl 2021;40(11):1349–79.

154. Torre-Cisneros J, Doblas A, Aguado JM, et al. Spanish Network for Research in Infectious Diseases. Tuberculosis after solid-organ transplant: incidence, risk factors, and clinical characteristics in the RESITRA (Spanish Network of Infection in Transplantation) cohort. Clin Infect Dis 2009;48(12):1657–65.

155. Nahid P, Dorman SE, Alipanah N, et al. Official American thoracic Society/centers for disease control and prevention/infectious diseases Society of America clinical practice guidelines: treatment of drug-susceptible tuberculosis. Clin Infect Dis 2016;63(7):e147–95.

156. Longworth SA, Daly JS. AST infectious diseases community of practice. Management of infections due to nontuberculous mycobacteria in solid organ transplant recipients- guidelines from the American Society of transplantation infectious diseases community of practice. Clin Transpl 2019;33(9):e13588.

157. Malouf MA, Glanville AR. The spectrum of mycobacterial infection after lung transplantation. Am J Respir Crit Care Med 1999;160(5 Pt 1):1611–6.

158. Keating MR, Daly JS, AST Infectious Diseases Community of Practice. Nontuberculous mycobacterial infections in solid organ transplantation. Am J Transpl 2013;13(Suppl 4):77–82.

159. Daley CL, Iaccarino JM, Lange C, et al. Treatment of nontuberculous mycobacterial pulmonary disease: an official ATS/ERS/SCMID/IDSA clinical practice guideline. Clin Infect Dis 2020;71(4):e1–36.

160. Hamad Y, Pilewski JM, Morrell M, et al. Outcomes in lung transplant recipeints with Mycobacterium abscessus infection: a 15-year experience from a large tertiary care center. Transpl Proc 2019;51(6):2035–42.

161. Perez AA, Singer JP, Schwartz BS, et al. Management and clinical outcomes after lung transplantation in patients with pre-transplant Mycobacterium abscessus infection: a single center experience. Transpl Infect Dis 2019;21(3):e13084.

162. Degiacomi G, Sammartino JC, Chiarelli LR, et al. Mycobacterium abscessus, an emerging and worrisome pathogen among cystic fibrosis patients. Int J Mol Sci 2019;20(23):E5868.
163. Furukawa BS, Flume PA. Nontuberculous mycobacteria in cystic fibrosis. Semin Respir Crit Care Med 2018;39(03):383–91.
164. Knoll BM, Kappagoda S, Gill RR, et al. Non-tuberculous mycobacterial infection among lung transplant recipients: a 15-year cohort study. Transpl Infect Dis 2012;14(5):452–60.
165. Chalermskulrat W, Sood N, Neuringer IP, et al. Non-tuberculous mycobacteria in end stage cystic fibrosis: implications for lung transplantation. Thorax 2006; 61(6):507–13.
166. Doucette K, Fishman JA. Nontuberculous mycobacterial infection in hematopoietic stem cell and solid organ transplant recipients. Clin Infect Dis 2004;38(10): 1428–39.
167. Griffith DE, Aksamit T, Brown-Elliott BA, et al. ATS Mycobacterial Disease Society of America. An official ATS/IDSA statement: diagnosis, treatment, and prevention of nontuberculous mycobacterial diseases. Am J Respir Crit Care Med 2007;175(04):367–416.
168. Aslam S. Bacteriophage therapy as a treatment option for transplant infections. Curr Opin Infect Dis 2020;33(4):298–303.

Novel Approaches to Multidrug-Resistant Infections in Cystic Fibrosis

Thomas S. Murray, MD, PhD[a,*], Gail Stanley, MD[b,c,d,*],
Jonathan L. Koff, MD[c,d,e,*]

KEYWORDS

- Cystic fibrosis • Multidrug-resistant organisms • Bacteriophage • Gallium

KEY POINTS

- Despite the introduction of cystic fibrosis transmembrane conductance regulator (CFTR) modulator therapy, multidrug-resistant organism (MDRO) pulmonary infections remain a significant problem for patients with cystic fibrosis (CF), and new therapeutic strategies are needed.
- Standard antibiotic dosing regimens may produce subtherapeutic levels for patients with CF, as the pharmacokinetics/pharmacodynamics often differ from patients without CF.
- Novel therapies, such as gallium and bacteriophage(s), are emerging as exciting options to treat MDRO infections but additional studies are required to determine the optimal dosing, and patient populations, which will benefit the most.

INTRODUCTION
Chronic Multidrug-Resistant Organism Infections in Cystic Fibrosis

Patients with cystic fibrosis (CF) are colonized early in life with bacteria and treated with repeated cycles of antibiotics. This leads to the emergence of pathogenic chronic multidrug-resistant organism (MDROs), defined as microorganisms resistant to one or more different classes of antibiotics.[1] Organisms that are problematic

This article was previously published in *Clinics in Chest Medicine* 43:4 December 2022.
[a] Department of Pediatrics, Section Infectious Diseases and Global Health, Yale University School of Medicine, PO Box 208064, 333 Cedar Street, New Haven, CT 06520-8064, USA; [b] Department of Internal Medicine, Section Pulmonary, Critical Care and Sleep Medicine, Yale University School of Medicine, PO Box 208057, 300 Cedar Street TAC-441 South, New Haven, CT 06520-8057, USA; [c] Adult Cystic Fibrosis Program; [d] Yale University Center for Phage Biology & Therapy; [e] Department of Internal Medicine, Section Pulmonary, Critical Care and Sleep Medicine, Yale University School of Medicine, PO Box 208057, 300 Cedar Street TAC-455A South, New Haven, CT 06520-8057, USA
* Corresponding authors.
E-mail addresses: Thomas.s.murray@yale.edu (T.S.M.); gail.stanley@yale.edu (G.S.); jon.koff@yale.edu (J.L.K.)

Infect Dis Clin N Am 38 (2024) 149–162
https://doi.org/10.1016/j.idc.2023.12.002
0891-5520/24/© 2023 Elsevier Inc. All rights reserved.

id.theclinics.com

include, but are not limited to, the gram-positive methicillin-resistant *Staphylococcus aureus* (MRSA), and a variety of gram-negative organisms that include *Pseudomonas aeruginosa*, *Burkholderia sp.*, *Stenotrophomonas maltophilia*, *Achromobacter xylosoxidans*, and nontuberculous mycobacteria (NTM). In 2019, 16.9% of *P. aeruginosa* infections in patients with CF were multidrug-resistant (MDR), while more than 50% of patients had a respiratory culture that grew MRSA.[2] As highly effective cystic fibrosis transmembrane conductance regulator (CFTR) modulator therapy is introduced at younger ages, there is optimism that this will reduce the incidence and/or severity of chronic infections and decrease the acquisition of new pathogens.[3,4] However, this is tempered by the observation that while the initiation of ivacaftor initially leads to decreases in *P. aeruginosa*, this effect is not maintained long term.[5] In addition, for some individuals with CF currently on CFTR modulator therapy, evidence suggests there is little change to the microbes in the airway.[6] Therefore, antibiotics remain integral to treatment regimens during pulmonary exacerbations,[4] and novel antimicrobial approaches or interventions are needed to treat these infections.

Several different therapeutic approaches have been tried in recent years to improve outcomes for patients with CF with chronic MDRO pulmonary infection (**Table 1**). One such approach is to improve the efficacy of existing antibiotics by optimizing the pharmacokinetics/pharmacodynamics (PK/PD), which may be achieved by altering the dosing regimen.[7] Another strategy to extend the benefits of a currently available drug (eg, vancomycin, ciprofloxacin, levofloxacin, and amikacin), is to develop an inhaled formulation that allows for higher concentrations in the lung while reducing systemic adverse effects.[8–10] Finally, existing beta-lactam drugs, such as ceftazidime and meropenem, have been combined with novel beta-lactamase inhibitors to create new drugs that target gram-negative MDROs that produce extended-spectrum beta-lactamases (ESBLs) and carbapenemases.[11]

While optimizing the delivery of existing drugs has been helpful, it is not surprising that resistant organisms continue to emerge. The above approaches also highlight the limitation of the existing antibiotic pipeline where few new drugs with novel mechanisms of action have been introduced in recent years. The result is innovative therapies currently being studied that either: (1) target the host to improve the immune response to infection [for example, granulocyte macrophage-colony stimulating factor (GM-CSF)] or (2) target the organism with a completely different class of molecule(s) that have antimicrobial activity (eg, gallium or bacteriophages).

DISCUSSION
Optimizing the Pharmacokinetics/Pharmacodynamics of Available Antibiotics

Based on pancreatic insufficiency and impaired gastrointestinal tract absorption, increased renal and hepatic drug clearance, and increased volume of distribution of hydrophilic drugs[12–14] standard antimicrobial dosing may not be appropriate for patients with CF as they require higher and/or more frequent drug administration to achieve therapeutic levels.[15–17] One review of anti-MRSA agents found that for both intravenous (IV) and oral administration, none of the currently recommended doses for any of the studied drugs achieved therapeutic levels for a sufficient time.[15] In each case either a higher dose or more frequent dosing was recommended to achieve the required minimum inhibitory concentrations (MICs) for the appropriate time. For certain beta-lactam antibiotics, such as meropenem, continuous infusions increase the time the drug concentration is above the MIC, which increases drug activity against isolates with higher MICs.[17,18] These data highlight the importance of studying

Table 1
Novel approaches to treat MDRO infections in patients with CF

Strategy	Examples	Advantages	Disadvantages
Extended antibiotic infusion/ increased dosing	Meropenem	Optimizes existing drugs based on PK/PD studies in patients with CF	Daily activities hampered by long times with IV infusion, potential for adverse effects with higher dosing
Newer antimicrobial agents (eg, novel b-lactam/b-lactamase combinations)	Ceftazidime/avibactam Ceftolozane/tazobactam	Additional efficacy against organisms that produce B-lactamases.	Emergence of resistant organisms
Inhaled existing antimicrobials	Vancomycin	Avoid systemic adverse effects while achieving higher concentrations at the infection site	Limited efficacy data for most new formulations.
Novel inhaled antimicrobial Inhaled agents that enhance the immune response	Nitric oxide Granulocyte monocyte-colony stimulating factor	May provide benefit for difficult-to-treat organisms such as M. abscessus	Limited data from clinical studies. Optimal dosing not clear may require frequent dosing
Phage		No off-target effects on human cells, Has the potential to revert antibiotic resistance	Phage-resistant bacteria are well-described
Gallium		IV therapy is well-tolerated	Only IV administration has been studied to date

Abbreviations: IV, Intravenous; MDRO, multidrug-resistant organism; PK/PD, pharmacokinetics/pharmacodynamics.

the PK/PD of novel antimicrobials in CF children and adults as they come to market because suboptimal dosing will potentially select for resistant strains.[19]

CLINICS CARE POINTS

- When prescribing CF antimicrobial therapy, do not necessarily rely on "standard" dosing established for the general population;
- For a given drug, examine the literature for PK/PD data to determine the optimal therapeutic regimen and required drug monitoring in CF;
- Continuous infusions are an option for select beta-lactams.

Newer Systemic Antimicrobials for Multidrug-Resistant Organisms Therapy

Gram-negative organisms (eg, *P. aeruginosa, Burkholderia* sp)

Existing beta-lactam antibiotics combined with novel beta-lactamase inhibitors have produced a number of newer drugs with potent *in vitro* activity against select MDR isolates when a primary driver of antimicrobial resistance is the production of ESBLs or carbapenemases.[11] Two examples that have been used in CF to treat MDR organisms are ceftazidime-avibactam and ceftolozane-tazobactam.[19–25] A case series of 8 adults with advanced CF lung disease complicated by MDR *P. aeruginosa* and/or *Burkholderia* infection who received 15 courses of ceftazidime-avibactam showed a clinical response in 13/15 (86.7%) patients with no serious adverse events reported.[24] However, *in vitro P. aeruginosa* resistance to ceftazidime-avibactam is well described and should be considered before using this agent.[21,23,26]

Ceftolozane-tazobactam has prominent *P. aeruginosa* activity with higher rates of *in vitro* susceptibility compared with ceftazidime-avibactam.[11] A study of 21 patients with MDR *P. aeruginosa* treated with ceftolozane-tazobactam with or without additional anti-pseudomonal antibiotics included 6 patients with CF. Of these patients with CF, 5 (83%) demonstrated a successful clinical response; the one patient who did not improve had ceftolozane-tazobactam-resistant isolates.[27] Additional individual case reports have suggested success with ceftolozane-avibactam for CF adults who have pulmonary exacerbations and respiratory cultures with MDR gram-negative bacteria.[28–30] While the existing data are generally in adults, ceftolozane-avibactam has also been proposed as an option for children with MDR *P. aeruginosa* refractory to standard therapies.[20]

Meropenem-vaborbactam is another new beta-lactam/beta-lactamase inhibitor combination. It differs from those previously discussed in that it does not provide additional activity against meropenem-resistant *P. aeruginosa*. However, it is efficacious against other MDR CF pathogens such as *Burkholderia* sp and *S. maltophilia*,[31] but there are little data on its clinical use for patients with CF. Additional combinations of beta-lactams and beta-lactamase inhibitors have been approved or are at various stages of clinical development.[11] An alternative novel approach is to use a beta-lactamase inhibitor from one of these new combinations to restore susceptibility of a different beta-lactam. For example, piperacillin susceptibility can be restored by the avibactam from ceftazidime-avibactam for MDR *Burkholderia* CF isolates resistant to piperacillin.[32] The relebactam from imipenem-relebactam can restore amoxicillin susceptibility to the resistant NTM, *Mycobacterium abscessus,* by inhibiting the mycobacterial beta-lactamases that degrade amoxicillin.[33]

Cefiderocol is a novel cephalosporin/siderophore that enters bacteria through the iron-uptake system and has activity against MDR gram negatives including *P. aeruginosa*.[34] It has been proposed as a potential salvage therapy for MDR gram negatives but very little data are available to support its use in CF.[35] One study of 8 patients with CF who received 12 courses of cefiderocol for MDR *A. xylosoxidans* noted a clinical response after 11/12 (91.7%) courses, but only one patient cleared the infection.[36] Additional studies are needed to determine if there is a role for cefiderocol when other agents have failed to generate a clinical response.

Although the correlation between *in vitro* antibiotic resistance and clinical outcomes is often absent in CF,[37,38] it is important to note that variable rates of *in vitro* resistance have been described for all of the above antibiotics.[11,25,27,39] Mechanisms of resistance to these agents include, but are not limited to, increased activity of efflux pumps, porin mutations, and overexpression of the AmpC beta-lactamase.[11,40] Additionally, none of the currently available new beta-lactam/beta-lactamase inhibitors bind class B metalloprotease b-lactamases, such that isolates with these enzymes will remain resistant.[11]

CLINICS CARE POINTS

- There are several new combinations of cephalosporins and beta-lactamase inhibitors for different MDR gram-negative pathogens.
- Based on the mechanism of action of specific drugs and the resistance mechanisms of some bacteria, antibiotic efficacy varies.
- While *in vitro* susceptibility testing does not correlate with clinical outcomes in CF, resistance to these new agents is described and worth monitoring.

Methicillin-Resistant S. aureus

Fewer new agents have been developed in recent years for MRSA treatment. Ceftaroline is a fifth-generation IV cephalosporin that targets the penicillin-binding protein 2A, which confers methicillin resistance to *S. aureus*. As with other antimicrobials, the PK/PD of ceftaroline in CF may require nonstandard dosing to achieve therapeutic levels.[15,41] There are little data for the use of ceftaroline to treat MRSA-associated pulmonary exacerbations.[42,43] One retrospective study of 90 patients with CF who received ceftaroline compared with 90 patients treated with vancomycin showed no difference in forced expiratory volume in 1 second (FEV1), which suggested equivalence between the 2 drugs.[42] Thus, ceftaroline may be an option for patients with renal dysfunction or those who are unable to tolerate vancomycin for other reasons. Importantly, carbapenem use in patients with CF has been linked to ceftaroline resistance, which makes susceptibility testing a consideration for patients who have previously received carbapenems for MDR gram-negative organisms.[44]

Novel Inhaled Therapies in Development

Inhaled delivery of existing antimicrobials. Concerns about the systemic toxicity of commonly used antimicrobials have led to the study of inhaled formulations that allow for high concentrations of drug delivery to the lungs with fewer systemic side effects.[9,10,45] A number of currently available antibiotics are being studied as inhalation therapy to address unmet needs for patients with CF. Phase 1 safety and PK studies of dry powder inhaled vancomycin in healthy adults and patients with CF elicited optimism. However, subsequent studies including a phase III randomized, multicenter, double-blinded, placebo-controlled study to evaluate the effectiveness of inhaled vancomycin in patients with CF ages 6 and older with MRSA (clinicaltrials.gov NCT03181932), did not meet the primary endpoints: improved lung function (FEV1% predicted) and decreased frequency of pulmonary exacerbations when compared with placebo.[46] In addition, a strategy to investigate the use of inhaled vancomycin for MRSA eradication was studied (clinicaltrials.gov NCT01594827). This trial enrolled 29 subjects; there were no differences in the rates of MRSA eradication, and inhaled vancomycin may be associated with increased rates of bronchospasm.[47] A recently completed phase I dose-escalation study examined inhaled teicoplanin, another anti-MRSA drug in patients with CF; the study results are pending at this time (clinicaltrials.gov NCT04176328).

For gram-negative organisms, an inhaled form of levofloxacin was evaluated in a phase III trial (clinicaltrials.gov NCT01180634). There was no difference between inhaled levofloxacin compared with placebo in the primary outcome of time to next pulmonary exacerbation. However, there was a statistically significant improvement in the treatment arm with respect to secondary outcomes of lung function and decreased microbial burden in the sputum.[48] Thus, inhaled levofloxacin has been approved in the European Union and Canada for adults.[49] Other antibiotics are also under development as inhaled therapy in areas with a significant clinical need. Oral clofazimine is a standard agent for the treatment of Mycobacterial infections that is being developed as an inhaled therapy, which has shown promise in a mouse model of NTM infection.[50]

Novel inhaled agents. In addition to new combinations and formulations of existing antibiotics, there are advances in developing inhaled administration of molecules integral to the host immune response to infection, especially for MDR *M. abscessus.*[51] These pathogens reside in host macrophages within the lung, thus there is a need to achieve high intracellular drug levels for treatment success. Two of the drugs furthest along in clinical development are inhaled nitric oxide (iNO) gas and GM-CSF.

NO as an antimicrobial. NO is a gas with both direct and indirect antimicrobial properties derived from L-arginine by iNO synthase, which is released by epithelial cells, macrophages, and other immune cells in response to infection. [52] NO production is reduced in CF, which is a potential mechanism for susceptibility to bacterial and viral infections.[53,54] Case reports describe the use of inhaled NO to decrease MDR-NTM numbers in the respiratory tract of patients that have failed traditional therapy, with an associated improvement in clinical symptoms.[55–57] A small phase 1 safety trial in patients with CF demonstrated that inhaled NO given five times daily (at 160 ppm) was safe when given over a 14-day period.[58] While there was an initial drop in the number of NTM recovered with improved lung function, sustained microbial clearance from the sputum was not achieved.[58] Another study looked at a higher inhaled NO dose in a single patient but was discontinued due to adverse effects.[55] While NTM clearance was not achieved, the patient had improved exercise tolerance and lung function.[55] A phase II clinical trial of inhaled NO in patients with CF (clinicaltrials.gov NCT02498535) was terminated due to COVID-19 thus, additional studies are required to determine appropriate dosing and confirm long-term benefits. Inhaled NO is also under investigation in patients with CF with *Pseudomonas, Staphylococcus,* or *Stenotrophomonas* (clinicaltrials.gov NCT02498535). A multi-center, randomized, placebo-controlled, phase II clinical trial has been completed and we await the reported results.[59]

GM-CSF as an antimicrobial. GM-CSF is released by alveolar macrophages in response to microbes, including NTM, and exogenous GM-CSF therapy is being studied as an antiinfective. Two patients with CF refractory to conventional therapy for *M abscessus* responded to inhaled GM-CSF, one in combination with antibiotics, and the other with GM-CSF alone.[60] A phase II clinical trial of inhaled GM-CSF for patients with CF with NTM (clinicaltrials.gov NCT03597347) was terminated early due to COVID-19 as well as changes in CF care that affected the primary outcome.[61] However, analysis of the primary outcome (sputum NTM culture conversion to negative after 48 weeks) showed that no significant sputum culture conversions occurred in the inhaled GM-CSF group. Based on these results, the use of inhaled GM-CSF in CF for NTM has been discontinued.

CLINICS CARE POINTS

- NO and GM-CSF are naturally produced by the immune system in response to infection.
- Inhaled NO and GM-CSF have been studied as adjuvant therapy for common CF bacterial infections, and highly resistant organisms such as NTM.
- Additional clinical studies are needed to establish the correct dosing and to determine whether there is a clinical benefit.

Novel Molecules with Antimicrobial Activity

Gallium is a metal that is used commercially in electronic circuits and semiconductors and is approved for clinical use in diagnostic procedures, and as a therapeutic in cancer and bone metabolism. Iron is an essential element for bacteria growth and metabolism. Bacteria use siderophores to scavenge iron from the environment. Gallium (Ga $^{3+}$) is similar enough in structure to ferric ion (Fe $^{3+}$), and will bind bacteria siderophores with high affinity.[62] However, Ga3+ cannot be reduced under physiologic conditions, rendering gallium-loaded enzymes inactive. Thus, gallium offers an opportunity to be used to disrupt bacterial iron metabolism,[63] which has been described as a "Trojan horse" strategy.[64] This potential use is particularly relevant in CF because gallium's antibacterial activity has been observed against *P. aeruginosa* and NTM,[63] and has an advantage for therapy because it is already FDA approved for clinical use for other conditions.

A phase II study (IGNITE; clinicaltrials.gov NCT02354859) investigated the safety and efficacy of IV gallium nitrate for 5 consecutive days in CF adults with chronic *P. aeruginosa*. While there was not a change in lung function (by 5% percent predicted), there was a significant decrease in *P. aeruginosa*, and gallium was well tolerated (CFF.org Clinical Trial Finder & clinicaltrials.gov NCT02354859), although we wait peer-reviewed published results. A limitation of this approach is the use of IV therapy in individuals with chronic *P. aeruginosa*, which would potentially require long-term IV access. However, in this patient population, IV therapies are already commonly used. Investigating the role of gallium during acute pulmonary exacerbations may be warranted. In addition, the potential for an inhaled formulation may be more appealing. Gallium was also found to be effective against NTM.[65] The ABATE trial (clinicaltrials.gov NCT04294043) is currently enrolling to study the safety and tolerability of inhaled gallium for NTM (*Mycobacterium avium* or *abscessus*) in an open-label multi-center trial.

Bacteriophages (phages) are viruses that infect and kill bacteria. Phage therapy is the application of lytic phages to treat bacterial infections.[66] Here, the strategy of using a natural competitor of bacteria, especially an MDRO or emerging pan-drug-resistant bacteria, could be described as "the enemy of my enemy is my friend."

The biosphere contains an estimated 10^{31} phages,[67] which means that natural exposure to phages occurs continuously throughout human life via contact with the environment (eg, food consumption and inhalation of particles suspended in the air). Phages are present on human skin[68] and in the gut,[69] and because humans have evolved with constant phage exposure, phages have generally been accepted as safe, provided they have been produced in a pharmaceutical-grade manner and are free of host bacteria endotoxins.[70,71] As phages are the most numerous organisms on the planet, there are estimated to be 10:1 more phages than bacteria[67] which suggests an opportunity to find naturally occurring phages that infect bacterial pathogens of interest. In addition, phages can be genetically engineered to be used therapeutically.[72]

It is important to note that there are limited data on the safety and efficacy of phage therapy in traditionally defined clinical studies. However, the Eliava Institute in Georgia and the Ludwik Hirszfeld Institute in Poland have provided phage therapy to many patients.[73] There is an increasing experience in the United States with FDA-approved compassionate cases and clinical trials,[70] although early attempts to show phage therapy efficacy in randomized clinical trials have been largely unsuccessful. The lack of efficacy in clinical trials may be attributed to poor study design, challenges in phage stabilization, or administration of phage at concentrations too low to be therapeutically active. One hypothetical concern with phage therapy is a toxic response caused by target pathogen lysis that releases bacterial toxins (eg, lipopolysaccharides and other virulence factors) that could trigger an inflammatory response. It is important to highlight that this effect has not been observed in animal studies of phage therapy. Notably, studies have shown that exposure to clinically relevant beta-lactam antibiotics leads to a higher release of bacterial endotoxin compared with phages.[74]

Specific to CF, there are case reports of the addition of phage therapy to standard clinical care in compassionate cases.[75] These include pediatric and adult patients whereby phage therapy was delivered either via nebulization or IV to target bacteria such as *P. aeruginosa*, *S. aureus*, or *A. xylosoxidans*.[75] Since the publication of these reports, interest in phage therapy in the United States has increased with several phage therapy programs starting or expanding [Tailored Antibacterials & Innovative Laboratories for Phage Research (TAILφR) at Baylor University, Army & Navy Laboratories, Mayo Clinic, Center for Phage Technology (CPT) at Texas A&M University, Center for Innovative Phage Applications & Therapeutics (IPATH) at University of California, San Diego, University of Pittsburgh (expertise in NTM phage), Center for Phage Biology & Therapy at Yale University]. Current or planned clinical trials to investigate phage therapy to treat *P. aeruginosa* are independently investigating single phage (clinicaltrials.gov NCT04684641) or phage cocktails (multiple phages given at the same time; clinicaltrials.gov NCT04596319 & NCT05010577), and different routes of administration (eg, nebulized vs IV).

It will be important to study each of these approaches. For example, while phage cocktails may provide a broader range of coverage for a specific bacterium, there is evidence that cocktails may increase genetic mutations in *P. aeruginosa* that could result in increased virulence.[76] Such an effect will need to be investigated in clinical strains of *P. aeruginosa* and other bacteria. In addition, there is evidence that multiple phages may interfere with phage replication within the same bacteria, potentially reducing the effectiveness of phage therapy.[77] However, single phage therapy may be limited by evolving bacterial resistance.[78] Recognizing that bacteria continue to evolve resistance to phage(s), investigators have developed a strategy to identify phages that target specific virulence factors on bacteria so that the result of phage therapy are surviving bacteria mutants with decreased expression or production of such virulence factors.[66] For example, phage therapy targeting *P. aeruginosa* antibiotic efflux pumps, responsible for resistance to multiple antibiotics, restored antibiotic susceptibility[79] and was reported in a compassionate use case to treat an infected aortic graft.[80] Compassionate use of phage therapy in patients with CF is performed by a few centers in the United States targeting MDR *P. aeruginosa*, *A. xylosoxidans* and NTM.[72] Currently a phase 2 randomized, double-blinded, single-site clinical trial studying the safety and effectiveness of single nebulized phage therapy is enrolling patients with CF with *P. aeruginosa* (clinicaltrials.gov NCT04684641).

Understanding bacteria and phage evolution will be essential to the development of future phage therapy. Approaches using phage cocktails may be relevant to treat pulmonary exacerbations, while single phage therapy may be an option for chronic treatment. Different approaches to phage delivery are also under investigation because of the potential for individual patient adaptive immune antibody responses to phage therapy to decrease the effectiveness of subsequent phage therapy.[81] It is hypothesized that IV administration will induce increased host adaptive immunity compared with nebulization, but this concern remains to be studied in clinical trials.

CLINICS CARE POINTS

- Gallium and phage therapy are examples of additional strategies to treat MDR bacteria.
- Continued well-designed and executed clinical trials are required to confirm initial observations.
- Compassionate treatment may be available for these types of therapies for carefully selected candidates.

SUMMARY

While MDRO infections have recently been recognized as an emerging global threat, individuals with CF, and their care teams, have been challenged with the complexities involved in the clinical care of MRSA, *P. aeruginosa*, *Burkholderia* sp., *S. maltophilia*, *A. xylosoxidans*, and NTM for far too long. While we await the discovery and development of additional antimicrobials with novel mechanisms of action, this article summarizes approaches that have been used to: (1) optimize the PK/PD of existing antibiotics, (2) administer new antibiotic combinations, and (3) repurpose existing antibiotics into inhaled formulations. However, because MDROs continue to evolve, additional approaches are required beyond the existing antibiotic pipeline. Novel approaches include: (1) targeting the host to improve the immune response(s) to infection [for example, GM-CSF] or (2) targeting the pathogen with a completely different class of molecule(s) that have antimicrobial activity (eg, gallium or bacteriophages). These approaches require additional clinical studies before they can be considered for routine clinical use.

FINANCIAL SUPPORT

There was no financial support provided for this article.

DISCLOSURE

T.S. Murray-none. J.L. Koff is the PI for bacteriophage clinical trial NCT04684641 and a national Co-PI for bacteriophage clinical trial NCT05010577. J.L. Koff & G.L. Stanley: Colleagues at Yale University have licensed intellectual property related to bacteriophage therapy to a company although neither J.L. Koff nor G.L. Stanley has a financial interest in this process.

REFERENCES

1. Centers for disease control and prevention https://www.cdc.gov/infectioncontrol/guidelines/mdro/. updated February 2017 Accessed July 7, 2022.

2. Cystic Fibrosis Foundation Patient Registry 2020 Annual Data Report Bethesda, Maryland ©2021 Cystic Fibrosis Foundation.
3. Rogers GB, Taylor SL, Hoffman LR, et al. The impact of CFTR modulator therapies on CF airway microbiology. J Cyst Fibros 2020;19(3):359–64.
4. Saiman L. Improving outcomes of infections in cystic fibrosis in the era of CFTR modulator therapy. Pediatr Pulmonol 2019;54(Suppl 3):S18–26.
5. Hisert KB, Heltshe SL, Pope C, et al. Restoring Cystic Fibrosis Transmembrane Conductance Regulator Function Reduces Airway Bacteria and Inflammation in People with Cystic Fibrosis and Chronic Lung Infections. Am J Respir Crit Care Med 2017;195(12):1617–28.
6. Harris JK, Wagner BD, Zemanick ET, et al. Changes in Airway Microbiome and Inflammation with Ivacaftor Treatment in Patients with Cystic Fibrosis and the G551D Mutation. Ann Am Thorac Soc 2020;17(2):212–20.
7. Epps QJ, Epps KL, Young DC, et al. State of the art in cystic fibrosis pharmacology optimization of antimicrobials in the treatment of cystic fibrosis pulmonary exacerbations: III. Executive summary. Pediatr Pulmonol 2021;56(7):1825–37.
8. Smith S, Rowbotham NJ, Regan KH. Inhaled anti-pseudomonal antibiotics for long-term therapy in cystic fibrosis. Cochrane Database of Systematic Reviews 2018;(3).
9. Elborn JS, Vataire AL, Fukushima A, et al. Comparison of Inhaled Antibiotics for the Treatment of Chronic Pseudomonas aeruginosa Lung Infection in Patients With Cystic Fibrosis: Systematic Literature Review and Network Meta-analysis. Clin Ther 2016;38(10):2204–26.
10. Wenzler E, Fraidenburg DR, Scardina T, et al. Inhaled Antibiotics for Gram-Negative Respiratory Infections. Clinical microbiology reviews 2016;29(3):581–632.
11. Yahav D, Giske CG, Grāmatniece A, et al. New β-Lactam-β-Lactamase Inhibitor Combinations. Clin Microbiol Rev 2020;34(1).
12. Parker AC, Pritchard P, Preston T, et al. Enhanced drug metabolism in young children with cystic fibrosis. Arch Dis Child 1997;77(3):239–41.
13. Kearns GL. Hepatic drug metabolism in cystic fibrosis: recent developments and future directions. Ann Pharmacother 1993;27(1):74–9.
14. Prandota J. Clinical pharmacology of antibiotics and other drugs in cystic fibrosis. Drugs 1988;35(5):542–78.
15. Epps QJ, Epps KL, Young DC, et al. State of the art in cystic fibrosis pharmacology-Optimization of antimicrobials in the treatment of cystic fibrosis pulmonary exacerbations: I. Anti-methicillin-resistant Staphylococcus aureus (MRSA) antibiotics. Pediatr Pulmonol 2020;55(1):33–57.
16. Epps QJ, Epps KL, Zobell JT. Optimization of anti-pseudomonal antibiotics for cystic fibrosis pulmonary exacerbations: II. Cephalosporins and penicillins latest update. Pediatr Pulmonol 2021;56(6):1784–8.
17. Magreault S, Roy C, Launay M, et al. Pharmacokinetic and Pharmacodynamic Optimization of Antibiotic Therapy in Cystic Fibrosis Patients: Current Evidences, Gaps in Knowledge and Future Directions. Clin Pharmacokinet 2021;60(4):409–45.
18. Prescott WA Jr, Gentile AE, Nagel JL, et al. Continuous-infusion antipseudomonal Beta-lactam therapy in patients with cystic fibrosis. P T 2011;36(11):723–63.
19. Bensman TJ, Wang J, Jayne J, et al. Pharmacokinetic-Pharmacodynamic Target Attainment Analyses To Determine Optimal Dosing of Ceftazidime-Avibactam for the Treatment of Acute Pulmonary Exacerbations in Patients with Cystic Fibrosis. Antimicrob Agents Chemother 2017;61(10).

20. Garazzino S, Altieri E, Silvestro E, et al. Ceftolozane/Tazobactam for Treating Children With Exacerbations of Cystic Fibrosis Due to Pseudomonas aeruginosa: A Review of Available Data. Front Pediatr 2020;8:173.

21. Forrester JB, Steed LL, Santevecchi BA, et al. Vitro Activity of Ceftolozane/Tazobactam vs Nonfermenting, Gram-Negative Cystic Fibrosis Isolates. Open Forum Infect Dis 2018;5(7):ofy158.

22. Nguyen TT, Condren M, Walter J. Ceftazidime-avibactam for the treatment of multidrug resistant Burkholderia cepacia complex in a pediatric cystic fibrosis patient. Pediatr Pulmonol 2020;55(2):283–4.

23. Nolan PJ, Jain R, Cohen L, et al. In vitro activity of ceftolozane-tazobactam and ceftazidime-avibactam against Pseudomonas aeruginosa isolated from patients with cystic fibrosis. Diagn Microbiol Infect Dis 2021;99(2):115204.

24. Spoletini G, Etherington C, Shaw N, et al. Use of ceftazidime/avibactam for the treatment of MDR Pseudomonas aeruginosa and Burkholderia cepacia complex infections in cystic fibrosis: a case series. J Antimicrob Chemother 2019;74(5): 1425–9.

25. Sader HS, Duncan LR, Doyle TB, et al. Antimicrobial activity of ceftazidime/avibactam, ceftolozane/tazobactam and comparator agents against Pseudomonas aeruginosa from cystic fibrosis patients. JAC Antimicrob Resist 2021;3(3): dlab126.

26. Van Dalem A, Herpol M, Echahidi F, et al. Vitro Susceptibility of Burkholderia cepacia Complex Isolated from Cystic Fibrosis Patients to Ceftazidime-Avibactam and Ceftolozane-Tazobactam. Antimicrob Agents Chemother 2018;62(9).

27. Haidar G, Philips NJ, Shields RK, et al. Ceftolozane-Tazobactam for the Treatment of Multidrug-Resistant Pseudomonas aeruginosa Infections: Clinical Effectiveness and Evolution of Resistance. Clin Infect Dis 2017;65(1):110–20.

28. Romano MT, et al. Ceftolozane/tazobactam for pulmonary exacerbation in a 63-year-old cystic fibrosis patient with renal insufficiency and an elevated MIC to Pseudomonas aeruginosa. IDCases 2020;21:e00830.

29. Stokem K, et al. Use of ceftolozane-tazobactam in a cystic fibrosis patient with multidrug-resistant pseudomonas infection and renal insufficiency. Respir Med Case Rep 2018;23:8–9.

30. Vickery SB, McClain D, Wargo KA. Successful Use of Ceftolozane-Tazobactam to Treat a Pulmonary Exacerbation of Cystic Fibrosis Caused by Multidrug-Resistant Pseudomonas aeruginosa. Pharmacotherapy 2016;36(10):e154–9.

31. Belcher R, Zobell JT. Optimization of antibiotics for cystic fibrosis pulmonary exacerbations due to highly resistant nonlactose fermenting Gram negative bacilli: Meropenem-vaborbactam and cefiderocol. Pediatr Pulmonol 2021;56(9): 3059–61.

32. Zeiser ET, Becka SA, Wilson BM, et al. Switching Partners": Piperacillin-Avibactam Is a Highly Potent Combination against Multidrug-Resistant Burkholderia cepacia Complex and Burkholderia gladioli Cystic Fibrosis Isolates. J Clin Microbiol 2019;57(8).

33. Lopeman RC, Harrison J, Rathbone DL, et al. Effect of Amoxicillin in combination with Imipenem-Relebactam against Mycobacterium abscessus. Sci Rep 2020; 10(1):928.

34. Zhanel GG, Golden AR, Zelenitsky S, et al. Cefiderocol: A Siderophore Cephalosporin with Activity Against Carbapenem-Resistant and Multidrug-Resistant Gram-Negative Bacilli. Drugs 2019;79(3):271–89.

35. Gavioli EM, Guardado N, Haniff F, et al. Does Cefiderocol Have a Potential Role in Cystic Fibrosis Pulmonary Exacerbation Management? Microb Drug Resist 2021 Dec;27(12):1726–32.

36. Warner NC, Bartelt LA, Lachiewicz AM, et al. Cefiderocol for the Treatment of Adult and Pediatric Patients With Cystic Fibrosis and Achromobacter xylosoxidans Infections. Clin Infect Dis 2021;73(7):e1754–7.

37. Hurley MN, Ariff AH, Bertenshaw C, et al. Results of antibiotic susceptibility testing do not influence clinical outcome in children with cystic fibrosis. J Cyst Fibros 2012;11(4):288–92.

38. Aaron SD, Vandemheen KL, Ferris W, et al. Combination antibiotic susceptibility testing to treat exacerbations of cystic fibrosis associated with multiresistant bacteria: a randomised, double-blind, controlled clinical trial. Lancet 2005; 366(9484):463–71.

39. Choby JE, Ozturk T, Satola SW, et al. Widespread cefiderocol heteroresistance in carbapenem-resistant Gram-negative pathogens. Lancet Infect Dis 2021;21(5): 597–8.

40. Chalhoub H, Saenz Y, Nichols WW, et al. Loss of activity of ceftazidime-avibactam due to MexAB-OprM efflux and overproduction of AmpC cephalosporinase in Pseudomonas aeruginosa isolated from patients suffering from cystic fibrosis. Int J Antimicrob Agents 2018;52(5):697–701.

41. Barsky EE, Pereira LM, Sullivan KJ, et al. Ceftaroline pharmacokinetics and pharmacodynamics in patients with cystic fibrosis. J Cyst Fibros 2018;17(3):e25–31.

42. Branstetter J, Searcy H, Benner K, et al. Ceftaroline vs vancomycin for the treatment of acute pulmonary exacerbations in pediatric patients with cystic fibrosis. Pediatr Pulmonol 2020;55(12):3337–42.

43. Molloy L, Snyder AH, Srivastava R, et al. Ceftaroline Fosamil for Methicillin-Resistant Staphylococcus aureus Pulmonary Exacerbation in a Pediatric Cystic Fibrosis Patient. J Pediatr Pharmacol Ther 2014;19(2):135–40.

44. Varela MC, Roch M, Taglialegna A, et al. Carbapenems drive the collateral resistance to ceftaroline in cystic fibrosis patients with MRSA. Commun Biol 2020; 3(1):599.

45. Nichols DP, Durmowicz AG, Field A, et al. Developing Inhaled Antibiotics in Cystic Fibrosis: Current Challenges and Opportunities. Ann Am Thorac Soc 2019;16(5):534–9.

46. Waterer G, Lord J, Hofmann T, et al. Phase I, Dose-Escalating Study of the Safety and Pharmacokinetics of Inhaled Dry-Powder Vancomycin (AeroVanc) in Volunteers and Patients with Cystic Fibrosis: a New Approach to Therapy for Methicillin-Resistant Staphylococcus aureus. Antimicrob Agents Chemother 2020;64(3).

47. Dezube R, Jennings MT, Rykiel M, et al. Eradication of persistent methicillin-resistant Staphylococcus aureus infection in cystic fibrosis. Journal of Cystic Fibrosis 2019;18(3):357–63.

48. Flume PA, VanDevanter DR, Morgan EE, Dudley MN, Loutit JS, Bell SC, et al. A phase 3, multi-center, multinational, randomized, double-blind, placebo-controlled study to evaluate the efficacy and safety of levofloxacin inhalation solution (APT-1026) in stable cystic fibrosis patients. J Cyst Fibros 2016;15(4): 495–502.

49. Cystic Fibrosis Foundation. Drug development pipeline: inhaled levofloxacin (Quinsair). 2022. Available at: https://apps.cff.org/trials/pipeline/details/9/Inhaled-Levofloxacin-Quinsair. Accessed July 7 ,2022.

50. Banaschewski B, Verma D, Pennings LJ, et al. Clofazimine inhalation suspension for the aerosol treatment of pulmonary nontuberculous mycobacterial infections. J Cyst Fibros 2019;18(5):714–20.
51. Waterer G. Beyond antibiotics for pulmonary nontuberculous mycobacterial disease. Curr Opin Pulm Med 2020;26(3):260–6.
52. Bogdan C. Nitric oxide synthase in innate and adaptive immunity: an update. Trends Immunol 2015;36(3):161–78.
53. Meng QH, Springall DR, Bishop AE, et al. Lack of inducible nitric oxide synthase in bronchial epithelium: a possible mechanism of susceptibility to infection in cystic fibrosis. J Pathol 1998;184(3):323–31.
54. Zheng S, De BP, Choudhary S, et al. Impaired innate host defense causes susceptibility to respiratory virus infections in cystic fibrosis. Immunity 2003;18(5):619–30.
55. Bogdanovski K, Chau T, Robinson CJ, et al. Antibacterial activity of high-dose nitric oxide against pulmonary Mycobacterium abscessus disease. Access Microbiol 2020;2(9). acmi000154.
56. Goldbart A, Gatt D, Golan Tripto I. Non-nuberculous mycobacteria infection treated with intermittently inhaled high-dose nitric oxide. BMJ Case Rep 2021;14(10).
57. Yaacoby-Bianu K, Gur M, Toukan Y, et al. Compassionate Nitric Oxide Adjuvant Treatment of Persistent Mycobacterium Infection in Cystic Fibrosis Patients. Pediatr Infect Dis J 2018;37(4):336–8.
58. Bentur L, Gur M, Ashkenazi M, et al. Pilot study to test inhaled nitric oxide in cystic fibrosis patients with refractory Mycobacterium abscessus lung infection. J Cyst Fibros 2020;19(2):225–31.
59. Cystic Fibrosis Foundation https://apps.cff.org/Trials/Pipeline/details/10122/Inhaled-Nitric-Oxide-Thiolanox. Accessed July 7, 2022.
60. Scott JP, Ji Y, Kannan M, et al. Inhaled granulocyte-macrophage colony-stimulating factor for Mycobacterium abscessus in cystic fibrosis. Eur Respir J 2018;51(4).
61. Cystic Fibrosis Foundation. https://apps.cff.org/Trials/Pipeline/details/10165/Inhaled-Molgramostim. Accessed July 7, 2022.
62. Chitambar CR, Narasimhan J. Targeting iron-dependent DNA synthesis with gallium and transferrin-gallium. Pathobiology 1991;59(1):3–10.
63. Goss CH, Kaneko Y, Khuu L, et al. Gallium disrupts bacterial iron metabolism and has therapeutic effects in mice and humans with lung infections. Sci Transl Med 2018;10(460).
64. Kaneko Y, Thoendel M, Olakanmi O, et al. The transition metal gallium disrupts Pseudomonas aeruginosa iron metabolism and has antimicrobial and antibiofilm activity. J Clin Invest 2007;117(4):877–88.
65. Abdalla MY, Switzer BL, Goss CH, et al. Gallium Compounds Exhibit Potential as New Therapeutic Agents against Mycobacterium abscessus. Antimicrob Agents Chemother 2015;59(8):4826–34.
66. Kortright KE, Chan BK, Koff JL, et al. Phage Therapy: A Renewed Approach to Combat Antibiotic-Resistant Bacteria. Cell Host & Microbe 2019;25(2):219–32.
67. Wommack KE, Colwell RR. Virioplankton: viruses in aquatic ecosystems. Microbiology and molecular biology reviews : MMBR 2000;64(1):69–114.
68. Oh J, Byrd AL, Deming C, et al. Biogeography and individuality shape function in the human skin metagenome. Nature 2014;514(7520):59–64.
69. Reyes A, Haynes M, Hanson N, et al. Viruses in the faecal microbiota of monozygotic twins and their mothers. Nature 2010;466(7304):334–8.

70. Abedon ST. Bacteriophage Clinical Use as Antibacterial "Drugs": Utility and Precedent. Microbiol Spectr 2017;5(4).

71. Abdelkader K, Gerstmans H, Saafan A, et al. The Preclinical and Clinical Progress of Bacteriophages and Their Lytic Enzymes: The Parts are Easier than the Whole. Viruses 2019;11(2).

72. Dedrick RM, Guerrero-Bustamante CA, Garlena RA, Russell DA, et al. Engineered bacteriophages for treatment of a patient with a disseminated drug-resistant Mycobacterium abscessus. Nat Med 2019;25(5):730–3.

73. Luong T, Salabarria A-C, Roach DR. Phage Therapy in the Resistance Era: Where Do We Stand and Where Are We Going? Clinical Therapeutics 2020;42(9): 1659–80.

74. Dufour N, Delattre R, Ricard JD, et al. The Lysis of Pathogenic Escherichia coli by Bacteriophages Releases Less Endotoxin Than by β-Lactams. Clin Infect Dis 2017;64(11):1582–8.

75. Chan BK, Stanley G, Modak M, et al. Bacteriophage therapy for infections in CF. Pediatr Pulmonol 2021;56(Suppl 1). S4–s9.

76. Wright RCT, Friman VP, Smith MCM, et al. Resistance Evolution against Phage Combinations Depends on the Timing and Order of Exposure. mBio 2019 Sep 24;10(5). e01652–19.

77. Dennehy JJ, Turner PE. Reduced fecundity is the cost of cheating in RNA virus phi6. Proc Biol Sci 2004;271(1554):2275–82.

78. Labrie SJ, Samson JE, Moineau S. Bacteriophage resistance mechanisms. Nat Rev Microbiol 2010;8(5):317–27.

79. Chan BK, Sistrom M, Wertz JE, et al. Phage selection restores antibiotic sensitivity in MDR Pseudomonas aeruginosa. Sci Rep 2016;6:26717.

80. Chan BK, Turner PE, Kim S, et al. Phage treatment of an aortic graft infected with Pseudomonas aeruginosa. Evol Med Public Health 2018;2018(1):60–6.

81. Dedrick RM, Freeman KG, Nguyen JA, et al. Potent antibody-mediated neutralization limits bacteriophage treatment of a pulmonary Mycobacterium abscessus infection. Nat Med 2021;27(8):1357–61.

Viral Pneumonias

Jennifer Febbo, MD[a],*, Jonathan Revels, DO[a], Loren Ketai, MD[b]

KEYWORDS

- Viral pneumonia • Tomography x-ray computed • Community-acquired infections
- Immunocompromised hosts

KEY POINTS

- Radiologic findings of influenza usually appear as bronchiolitis, bronchopneumonia, or manifestations of airway-centric infection. H1N1 influenza may have a similar appearance but can also cause an organizing pneumonia pattern.
- The respiratory syncytial virus, parainfluenza virus, and human metapneumovirus have a predilection for airway-centric infection. They usually cause mild symptoms in immunocompetent adults but more likely to cause bronchopneumonia in immunocompromised patients.
- Adenovirus causes nonsegmental consolidation, particularly in the setting of outbreaks of novel serotypes. In the setting of other viral lower respiratory tract infections, lobar consolidation usually suggests bacterial superinfection.
- Cytomegalic virus (CMV) and herpes simplex virus in the respiratory tract of hospitalized patients represent reactivation of latent infection, which is not always pathogenic. When pathogenic, such as in the setting of lung transplants, CMV often causes ground-glass opacities and micronodules.

INTRODUCTION

Viral pneumonia upended the world in 1918 and again in 2020, but it has also been a major source of respiratory illness in the intervening century. More than 200 species of virus are capable of infecting humans and 3 to 4 new human viruses are discovered each year.[1] A handful of these viruses infect the lower respiratory tract, causing significant morbidity and mortality among humans and resulting in over $6.4 billion in hospital stays.[2] Although many pathogens causing community-acquired pneumonias still go undiagnosed, the development of real-time polymerase chain reactions (PCRs) for numerous respiratory viruses has dramatically increased the documentation of viral pneumonias over the last 2 decades.[3] Recognition of radiologic features that prompt

This article was previously published in *Radiologic Clinics of North America* 60:3 May 2022.
[a] University of New Mexico, 2211 Lomas Boulevard NE, Albuquerque, NM 87106, USA;
[b] Department of Radiology, MSC 10 5530, 1 University of New Mexico, Albuquerque, NM 87131-0001, USA
* Corresponding author.
E-mail address: jfebbo@salud.unm.edu

Infect Dis Clin N Am 38 (2024) 163–182
https://doi.org/10.1016/j.idc.2023.12.009
0891-5520/24/© 2023 Elsevier Inc. All rights reserved.

testing for viral pathogens could reduce the use of unnecessary antibiotics, and in selected cases prompt institution of antiviral agents.[4,5]

Most viral pneumonias are community-acquired; however, a few are associated with health care settings. Immunocompromised patients are often infected with these community-acquired viruses, but are at greater risk of severe infection, including with those which are typically indolent. This article will review the imaging of community-acquired and health care–associated viral pneumonia, as well as viral pneumonia in the immunocompromised host. COVID-19 is specifically discussed by Sing and colleagues elsewhere in this issue.

COMMUNITY-ACQUIRED VIRAL PNEUMONIA

The overwhelming majority of viral pneumonias are community acquired. Some of these viruses, such as RSV and parainfluenza, are acquired as children and result in mild, self-limited illness. Among adults with pneumonia in whom a pathogen can be detected, viruses are the primary or coinfecting pathogen in 26% of cases requiring hospitalization.[4] Immunocompetent patients requiring hospitalization are generally elderly and often have underlying conditions such as chronic obstructive pulmonary disease (COPD).[5] The main pathogens comprising community-acquired viral pneumonia are influenza, human metapneumovirus (HMPV), respiratory syncytial virus (RSV), adenovirus, and rhinovirus. Hantavirus pulmonary infections are much less common, but are clinically important because they can cause severe, often fatal, respiratory failure in otherwise healthy, young adults.

INFLUENZA

Before the COIVD-19 pandemic, influenza was the principal cause of severe viral pneumonia in the world. Influenza can be broadly categorized into one of the multiple groups (A, B, C, or D), influenza A is most predominant.[6] In the United States, between the years 2010 and 2018, 4 to 23 million medical visits and 12,000 to 79,000 deaths occurred each year due to influenza.[7] Cases decreased dramatically in 2020 likely due to personal public health measures (eg, mask wearing) and reduced medical office visits instituted to minimize the spread of COVID-19.[8]

Most patients with influenza experience a self-limited upper respiratory infection of the airways, which only occasionally progresses to the lower respiratory tract.[6,9,10] Influenza pneumonia is typically mild, but in pregnant patients,[11] elderly patients, and/or those with chronic underlying disease, such as heart failure or COPD, the pneumonia can be severe and sometimes fatal.[10,12,13]

Influenza is predominantly an airway-centric infection and imaging manifestations often reflect this (**Table 1**). In severe infections, however, diffuse disease can obscure the underlying airway findings. Radiographs typically demonstrate ill-defined reticulonodular opacities in a central distribution (in contrast to peripheral/subpleural reticular opacities seen in edema), reflecting the airway-centric process. Less commonly, radiographs can also show multifocal consolidation. On computed tomography (CT), features of bronchitis (bronchial wall thickening) and bronchiolitis (tree-in-bud opacities) may be present[6,9] (**Fig. 1**). When airspace opacities occur, ground-glass opacities and multifocal consolidation are more common than localized consolidation, and often occur in a peribronchial distribution[9] (**Figs. 2** and **3**). Pleural effusions are rarely seen in the pneumonias caused by influenza as the sole pathogen.[6,9] Secondary infections are common in severe cases of influenza, and are suggested by radiological features such as focal lobar consolidation or worsening opacities following initial improvement.[6,9] In a series of patients accrued before 2009, diffuse airspace disease was only rarely

Table 1
Imaging patterns of viral pneumonia by etiology

	Diffuse Ground Glass	Consolidation—Not Bronchocentric	Consolidation—Bronchocentric	Organizing Pneumonia	Tree-In-Bud Micronodules	Micronodules, Not Tree-In-Bud	Linear/Interstitial
Seasonal influenza	+	+	++		++	+	
H1N1	++	+	++	++	+	+	
Adenovirus	+	+++	+		+	+	
HMPV	+		+		+++	+	
RSV	+		+		+++	+	
Parainfluenza	+		++		+++	+	
Hantavirus	+++	++					+++
HSV	++		++			+	+
CMV	+++	++	+		+	++	
VZV	+	+	+			+++	

Increasing + indicates increasing relative frequency of the associated pattern. The purpose of this table is to indicate general trends; the absence of a + is not to suggest a complete absence of this finding on all imaging.

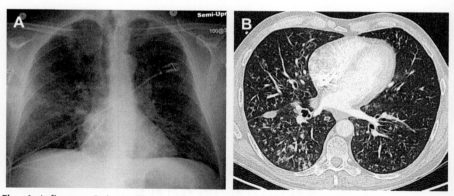

Fig. 1. Influenza B in a 60-year-old man. (*A*) Frontal chest radiograph demonstrates perihilar-predominant bilateral reticulonodular opacities with bronchial wall thickening. (*B*) Axial chest CT shows extensive bilateral centrilobular nodules, including tree-in-bud distribution, and bronchial wall thickening indicating bronchiolitis and bronchitis, airway-centric disease. Incidental focal fluid within the right major fissure.

caused by influenza and was more typical of bacterial pneumonia.[9] Acute respiratory distress syndrome (ARDS), however, is seen in other variants of influenza (see below, H1N1).

New strains arise as influenza viruses circulate in swine, birds, and humans, and genetic reassortment occurs between viruses from different animals.[14] One such reassortment resulted in the swine-origin H1N1 pandemic in 2009. This influenza A subtype was classified as H1N1 based on the surface glycoproteins hemagglutinin (H) and neuraminidase (N), which promote propagation of the virus into lower respiratory tract cells.[14] Similar to seasonal influenza infections, most patients experienced an uncomplicated clinical course, but a small percentage of patients developed severe respiratory distress.[15] Although the overall mortality from H1N1 influenza was not increased markedly compared with circulating strains, there was a dramatic shift in mortality toward younger patients, such that 87% of fatalities occurred in patients younger than 65 years.[16]

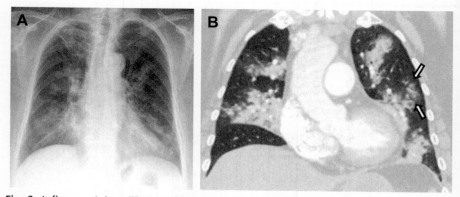

Fig. 2. Influenza A in a 73-year-old woman. (*A*) Frontal chest radiograph shows bilateral centrally distributed hazy opacities. (*B*) Coronal chest CT demonstrates bilateral peribronchovascular consolidation consistent with bronchopneumonia. There are also small acinar nodules in the left upper lobe (*arrows*).

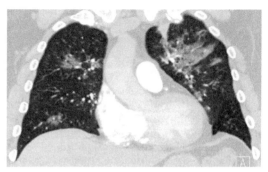

Fig. 3. Bronchopneumonia caused by H3N1 influenza A in a 66-year-old man. Coronal chest CT demonstrates bilateral peribronchovascular ground-glass opacities with interlobular septal thickening.

Although radiographs in swine-origin H1N1 infections are usually normal. Chest radiographs and CTs in swine-origin H1N1 that progresses to pneumonia often include features of consolidation within multiple lobes, with lower lobe predominance.[17] H1N1 can also result in an organizing pneumonia pattern, with peribronchovascular and peripheral/subpleural ground-glass opacities and consolidation[18,19] (**Fig. 4**). Finally, H1N1 can progress to ARDS (**Fig. 5**). Compared with ARDS by other types of severe community-acquired pneumonia, H1N1-related ARDS may lead to worse oxygen exchange and increased use of extracorporeal membrane oxygenation.[20]

Some animal-origin influenza viruses can replicate in human cells but have not yet acquired genetic constituents that enable efficient human-to-human transmission. Two such viruses include H5N1 and H7N9 influenza. Together, over 2,000 human infections have been reported with these organisms, accompanied by a high mortality rate.[21] Reports of imaging are limited to very small series. In general consolidation and ground-glass opacities were multifocal at the time at initial imaging and commonly progressed to bilateral disease within several days.[22,23] Pleural effusions were reported to be more frequent in H5N1 than usually seen in human influenza, but remained rare in H7N9 influenza. Occasional pneumatoceles and cavities were also reported with H5N1 pneumonia.[22]

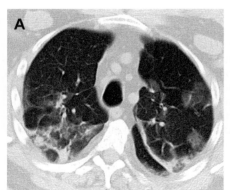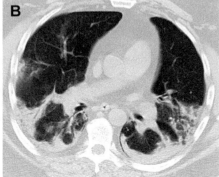

Fig. 4. H1N1 in a 44-year-old man. (*A, B*) Axial chest CT images show bilateral peribronchovascular and peripheral ground-glass opacities and consolidation in an organizing pneumonia pattern.

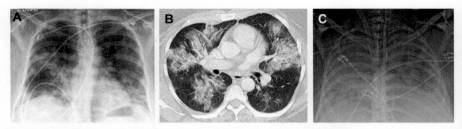

Fig. 5. Forty-three-year-old otherwise healthy woman with H1N1 infection demonstrating progression from bronchopneumonia to ARDS. (*A*) Initial frontal chest radiograph demonstrates bilateral hazy perihilar and basilar airspace opacities. (*B*) Axial chest CT on the same day shows bilateral peribronchovascular ground-glass opacities, with areas of interlobular septal thickening. (*C*) Frontal chest radiograph 11 days later shows near-complete opacification of both lungs and an extracorporeal membrane oxygenation (ECMO) catheter.

Testing for influenza can be performed by a variety of means including nasal swab, respiratory aspirate, or respiratory lavage. The rapid influenza detection method can return results in less than 15 minutes, has a high specificity for the detection of influenza (>98%), but the sensitivity ranges between 50% and 70%.[7] Reverse transcription–polymerase chain reaction (RT-PCR) has a higher sensitivity for detection of influenza and it should be performed in cases where there is clinical suspicion for influenza infection but a negative rapid test.[7] Viral cultures may be performed when there is clinical concern for possible drug resistance or a variant influenza that may be related to an emerging pandemic.[7]

Treatment of seasonal influenza with one of four antiviral medications: oseltamivir, peramivir, baloxavir, or zanamivir is recommended within 24 to 48 hours of the onset of symptoms.[23,24] Oseltamivir or zanamivir are used in the treatment of swine-origin H1N1 influenza.[23]

ADENOVIRUS

Adenovirus is spread through fecal-oral route in children and aerosolized droplets among adults. Its overall incidence peaks in summer months; however, epidemics are typically seen in winter or early spring.[25–27] Most adenovirus infections (80%) that occur in children are mild; however, pneumonia can occur in up to 20% of infants.[27] Among immunocompetent adults, lower respiratory tract infections occur in small epidemic outbreaks within closely confined groups of adults such as within the military. There are numerous serotypes of adenovirus, with serotypes −1 through 7, −21, and −14 responsible for most febrile respiratory illnesses in adults. Serotype 14, one of the newer serotypes to affect North America manifested as a military base outbreak of pneumonia in 2006. Likely abetted by limited humoral immunity in the populace, the serotype rapidly spread to over 15 states by 2007.[27]

Chest radiographs of adenovirus pneumonia are similar to nonviral community-acquired pneumonia, and are less likely to produce a dominant airway centric pattern compared with the virus described in the next section. Radiographs may show unilateral or bilateral consolidation, and patchy hazy opacities.[28,29] On chest CT, most patients demonstrate unilateral or bilateral consolidation[9,29,30] (**Fig. 6**). Patchy ground-glass opacities are less common and nodules are infrequent. Although pleural effusions are uncommon on chest radiographs, they have been seen on CT in up to three-fourths of patients.[30] Lymphadenopathy is seen in approximately one-third of patients who undergo CT scanning.

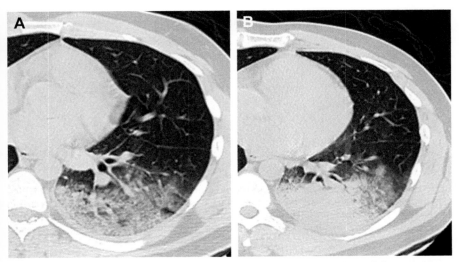

Fig. 6. Adenovirus in an otherwise healthy man in his early 20s. (*A, B*) Axial chest CT images demonstrate focal left lower lobe mixed consolidation and ground-glass opacities.

Diagnosis of adenovirus pneumonia can be achieved through PCR, immunohistochemical staining, or culture of bronchoalveolar lavage (BAL) fluid. Outbreaks of adenovirus pneumonia have led to oral immunization against adenovirus by the military; however, immunization is not currently available for civilians. There is no specific antiviral drug approved to target adenovirus. As adenovirus is a DNA virus, some patients with severe pneumonia are treated with cidofovir, an antiviral agent that inhibits DNA polymerase.[27]

HMPV, RSV, AND PARAINFLUENZA

RSV and parainfluenza virus have long been recognized as causing lower respiratory tract infections. HMPV is a relatively newly discovered pathogen, first classified as a paramyxovirus in 2001. More recently, HMPV and RSV have been moved to the family Pneumoviridae. Nevertheless, both share many characteristics with parainfluenza virus, particularly the propensity for airway infection.[6,31,32] These viruses are typically acquired as children; however, reactivation or reinfection can occur in adulthood secondary to waning immunity.[5] HMPV, RSV, and parainfluenza viruses have been detected in 4%, 3%, and 2% of hospitalized adults with community-acquired pneumonia, respectively.[4]

Among immunocompromised hosts, these viruses are important pathogens. Infections occur in 5% to 10% of hematopoietic stem cell transplant (HSCT) and transplant patients in the first 100 days posttransplant, and affect the lower tract in approximately 5% to 50% of these cases.[33,34] RSV, HMPV, and parainfluenza can all result in rapidly fatal pneumonia in immunocompromised patients.[5,6,25,32,35]

HMPV, RSV, and parainfluenza pulmonary infections have a propensity for airway-centric involvement secondary to preferential infection of ciliated respiratory epithelial cells.[31] Airway centric infection manifests as centrilobular nodules with and without tree-in-bud configuration, bronchial wall thickening, and as peribronchiolar ground-glass opacities or consolidation[6,9,31,34,36] (**Figs. 7–9**). In a retrospective evaluation of 100 (both immunocompetent and immunocompromised) patients diagnosed with

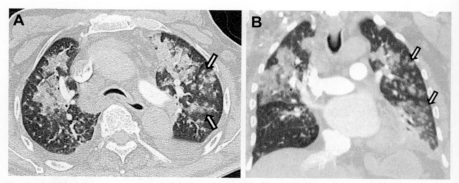

Fig. 7. Human metapneumovirus in a 63-year-old man. (*A*) Axial and (*B*) coronal chest CT images demonstrate bilateral peribronchovascular consolidation and ground-glass opacities indicative of bronchopneumonia. Centrilobular nodules (*arrows*) are also consistent with airway-centric disease. Incidental note of probable tracheomalacia on (*A*).

HMPV, the most commonly observed radiographic abnormality was bilateral, peribronchovascular airspace opacities.[32] CTs were performed only a minority of the cohort, most commonly demonstrating bilateral, ground-glass opacities. Centrilobular nodules were present in slightly less than half of these patients.[32] Although findings of small airway disease can be obscured in cases of extensive pneumonia in immunocompromised hosts, in a small series of patients with either HSCT or lung transplant, small nodules or tree in bud opacities were still observed on CTs in more than a third of patients.[37]

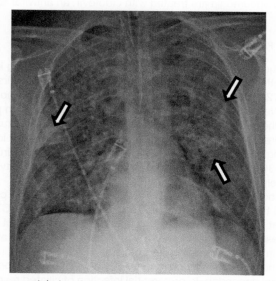

Fig. 8. Respiratory syncytial virus in a 29-year-old man with acute myelogenous leukemia status poststem cell transplant. Frontal chest radiograph demonstrates bilateral reticulonodular opacities and bronchial wall thickening compatible suggesting bronchiolitis and bronchitis. There are more focal airspace opacities in the right mid and lower lung, and left perihilar lung (*arrows*) likely representing associated pneumonia.

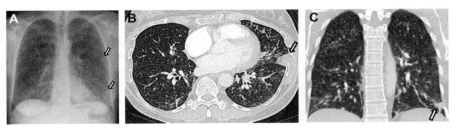

Fig. 9. Parainfluenza in a 61-year-old woman with multiple myeloma on chemotherapy. (*A*) Frontal chest radiograph shows bronchial wall thickening central reticulonodular opacities. There are also patchy airspace opacities in the left mid and lower lung (*arrows*). (*B*) Axial and (*C*) coronal CT images demonstrate bilateral solid and ground-glass centrilobular nodules, as well as localized consolidation in the lingula and left lower lobe (*arrow*).

Most CT findings of RSV and parainfluenza are similar to those seen with HMPV. Both demonstrate tree-in-bud opacities and bronchial wall thickening on CT in most patients.[38] Ground-glass opacities or consolidation are seen in one-fourth to one-third of patients.[9] Parainfluenza may be more likely than RSV to cause patchy basilar multifocal consolidation.[39] Pleural effusions occasionally occur in RSV pneumonia, which differs from parainfluenza and HMPV pneumonia in which associated effusions are rare.[6,9]

Imaging cannot confidently differentiate HMPV, RSV, and parainfluenza pneumonias from other common community-acquired pathogens causing airway centric infections, such as mycoplasma or Hemophilus influenza (**Fig. 10**). In addition, HMPV can cause nodular consolidation in approximately a third of cases, a feature more often considered to be associated with bacterial pneumonia.[32] Accordingly, specific diagnosis of these airway-centric infections is usually based on RT-PCR or serology. Therapy in symptomatic adults is supportive as there are no current targeted therapies.[5]

RHINOVIRUS

Rhinovirus, a primary respiratory-tract pathogen, which peaks in incidence in summer and fall, is best known for causing, "the common cold," a syndrome of upper

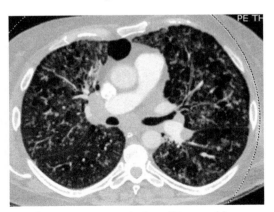

Fig. 10. Haemophilus influenzae pneumonia in a 50-year-old woman with emphysema. Axial chest CT demonstrates numerous centrilobular nodules throughout both lungs, some of which have tree-in-bud morphology, consistent with infectious bronchiolitis imaging appearance is very similar to the previous cases of parainfluenza pneumonia.

respiratory symptoms including rhinorrhea and cough.[40,41] In addition, rhinovirus is increasingly recognized as a cause of community-acquired pneumonia, albeit more frequently among immunocompromised than immunocompetent patients. In the former, it may be more common than the airway-centric viruses (eg, RSV, HMPV) infections described earlier. Coinfections with other viruses or with bacterial pathogens are common in both patient groups.[40,42]

There are relatively few studies depicting the radiologic appearance of rhinovirus pneumonia. A selected series of patients in which BAL was performed, focused predominantly on immunocompromised patients. Imaging demonstrated bilateral opacities in most cases, approximately half of which were predominantly peribronchial.[42] Nodules were also present, but were less common (**Fig. 11**). Mortality from rhinovirus-associated pneumonia and influenza pneumonia were similar in this cohort. In general, however, in the absence of bacterial coinfection, rhinovirus may be less likely to cause severe symptoms than the viruses discussed earlier. This observation and the current lack of an effective antiviral agent targeting rhinovirus render its detection of uncertain clinical importance. Treatment is currently supportive or should be directed at the copathogen.

HANTAVIRUS

Hantavirus is a potential cause for fulminant pneumonia in an otherwise healthy adult with a relevant environmental exposure. It is a zoonotic infection acquired through inhaling aerosolized rodent excreta. "New World" hantaviruses have resulted in several small outbreaks in the western United States, the first in the Four Corners area in 1993.[43,44] (In contrast to New World hantaviruses, "Old World" viruses in Asia and Europe and most commonly result in hemorrhagic fever with renal syndrome.). In North and South America, New World hantavirus can manifest as cardiovascular and respiratory failure referred to as Hantavirus Pulmonary Syndrome (HPS). In these patients, hantavirus directly infects lung endothelial cells and macrophages, which leads to extensive pulmonary edema and shock.[43]

Radiologically, HPS may mimic cardiogenic pulmonary edema; albeit, with a normal cardiac silhouette. Early findings include Kerley B lines and peribronchial cuffing, all suggesting interstitial edema[45,46] (**Fig. 12**). Most patients rapidly progress to extensive

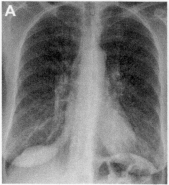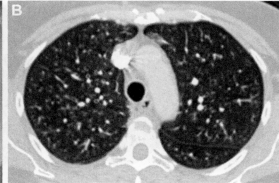

Fig. 11. Fifty-nine-year-old woman with productive cough and positive rhinovirus PCR. (*A*) Frontal chest radiograph shows subtle bilateral micronodules throughout both lungs. (*B*) Axial chest CT confirms bilateral 2-3 mm centrilobular tree-in-bud nodules in the upper lobes.

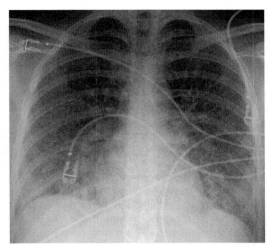

Fig. 12. Linear reticular pattern of early hantavirus in a 26-year-old woman. Frontal chest radiograph demonstrates fine reticular and hazy opacities with lower lung predominance.

bilateral predominantly perihilar or bibasilar hazy airspace opacities on chest radiographs (**Fig. 13**). Reports of CT findings in hantavirus are limited to small case series or case reports, and may be skewed toward less severely affected patients who are hemodynamically stable. Available reports have shown bilateral central or basilar-predominant ground-glass opacities with smooth interlobular septal thickening, occasionally with concurrent small ill-defined nodules or focal consolidation.[47,48] The majority of patients have small pleural effusions.

Diagnosis can be confirmed serologically through positive IgM and IgG analysis, or through reverse transcriptase PCR for the viral genome. Hantavirus is associated with a high morbidity rate, 40% worldwide; however, treatment is primarily supportive and no FDA-approved methods are currently available.[43]

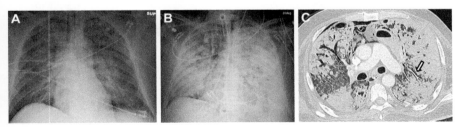

Fig. 13. Progression of hantavirus to ARDS in a 54-year-old man. (*A*) AP chest radiograph demonstrates bilateral perihilar hazy opacities in a "bat wing," pattern as well as Kerley B lines, with normal size of the cardiac silhouette and no pleural effusions. (*B*) AP frontal chest radiograph 3 days later demonstrates extensive bilateral consolidation and hazy opacities which obscure the cardiac silhouette. There is a small right pneumothorax, and lucencies along the right mediastinum and right heart border representing pneumomediastinum. ECMO cannula is in place. (*C*) Chest CT shows extensive bilateral consolidation. Pneumomediastinum and Macklin effect in the left lower lobe suggest barotrauma (*arrow*).

HOSPITAL-ASSOCIATED VIRAL PNEUMONIA

Although most viral infections are community-acquired, a few viruses such as Herpes simplex virus (HSV) contribute to morbidity and mortality in immunocompetent adults in the hospital setting. HSV infection can produce bronchopneumonia secondary to reactivation of existing virus within immunocompromised patients (eg, with hematologic malignancies) and in some immunocompetent patients with underlying conditions (eg, burns, major surgeries, diabetes, and prolonged mechanical ventilation.).[49,50]

Because the incidence of HSV infection is low, studies of radiologic findings combine immunocompetent and immunocompromised patients. In one study of 23 patients, all demonstrated multifocal patchy or segmental airspace opacities on radiographs, which were both central and peripheral in the majority.[50] Approximately half of patients had pleural effusions. Chest CT findings of multifocal ground-glass opacities combined with areas of peribronchiolar consolidation and interlobular septal and bronchial wall thickening have been reported in most patients.[50,51] Nodules are less common in HSV infection than in varicella, but may be present on CT in 30% of patients (see Brixey and colleagues' article, "Non-Imaging Diagnostic Tests For Pneumonia,"in this issue). These may be centrilobular ground-glass nodules or discrete nodules larger than 5 mm, some of which can manifest a halo sign. Pleural effusions may be seen but lymphadenopathy is uncommon. In critically ill patients, oral and BAL positivity for HSV is nonspecific and by itself is not proof of HSV pneumonia (**Fig. 14**). For example, HSV has been detected in up to 71% of respiratory samples from ARDS patients.[52]

Several other viruses have been implicated in nosocomial infections, but their role remains uncertain. Like HSV, CMV can reactivate after latent infection and has been implicated as another source of ventilator-acquired pneumonia (see below). Controversy exists regarding whether CMV positivity actually worsens clinical outcomes or contributes to lung injury.[53,54] Acanthamoeba polyphaga mimivirus (mimivirus) is an ameba-associated virus, which has recently been isolated within the lower respiratory

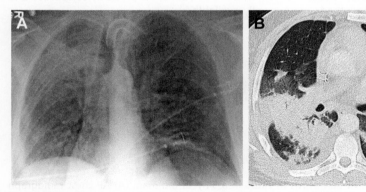

Fig. 14. Forty-four-year-old man with pseudomonas pneumonia. Herpes virus demonstrated on bronchoscopy performed on during after 2 weeks of hospitalization. (A) Frontal chest radiograph shows a right upper lung consolidation, more suggestive of bacterial pneumonia. (B) Axial chest CT demonstrates extensive consolidation in the superior segment of the right lower lobe, and additional smaller foci of consolidation in the left lower lobe. The multifocal consolidation is most consistent with a bacterial pneumonia. Presence of HSV virus on bronchoscopy may be incidental and not contribute significantly to the patient's pneumonia.

tract of hospitalized adults and adults in long-term care facilities.[55] However, its status as a true pathogen is controversial, and suspected cases of mimivirus pneumonia are limited to case reports.[56,57]

VIRAL PNEUMONIA IN THE IMMUNOCOMPROMISED PATIENT

Community-acquired viral respiratory infections also commonly affect immunocompromised individuals. Viruses that usually result in limited symptoms in immunocompetent hosts can cause severe pneumonia in those patients. Immunocompromised hosts most at risk for severe viral pneumonia include those following HSCT, or solid organ transplantation.[6] Radiologic studies of community-acquired pneumonia frequently combine both immunocompetent and immunocompromised patients to increase sample size, and therefore in the case of several pathogens, the imaging appearance in both patient groups has been reviewed above. Cytomegalovirus (CMV) is a ubiquitous pathogen whose association with pneumonia is largely confined to immunocompromised adults. Varicella pneumonia is most common in immunocompromised patients but remains a cause of severe pneumonia in immunocompetent adults in countries without universal varicella vaccination.

CYTOMEGALOVIRUS

CMV causes a systemic infection that can present acutely with mononucleosis, pharyngitis, fever, and lymphadenopathy.[58] The virus commonly establishes chronic, latent infection that can reactivate in immunocompromised hosts such as after HSCT, solid organ transplant (particularly lung transplant), and among those with acquired immunodeficiency syndrome (AIDS). Although it is not specifically a respiratory pathogen, it can cause severe pneumonia in these patients. CMV prophylaxis is very effective in the setting of HSCT, reducing infection from 20% to 70% to 1% to 3%, but is less so in lung transplant recipients (see Michelle Hershman and Scott Simpson's article "Thoracic Infections in Solid Organ Transplants; Radiological Features and Approach to Diagnosis," in this issue).[59]

Because CMV within the lungs usually represents reactivation of a systemic infection rather than inhaled pathogen its manifestations in the lung are pleomorphic and not confined to airway disease. The most common abnormality on chest radiographs is bilateral hazy opacities, which manifest as bilateral ground-glass opacities on chest CT.[60–62] Multiple centrilobular micronodules are also a common finding. In severe cases, multifocal consolidation can predominate or be intermixed with ground-glass opacities (**Figs. 15** and **16**). Interlobular septal thickening and pleural effusions are less common findings. Nodules with halo sign are uncommon and cavitary nodules have been reported but are rare.[60,62,63]

CMV is the most common viral infection among patients living with HIV, but has become much less prevalent following the advent of HAART. In the setting of HIV findings, CMV infection findings are similar to those described earlier. Radiographs commonly demonstrate bilateral hazy opacities seen as ground-glass opacities on CT. Consolidation, discrete masses, and nodules can also occur, and airway abnormalities (bronchiectasis and bronchial wall thickening) can be seen on CT.[64] Pneumocystis jiroveci pneumonia (PJP) can be difficult to distinguish from CMV as both infections are seen in patients with very low CD4 counts and can manifest as diffuse ground-glass opacities. However, CMV infection is associated with micronodules and macronodules more frequently than pneumocystis.[62] Consolidation and the halo sign have also been seen in CMV to a significantly higher degree. The relative likelihood of

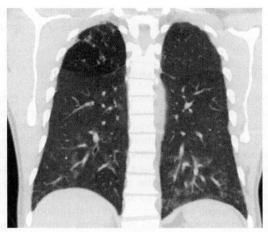

Fig. 15. Cytomegalovirus in a 52-year-old man status postrenal transplant. Coronal chest CT with dominant findings of bilateral lower lobe peribronchovascular ground-glass opacities. There are a few nodules in the right lung apex. (*Courtesy of* Brent P. Little, MD, Jacksonville, Florida.).

CMV versus PJP is also highly dependent on viral/and or pneumocystis prophylaxis, respectively.

Diagnosis of CMV pneumonitis is difficult, similar to HSV pulmonary infection (see above, "hospital-associated viral pneumonias"). As with other latent infections, the presence of CMV virus on viral cultures of BAL fluid is not proof of pathogenic CMV infection.[54,64] More definitive diagnosis can be made by BAL cytology or other

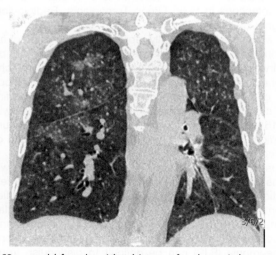

Fig. 16. CMV in a 62-year-old female with a history of orthotopic heart transplant for non-ischemic cardiomyopathy. Her CMV prophylaxis was stopped early on posttransplant due to thrombocytopenia/anemia. Coronal chest CT demonstrates diffuse bilateral nodules with mild peribronchovascular ground-glass opacities. (*Courtesy of* Farouk Dako, MD, MPH, Philadelphia, Pennsylvania.).

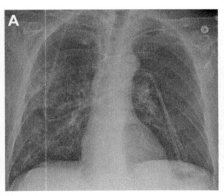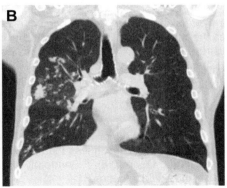

Fig. 17. Varicella pneumonia in a 72-year-old man with multiple myeloma status postautologous transplant complicated. (*A*) Frontal radiograph demonstrates multiple nodules in the right lung. (*B*) Coronal chest CT demonstrates a focal area of nodular consolidation with clustered adjacent centrilobular micronodules. Fewer micronodules are present in the lower lobe. (*Courtesy of* Shamus Moran, MD, Seattle, Washington.).

methods (see Brixey et al.).[64] First-line treatment is with the systemic antiviral intravenous ganciclovir. Foscarnet and cidofovir are antivirals which may be used for resistant infections.[5]

VARICELLA

Varicella, member of the herpes family, can cause severe pneumonia in immunocompromised patients and unvaccinated immunocompetent adults. Most children in the United States are vaccinated against the varicella virus after 12 months of age;[65] however, vaccination is only widespread in predominantly high socioeconomic countries.[66] Individuals who did not receive the vaccination and were not infected as children are at risk of contracting varicella as an adult, and between 5% to 15% of infected adults develop pneumonia.[65] Compared with children, varicella pneumonia

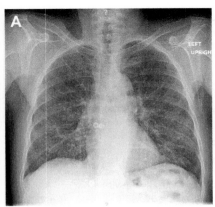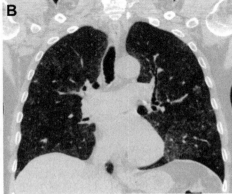

Fig. 18. Varicella pneumonia in a 54-year-old man with multiple myeloma, relapsed following HSCT. (*A*) Frontal chest radiograph shows diffuse bilateral reticular and micronodular opacities. (*B*) Coronal chest CT confirms the diffuse solid and ground-glass micronodules in a random distribution. The distribution suggests a hematogenous component of spread of infection. (*Courtesy of* Shamus Moran, MD, Seattle, Washington.).

in adults is associated with a 4 to 50 fold greater risk of hospitalization and a 174 fold greater risk of death.[66] Severe pneumonia typically develops an average of 3 days after the characteristic varicella rash and can rapidly progress to acute respiratory distress syndrome.[67] Mortality of intubated patients reaches 50%.[65]

Chest radiographs demonstrate ill-defined nodules measuring less than 1 cm, which may coalesce. Occasional findings include consolidation, hilar lymphadenopathy, or pleural effusions.[6,67] Chest CT in immunocompetent hosts often display 1 to 10 mm centrilobular nodules with and without ground glass halos, as well as randomly-distributed nodules.[68,69] CTs of immunocompetent and immunosuppressed patients with severe pneumonia contain centrilobular nodules in 50%, consolidation and ground-glass opacities in less than half, and effusions in approximately one-third of cases (**Figs. 17** and **18**).[68] Randomly distributed 2 to 3 mm calcified nodules are typical of healed infection.[6]

First-line therapy of varicella is the antiviral acyclovir, administered intravenously. In the setting of typical skin rash and exposure history, therapy is often initiated before the diagnosis is confirmed with PCR.[5]

SUMMARY

Viral pneumonia is prevalent among both immunocompetent and immunocompromised hosts, typically causing more severe disease in the latter. Several viral pneumonias, such as influenza, HMPV, RSV, and parainfluenza demonstrate similar airway-centric distribution, the likelihood of a specific organism often dependent on seasonal epidemics. Other viral pneumonias, such as adenovirus, frequently cause pneumonias with imaging findings indistinguishable from community-acquired bacterial pneumonias. For a few organisms, additional factors are central to the likelihood of infection, for example, environmental exposure for Hantaviruses and vaccination status for Varicella. In organisms that typically cause chronic infections in humans, such as HSV and CMV, the relationship between infection and clinical pneumonia is complex and incompletely understood.

CLINICS CARE POINTS

- HMPV, RSV, and parainfluenza pulmonary infections have a propensity for airway centric involvement with associated imaging findings of bronchiolitis and bronchopneumonia. Since this imaging appearance can be mimicked by bacterial pathogens, diagnosis is usually based on PCR.

- Influenza is also an airway centric infection causing bronchiolitis and bronchopneumonia. Diffuse airspace disease is rare in most seasonal outbreaks but occurs more commonly with infection with novel influenza viruses, such as H1N1 and avian influenza.

- Adenovirus can cause lobar type consolidation, which in the setting of infection with other virus pathogens (including influenza) suggests bacterial co-infection.

- Both HSV and CMV infections represent systemic reactivation of a latent infection rather than an acute primary pulmonary infection and positive respiratory cultures are not proof of pneumonia. Among immunocompromised hosts (patients living with advanced AIDS), CMV most commonly presents with ground glass opacities and centrilobular micronodules.

- Varicella and Hantavirus can cause severe pneumonia in otherwise healthy adults, one in the absence of prior vaccination or childhood infection, the other following specific environmental exposure. Imaging is dominated by micronodules in the setting of varicella, and linear interstitial opacities in the setting of Hantavirus Pulmonary Syndrome (HPS).

DISCLOSURE

The authors have nothing to disclose.

REFERENCES

1. Woolhouse M, Scott F, Hudson Z, et al. Human viruses: discovery and emergence. Philos Trans R Soc Lond B Biol Sci 2012;367(1604):2864–71.
2. Liang L, Moore B, Soni A, Healthcare cost and utilization project: statistical brief #261Agency for Healthcare Research and Quality: Rockville, MD. National Inpatient Hospital Costs: The Most Expensive Conditions by Payer. 2017. Accessed. https://www.hcup-us.ahrq.gov/reports/statbriefs/sb261-Most-Expensive-Hospital-Conditions-2017.pdf. [Accessed 1 June 2021]. Available at.
3. Tiveljung-Lindell A, Rotzén-Ostlund M, Gupta S, et al. Development and implementation of a molecular diagnostic platform for daily rapid detection of 15 respiratory viruses. J Med Virol 2009;81(1):167–75.
4. Jain S, Self WH, Wunderink RG, et al, CDC EPIC Study Team. Community-acquired pneumonia requiring hospitalization among U.S. Adults. N Engl J Med 2015;373(5):415–27.
5. Dandachi D, Rodriguez-Barradas MC. Viral pneumonia: etiologies and treatment. J Investig Med 2018;66(6):957–65.
6. Koo HJ, Lim S, Choe J, et al. Radiographic and CT features of viral pneumonia. Radiographics 2018;38(3):719–39.
7. Chow EJ, Doyle JD, Uyeki TM. Influenza virus-related critical illness: prevention, diagnosis, treatment. Crit Care 2019;23(1):214.
8. Olsen SJ, Azziz-Baumgartner E, Budd AP, et al. Decreased influenza activity during the COVID-19 pandemic — United States, Australia, Chile, and South Africa, 2020. MMWR Morbidity Mortality Wkly Rep 2020;69(37):1305–9.
9. Miller WT, Mickus TJ, Barbosa E, et al. CT of viral lower respiratory tract infections in adults: comparison among viral organisms and between viral and bacterial infections. AJR Am J Roentgenol 2011;197(5):1088–95.
10. Oikonomou A, Müller NL, Nantel S. Radiographic and high-resolution CT findings of influenza virus pneumonia in patients with hematologic malignancies. Am J Roentgenology 2003;181(2):507–11.
11. ACOG Committee Opinion No. 753: Assessment and Treatment of Pregnant Women With Suspected or Confirmed Influenza. Obstet Gynecol 2018;132(4):e169–73.
12. Oliveira EC, Marik PE, Colice G. Influenza pneumonia. Chest 2001;119(6):1717–23.
13. McElhaney JE, Verschoor CP, Andrew MK, et al. The immune response to influenza in older humans: beyond immune senescence. Immun Ageing 2020;17(1).
14. Cheng VC, To KK, Tse H, et al. Two years after pandemic influenza A/2009/H1N1: what have we learned? Clin Microbiol Rev 2012;25(2):223–63.
15. Ajlan AM, Quiney B, Nicolaou S, et al. Swine-origin influenza A (H1N1) viral infection: radiographic and CT findings. Am J Roentgenology 2009;193(6):1494–9.
16. Shrestha SS, Swerdlow DL, Borse RH, et al. Estimating the burden of 2009 pandemic influenza A (H1N1) in the United States (April 2009-April 2010). Clin Infect Dis 2010;52(Supplement 1):S75–82.
17. Abbo L, Quartin A, Morris MI, et al. Pulmonary imaging of pandemic influenza H1N1 infection: relationship between clinical presentation and disease burden on chest radiography and CT. Br J Radiol 2010;83(992):645–51.

18. Cornejo R, Llanos O, Fernández C, et al. Organizing pneumonia in patients with severe respiratory failure due to novel A (H1N1) influenza. BMJ Case Rep 2010; 2010. bcr0220102708.
19. Torrego A, Pajares V, Mola A, et al. Influenza A (H1N1) organiZing pneumonia. BMJ Case Rep 2010;2010. bcr12.2009.2531.
20. Töpfer L, Menk M, Weber-Carstens S, et al. Influenza A (H1N1) vs non-H1N1 ARDS: analysis of clinical course. J Crit Care 2014;29(3):340–6.
21. Li YT, Linster M, Mendenhall IH, et al. Avian influenza viruses in humans: lessons from past outbreaks. Br Med Bull 2019;132(1):81–95.
22. Qureshi NR, Hien TT, Farrar J, et al. The radiologic manifestations of H5N1 avian influenza. J Thorac Imaging 2006;21(4):259–64.
23. Rewar S, Mirdha D, Rewar P. Treatment and prevention of pandemic H1N1 influenza. Ann Glob Health 2016;81(5):645.
24. Gaitonde DY, Moore FC, Morgan MK. Influenza: diagnosis and treatment. Am Fam Physician 2019;100(12):751–8.
25. Lee N, Qureshi ST. Other viral pneumonias: coronavirus, respiratory syncytial virus, adenovirus, hantavirus. Crit Care Clin 2013;29(4):1045–68.
26. Stefanidis K, Konstantelou E, Yusuf GT, et al. Radiological, epidemiological and clinical patterns of pulmonary viral infections. Eur J Radiol 2021;136:109548.
27. Lynch JP 3rd, Kajon AE. Adenovirus: epidemiology, global spread of novel serotypes, and advances in treatment and prevention. Semin Respir Crit Care Med 2016;37(4):586–602.
28. Cha MJ, Chung MJ, Lee KS, et al. Clinical features and radiological findings of adenovirus pneumonia associated with progression to acute respiratory distress syndrome: a single center study in 19 adult patients. Korean J Radiol 2016;17(6): 940–9.
29. Tan D, Fu Y, Xu J, et al. Severe adenovirus community-acquired pneumonia in immunocompetent adults: chest radiographic and CT findings. J Thorac Dis 2016;8(5):848–54.
30. Jiang J, Wan R, Pan P, et al. Comparison of clinical, laboratory and radiological characteristics between COVID-19 and adenovirus pneumonia: a retrospective study. Infect Drug Resist 2020;13:3401–8.
31. Marinari LA, Danny MA, Simpson SA, et al. Lower respiratory tract infection with human metapneumovirus: chest CT imaging features and comparison with other viruses. Eur J Radiol 2020;128:108988.
32. Keske Ş, Gümüş T, Köymen T, et al. Human metapneumovirus infection: diagnostic impact of radiologic imaging. J Med Virol 2019;91(6):958–62.
33. Gabutti G, De Motoli F, Sandri F, et al. Viral respiratory infections in hematological patients. Infect Dis Ther 2020;9(3):495–510.
34. Pochon C, Voigt S. Respiratory virus infections in hematopoietic cell transplant recipients. Front Microbiol 2019;9:3294.
35. El Chaer F, Shah DP, Kmeid J, et al. Burden of human metapneumovirus infections in patients with cancer: risk factors and outcomes. Cancer 2017;123(12): 2329–37.
36. Godet C, Le Goff J, Beby-Defaux A, et al. Human metapneumovirus pneumonia in patients with hematological malignancies. J Clin Virol 2014;61(4):593–6.
37. Shahda S, Carlos WG, Kiel PJ, et al. The human metapneumovirus: a case series and review of the literature. Transpl Infect Dis 2011;13(3):324–8.
38. Herbst T, Van Deerlin VM, Miller WT Jr. The CT appearance of lower respiratory infection due to parainfluenza virus in adults. AJR Am J Roentgenol 2013; 201(3):550–4.

39. Kim MC, Kim MY, Lee HJ, et al. CT findings in viral lower respiratory tract infections caused by parainfluenza virus, influenza virus and respiratory syncytial virus. Medicine (Baltimore) 2016;95(26):e4003.

40. To KKW, Yip CCY, Yuen KY. Rhinovirus - From bench to bedside. J Formos Med Assoc 2017;116(7):496–504.

41. Moriyama M, Hugentobler WJ, Iwasaki A. Seasonality of respiratory viral infections. Annu Rev Virol 2020;7(1):83–101.

42. Choi SH, Huh JW, Hong SB, et al. Clinical characteristics and outcomes of severe rhinovirus-associated pneumonia identified by bronchoscopic bronchoalveolar lavage in adults: comparison with severe influenza virus-associated pneumonia. J Clin Virol 2015;62:41–7.

43. Munir N, Jahangeer M, Hussain S, et al. Hantavirus diseases pathophysiology, their diagnostic strategies and therapeutic approaches: a review. Clin Exp Pharmacol Physiol 2020;48:20–34.

44. Centers for Disease Control. "Hantavirus: Outbreaks." Reviewed Jan 17, 2018. Available at: https://www.cdc.gov/hantavirus/outbreaks/index.html. Accessed May 25, 2021.

45. Ketai LH, Williamson MR, Telepak RJ, et al. Hantavirus pulmonary syndrome: radiographic findings in 16 patients. Radiology 1994;191(3):665–8.

46. Boroja M, Barrie JR, Raymond GS. Radiographic findings in 20 patients with Hantavirus pulmonary syndrome correlated with clinical outcome. AJR Am J Roentgenol 2002;178(1):159–63.

47. de Lacerda Barbosa D, Zanetti G, Marchiori E. Hantavirus Pulmonary Syndrome: High-resolution Computed Tomography Findings. Arch Bronconeumol 2017;53(1):35–6.

48. Gasparetto EL, Davaus T, Escuissato DL, et al. Hantavirus pulmonary syndrome: high-resolution CT findings in one patient. Br J Radiol 2007;80(949):e21–3.

49. Aquino SL, Dunagan DP, Chiles C, et al. Herpes simplex virus 1 pneumonia: patterns on CT scans and conventional chest radiographs. J Comput Assist Tomogr 1998;22(5):795–800.

50. Chong S, Kim TS, Cho EY. Herpes simplex virus pneumonia: high-resolution CT findings. Br J Radiol 2010;83(991):585–9.

51. Hammer MM, Gosangi B, Hatabu H. Human herpesvirus alpha subfamily (Herpes Simplex and Varicella Zoster) viral pneumonias: CT findings. J Thorac Imaging 2018;33(6):384–9.

52. Luyt CE, Combes A, Deback C, et al. Herpes simplex virus lung infection in patients undergoing prolonged mechanical ventilation. Am J Respir Crit Care Med 2007;175:935–42.

53. Papazian L, Fraisse A, Garbe L, et al. Cytomegalovirus. An unexpected cause of ventilator-associated pneumonia. Anesthesiology 1996;84(2):280–7.

54. Coisel Y, Bousbia S, Forel JM, et al. Cytomegalovirus and herpes simplex virus effect on the prognosis of mechanically ventilated patients suspected to have ventilator-associated pneumonia. PLoS One 2012;7(12):e51340.

55. La Scola B, Marrie TJ, Auffray JP, et al. Mimivirus in pneumonia patients. Emerg Infect Dis 2005;11(3):449–52.

56. Sakhaee F, Vaziri F, Bahramali G, et al. Pulmonary infection related to mimivirus in patient with primary ciliary dyskinesia. Emerg Infect Dis 2020;26(10):2524–6.

57. Saadi H, Reteno DG, Colson P, et al. Shan virus: a new mimivirus isolated from the stool of a Tunisian patient with pneumonia. Intervirology 2013;56(6):424–9.

58. de Melo Silva J, Pinheiro-Silva R, Dhyani A, et al. Cytomegalovirus and epstein-barr infections: prevalence and impact on patients with hematological diseases. Biomed Res Int 2020;2020:1627824.
59. Clausen ES, Zaffiri L. Infection prophylaxis and management of viral infection. Ann Transl Med 2020;8(6):415.
60. Franquet T, Lee KS, Müller NL. Thin-section CT findings in 32 immunocompromised patients with cytomegalovirus pneumonia who do not have AIDS. AJR Am J Roentgenol 2003;181(4):1059–63.
61. Moon JH, Kim EA, Lee KS, et al. Cytomegalovirus pneumonia: high-resolution CT findings in ten non-AIDS immunocompromised patients. Korean J Radiol 2000; 1(2):73–8.
62. Du CJ, Liu JY, Chen H, et al. Differences and similarities of high-resolution computed tomography features between pneumocystis pneumonia and cytomegalovirus pneumonia in AIDS patients. Infect Dis Poverty 2020;9:149.
63. Najjar M, Siddiqui AK, Rossoff L, et al. Cavitary lung masses in SLE patients: an unusual manifestation of CMV infection. Eur Respir J 2004;24(1):182–4.
64. McGuinness G, Scholes JV, Garay SM, et al. Cytomegalovirus pneumonitis: spectrum of parenchymal CT findings with pathologic correlation in 21 AIDS patients. Radiology 1994;192(2):451–9.
65. Denny JT, Rocke ZM, McRae VA, et al. Varicella pneumonia: case report and review of a potentially lethal complication of a common disease. J Investig Med High Impact Case Rep 2018;6. 2324709618770230.
66. Wutzler P, Bonanni P, Burgess M, et al. Varicella vaccination - the global experience. Expert Rev Vaccines 2017;16(8):833–43.
67. Mirouse A, Vignon P, Piron P, et al. Severe varicella-zoster virus pneumonia: a multicenter cohort study. Crit Care 2017;21(1):137.
68. Gasparetto EL, Warszawiak D, Tazoniero P, et al. Varicella pneumonia in immunocompetent adults: report of two cases, with emphasis on high-resolution computed tomography findings. Braz J Infect Dis 2005;9(3):262–5.
69. Kim JS, Ryu W, Lee SI, et al. High resolution CT findings of varicella-zoster pneumonia. Am J Roentgenology 1999;172(1):113–6.

Influenza and Viral Pneumonia

Rodrigo Cavallazzi, MD[a],*, Julio A. Ramirez, MD[b]

KEYWORDS

- Influenza • Virus • Pneumonia • Epidemiology • Antiviral • Symptoms
- Polymerase chain reaction

KEY POINTS

- Human influenza is an RNA virus that belongs to the Orthomyxoviridae family and is categorized into types A, B, and C based on its nucleoprotein and matrix protein.
- Most community-acquired respiratory viruses are RNA viruses except for adenovirus and human bocavirus, which are DNA viruses.
- Using molecular techniques, respiratory viruses are identified in approximately 25% of patients with community-acquired pneumonia.
- In addition to the community-acquired respiratory viruses, immunocompromised patients are particularly susceptible to viruses of the Herpesviridae family.
- It is difficult to diagnose influenza or other viral infections on clinical grounds.
- Patients with influenza pneumonia should be treated with a neuraminidase inhibitor.

INTRODUCTION

Respiratory viral infections cause a substantial burden. They are prevalent and tend to affect those who are more vulnerable such as children, elderly, and people living in developing areas such as sub-Saharan Africa and Southeast Asia.[1] The advent of molecular techniques has facilitated the identification of respiratory viruses in patients with pneumonia and has shed light on how commonly these viruses occur in patients with pneumonia. With the currently available diagnostic tools, viral pathogens are more often identified than bacterial pathogens in community-acquired pneumonia.[2] A large amount of effort is currently being dedicated to elucidate the pathogenicity of respiratory viruses and the interaction between viruses and bacteria in the setting of pneumonia. Since the last century, several devastating pandemics and outbreaks related

Funding: The authors have nothing to disclose.
Portions of this article were previously published in *Clinics in Chest Medicine* 39:4 December 2018.
[a] Division of Pulmonary, Critical Care, and Sleep Disorders, University of Louisville, Louisville, KY, USA; [b] Norton Infectious Diseases Institute, Norton Healthcare, Louisville, KY, USA
* Corresponding author. 550 South Jackson Street, ACB, A3R27, Louisville, KY 40202.
E-mail address: r0cava01@louisville.edu

Infect Dis Clin N Am 38 (2024) 183–212
https://doi.org/10.1016/j.idc.2023.12.010
0891-5520/24/© 2023 Published by Elsevier Inc.

id.theclinics.com

to respiratory viruses have occurred.[3,4] Recently, there has been a growing interest in the development of new antiviral medications for respiratory infection. In this article, we provide an overview of pneumonia caused by influenza and other respiratory viruses from the practicing clinician perspective with a focus on the adult population.

MICROBIOLOGY OVERVIEW

Human influenza is an RNA virus that belongs to the Orthomyxoviridae family and is categorized into types A, B, and C based on its nucleoprotein and matrix protein.[3] Influenza A virus is subcategorized into subtypes such as H1N1, H1N2, and H3N2 based on hemagglutinin (H) and neuraminidase (N) composition. Influenza B is subcategorized into the B/Yamagata and the B/Victoria lineages.[3,5,6] Most influenza infections are caused by types A and B.[7] Small genetic mutations that influenza undergoes every year are called antigenic drift and are responsible for seasonal outbreaks. Conversely, influenza pandemics are caused by antigenic shift, which occurs when new hemagglutinin or neuraminidase subtypes are acquired.[7]

Most community-acquired respiratory viruses are RNA viruses except for adenovirus and human bocavirus, which are DNA viruses.[8-15] The Paramyxoviridae family includes respiratory syncytial virus, human parainfluenza virus, and human metapneumovirus. A distinctive feature of the Paramyxoviridae family viruses is the presence of a fusion protein.[9,12,14] The fusion protein, which enables the integration of the virus with the cell membrane, allowing the introduction of the viral genome into the cell cytoplasm, is a target for vaccines and antivirals.[16] The Picornaviridae family of virus, which includes enterovirus and human rhinovirus, are characterized by a capsid that contains the viral genome. The capsid has a large cleft (or canyon) which binds to adhesion molecules on the cell surface, leading to the eventual entry of the viral genome into the cell. The capsid and the adhesion molecules are potential targets of antivirals.[17,18] The coronaviruses contain 2 important structural proteins: membrane protein M, which is expressed in large amounts, and the spike protein S.[13] The latter is a class I viral fusion protein and mediates the entry of the virus into the cell.[19] See **Table 1**.

INCIDENCE AND EPIDEMIOLOGY
Epidemiology of Viral Respiratory Infection in Community-Acquired Pneumonia

A systematic review included 31 observational studies that enrolled patients with community-acquired pneumonia who underwent viral polymerase chain reaction testing. The pooled proportion of patients with viral infection was 24.5% (95% CI 21.5%–27.5%; I2 = 92.9%).[20] Most of these studies were performed in the inpatient setting and viral polymerase chain reaction was obtained mostly from nasal or oropharyngeal swab. In the only study that was performed in the outpatient setting, the proportion of viral infection was 12.1% (95% CI 7.7%–16.5%; I2 = 0.0%).[21] The pooled proportion of viral infection was 44.2% (95% CI 35.1%–53.3%; I2 = 0%) from 2 studies of patients with community-acquired pneumonia admitted to the intensive care unit (ICU) and in which a lower respiratory sample was obtained in more than half of the patients.[22,23] The proportion of dual bacterial and viral infection was 10% (95% CI 8%–11%; I2 = 93.1%). Although the presence of a viral infection did not significantly increase the risk of short-term death, patients with dual bacterial-viral infection had twice the risk of death as compared with patients without dual infection.[20] A population-based study from Louisville estimated that 1,591,825 patients are admitted for community-acquired pneumonia each year in the United States.[24] Assuming a prevalence of viral infection of 24.5% among patients hospitalized for community-acquired pneumonia, it is estimated that around 390,000 patients each

Table 1
Characteristics and taxonomy of commonly identified respiratory viruses in patients with community-acquired pneumonia

Virus	Genome	Family	Important Antigenic Structures
Influenza	RNA	Orthomyxoviridae	Surface glycoproteins hemagglutinin (HA) and the neuraminidase (NA)[8]
Respiratory syncytial virus	RNA	Paramyxoviridae	Attachment glycoprotein (G) and fusion (F) glycoprotein[9]
Human rhinovirus	RNA	Picornaviridae	Viral capsid proteins VP1, VP2, VP3, and VP4[10]
Adenovirus	DNA	Adenoviridae	Capsid major structures: hexon (the building block of the capsid), penton base and polypeptides[11]
Human parainfluenza virus	RNA	Paramyxoviridae	Surface glycoproteins hemagglutinin-neuraminidase and fusion protein. Membrane protein[12]
Coronavirus	RNA	Coronaviridae	Membrane glycoprotein and spike protein[13]
Human metapneumovirus	RNA	Paramyxoviridae	Virus fusion (F) glycoprotein[14]
Human bocavirus	DNA	Parvoviridae	Capsid viral proteins (VPs), VP1 and VP2[15]

year are admitted to hospitals in the United States for viral community-acquired pneumonia. It is important to note that the identification of a viral pathogen in a patient with pneumonia does not necessarily mean that the virus has a pathogenic effect, particularly if the identification is via nasopharyngeal swab (**Fig. 1, Table 2**).

Epidemiology of Viral Respiratory Infection in Immunocompromised Patients

In immunocompromised patients with pneumonia, infection by respiratory viruses is exceedingly common. Surveillance studies show that a respiratory viral pathogen is identified in close to a third of hospitalized patients with leukemia or hematopoietic stem cell transplantation and respiratory symptoms. Pneumonia occurs in the majority of immunosuppressed patients infected with a respiratory viral pathogen.[25] Immunocompromised patients are commonly infected by the same respiratory viruses that cause infection in immunocompetent patients. However, viruses of the Herpesviridae family also tend to cause infection in immunocompromised patients. As an example, in an early series of patients who underwent allogenic bone marrow transplantation, cytomegalovirus was the most common viral pathogen.[26] Varicella zoster virus reactivation can occur in patients after hematopoietic stem cell transplantation with early series reporting incidences ranging from 22% to 41%[27,28] It is not unusual for the infection to present in a disseminated form in these patients, and pneumonia is one of the complications.[27–29]

Epidemiology of Hospital-Acquired Viral Respiratory Infection

Traditionally, hospital-acquired respiratory viral infection has been thought to be limited to immunocompromised patients. However, it is now known that this can also commonly occur in immunocompetent patients. This was highlighted by a prospective cohort study that included 262 patients with hospital-acquired pneumonia. The hospital-acquired pneumonia was established when patients developed clinical findings of pneumonia 48 hours or more after hospital admission. The median time from hospital admission to development of hospital-acquired pneumonia was 20 days. The proportion of viral infection was 36.1% in immunocompromised patients and 11.2% in nonimmunocompromised patients. The identified viruses were respiratory syncytial virus (6.1%), parainfluenza virus (6.1%), influenza virus (3.8%), cytomegalovirus (1.9%), human coronavirus (1.5%), bocavirus (0.8%), human metapneumovirus

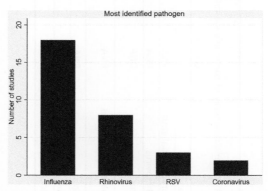

Fig. 1. Number of studies according to most commonly identified viral pathogen. Studies were conducted before the COVID-19 pandemic. (*Data from* Burk M, El-Kersh K, Saad M, Wiemken T, Ramirez J, Cavallazzi R. Viral infection in community-acquired pneumonia: A systematic review and meta-analysis. *Eur Respir Rev.* 2016;25(140):178-188.)

Table 2
Different scenarios for the effect of an identified viral pathogen in the setting of pneumonia

Virus is a "bystander" and does not have a pathogenic effect	Although uncommon in adults, asymptomatic carriage of respiratory viruses occurs[155]
Virus has a pathogenic effect and is causing pneumonia in isolation	Potential mechanisms include dysregulation of cytokines and chemokines, infection of epithelial cells in the lungs, and apoptosis[156]
Virus has a pathogenic effect and is causing pneumonia along with a bacterial pathogen	A study showed that the mortality for patients with community-acquired pneumonia and bacterial and viral coinfection is higher[20]
Virus caused a recent infection that prompted a secondary bacterial infection	This occurs particularly with *S pneumoniae* or *Staphylococcus aureus* infection following influenza infection[157]
	Lag time of 2–4 wk between the viral and bacterial infection[158]
	Polymerase chain reaction test may remain positive for up to 5 wk after a viral infection[159]

(0.8%), and adenovirus (0.4%).[30] These findings, which could be due to exposure visitors and health-care workers, underscore the importance of infection control measures in hospitalized patients. Conceivably, these findings could also be due exposure before hospital admission.

Pandemics and Outbreaks Before Coronavirus Disease 2019

Since the last century, there have been 5 influenza pandemics: 1918 to 1919 Spanish influenza, 1957 H2N2 Asian influenza, 1968 H3N2 Hong Kong influenza, 1977 H1N1 Russian influenza, and the 2009 H1N1 pandemic.[3,4] It is estimated that the 2009 H1N1 pandemic caused 201,200 respiratory deaths and 83,000 cardiovascular deaths. Most of these deaths occurred in patients aged younger than 65 years.[31] In 2003, a major outbreak of atypical pneumonia was reported. The cases initially clustered in China but were subsequently reported worldwide. The pneumonia often resulted in acute respiratory failure and was named severe acute respiratory syndrome.[32] Subsequently, the etiologic agent of this disease was identified as a novel coronavirus,[33,34] which was named the Urbani strain of severe acute respiratory syndrome-associated coronavirus.[33] In 2012, another novel coronavirus was isolated from a patient with pneumonia in Saudi Arabia.[35] The virus was subsequently named Middle East respiratory syndrome coronavirus.[36] Infection by this virus causes an illness that is clinically similar to that caused by severe acute respiratory syndrome-associated coronavirus but with higher mortality.[37] Cases of Middle East respiratory syndrome coronavirus were initially reported in Saudi Arabia but were subsequently reported in other countries, including the United States, typically in persons who had traveled from Arabian Peninsula.[38–40] Middle East respiratory syndrome coronavirus can be acquired by exposure to dromedary camels, products from animals, and humans. Cases continue to be identified particularly in Saudi Arabia but also in other countries in the Middle East. However, person-to-person transmission has been limited mostly to health-care facilities. As of November of 2022, there had been 2600 reported cases of Middle East respiratory syndrome coronavirus.[41]

Influenza

The incidence of influenza can vary substantially in different seasons. For example, the influenza activity was lower in the 2021 to 2022 compared with other seasons before the coronavirus disease 2019 (COVID-19) pandemic. In the 2021 to 2022 season, it is estimated there were 101,262 (95% CI: 82,653–185,191) admissions and 4601 (95% CI: 3769–20,814) deaths associated with influenza in the United States. Adults aged 65 years or older accounted for 51% of the hospitalizations and 83% of the deaths associated with influenza.[42]

Different studies showed that approximately one-third of hospitalized patients with laboratory-confirmed influenza have pneumonia.[43–45] In a study that included 4765 patients hospitalized with influenza, those with pneumonia were older than those without pneumonia (median age of 74 years vs 69 years; P<.01). In a multivariate analyses, the following factors were significant predictors of pneumonia in hospitalized patients with influenza: age older than 75 years (OR = 1.27 [95% CI: 1.10–1.46]), White race (OR = 1.24 [95% CI: 1.03–1.49]), nursing home residence (OR = 1.37 [95% CI: 1.14–1.66]), chronic lung disease (OR = 1.37 [95% CI: 1.18–1.59]), and immunosuppression (OR = 1.45 [95% CI: 1.19–1.78]). Asthma was associated with lower odds of pneumonia (OR = 0.76 [95% CI: 0.62–0.92]).[44] In another study of 579 adult patients hospitalized with laboratory-confirmed influenza, a multivariate analyses showed that the following factors were significantly associated with pneumonia: older age (OR = 1.026 [95% CI: 1.013–1.04]), higher C-reactive protein, milligram per deciliter (OR = 1.128 [95% CI: 1.088–1.17]), smoking (OR = 1.818 [95% CI: 1.115–2.965]), low albumin level (OR = 2.518 [95% CI: 1.283–4.9]), acute respiratory failure (OR = 4.525 [95% CI: 2.964–6.907]), and productive cough (OR = 8.173 [95% CI: 3.674–18.182]).[45]

During an influenza season, the attributed mortality to pneumonia and influenza in the United States ranges from 5.6% to 11.1%.[46] In a cohort study that included laboratory-confirmed cases of influenza admitted to the hospital, those with pneumonia, as compared with those without pneumonia, were more likely to require ICU admission (27% vs 10%), mechanical ventilation (18% vs 5%) and to die (9% vs 2%).[44] See **Fig. 2**.

Severe Acute Respiratory Syndrome Coronavirus 2

COVID-19, the disease caused by the coronavirus severe acute respiratory syndrome coronavirus 2 (SARS-CoV-2), was first recognized in a cluster of patients in December of 2019. It then spread throughout the world and caused a devastating pandemic. As

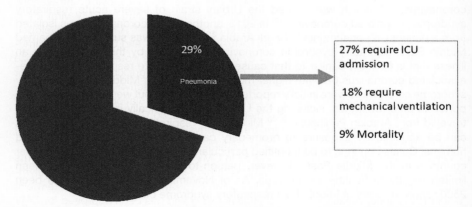

29%

Pneumonia

27% require ICU admission

18% require mechanical ventilation

9% Mortality

Fig. 2. Proportion of pneumonia and associated outcomes in patients admitted to the hospital with influenza infection. (*Data from* Garg S, Jain S, Dawood FS, et al. Pneumonia among adults hospitalized with laboratory-confirmed seasonal influenza virus infection-united states, 2005-2008. *BMC Infect Dis*. 2015;15:369-015-1004-y.)

of September of 2023, there have been close to 7 million deaths worldwide caused by COVID-19.[47] SARS-CoV-2 undergoes periodic mutations, which lead to different variants over time: Alpha, Delta, and Omicron. Currently, the variant predominantly circulating is the Omicron.[48] Clinical manifestations and severity of COVID-19 differ with each variant predominance, which may reflect not only the changing variant virulence but also the effects of increasing immunity in the population and restructuring of health care.[49] The risk of hospitalization during the Omicron period has been 1.9%.[50] For patients hospitalized primarily for COVID-19, the mortality risk was 13.1% in the early Omicron period (January–March 2022) and 4.9% in the later Omicron period (April–June 2022).[51] Risk factors for higher mortality include increasing age, presence of underlying medical conditions, and disability.[52] Racial and ethnic minorities have been disproportionally affected by COVID-19, likely a reflection of worse living conditions, less access of health care, and jobs that are often frontline or essential.[53] Unvaccinated status is also a major risk factor for mortality. During the late Omicron BA.4/BA.5 variant period (September 18–December 3, 2022) in the United States, unvaccinated persons had a mortality rate ratio that was 5 times higher compared with those who received monovalent vaccines only and 14 times higher compared with those who received bivalent booster.[54]

Respiratory Syncytial Virus

In older subjects, the burden of respiratory syncytial virus infection is similar to that of influenza. A study prospectively followed 2 outpatient cohorts during 4 seasons: 608 heathy elderly patients and 540 high-risk adults. High-risk status was defined as the presence of congestive heart failure or chronic pulmonary disease. Respiratory syncytial virus infection was diagnosed in 3% to 7% of healthy elderly subjects and 4% to 10% of high-risk subjects. This accounted for 1.5 respiratory syncytial virus infection per 100 person-months in high-risk adults and 0.9 in healthy elderly subjects.[55] In an analysis of hospitalization and viral surveillance data that encompassed several years, it was estimated that the respiratory syncytial virus-associated hospitalization rate per 100,000 person-years in the United States was 12.8 (95% CI: 2.4–73.9) for patients aged 50 to 64 years and 86.1 (95% CI: 37.3–326.2) for patients aged 65 years or older. In contrast to influenza-associated hospitalizations, the rates of respiratory syncytial virus-associated hospitalizations were relatively similar across the years.[56] In a cohort of 1388 hospitalized adults aged older than 65 years or with underlying cardiopulmonary diseases, respiratory syncytial virus infection was diagnosed in 8% to 13% of these patients depending on the year. Of the 132 hospitalized patients with respiratory syncytial virus infection, 41 (31%) had an infiltrate on chest radiograph, 20 (15%) required ICU admission, 17 (13%) required mechanical ventilation, and 10 (8%) died.[55]

Epidemiology of Other Respiratory Viruses

Rhinovirus

- Most common cause of common cold, a self-limited acute illness that occurs 2 to 4 times per year in adults.
- This infection is characterized by sneezing, nasal discharge, sore throat, and low-grade fever.[57]
- Rhinovirus tends to occur more often in the early fall or spring.[58]
- Rhinovirus is commonly identified in the upper respiratory tract of patients with community-acquired pneumonia via molecular techniques. In fact, rhinovirus was the most commonly identified pathogen in a large cohort of adult patients hospitalized with CAP conducted in the United States.[2]

Common human coronavirus

- Occurs more commonly in the winter and follows a seasonal pattern that resembles that of influenza.[59]
- Coronaviruses HCoV-229E, HCoV-NL63, HCoV-OC43, and HCoV-HKU1 have ubiquitous circulation and are a usual etiology of common cold.[37]
- Coronaviruses have also been commonly associated with lower respiratory tract symptoms.[59]
- Adult hospitalized patients with coronavirus infection are often immunocompromised, and pneumonia is a common occurrence.[60]
- Severe acute respiratory syndrome coronavirus and Middle East respiratory syndrome coronavirus caused outbreaks and pandemics of an acute respiratory illness, often leading to respiratory failure.[37]

Adenovirus

- Adenovirus is a common cause of upper respiratory tract symptoms and conjunctivitis.[61]
- Adult patients with adenovirus pneumonia are relatively young.
- Different studies have reported that patients with community-acquired pneumonia and adenovirus infection have mean age that ranges from 30 to 38 years.[62,63]
- Adenovirus also causes serious infection in immunocompromised patients. The adenovirus species found in immunocompromised patients are not typically found in the community, which indicates endogenous viral reactivation in these patients.[64]
- No clear seasonality although cases may spike in some months.[65]
- Several outbreaks caused by adenovirus have been reported. Some examples include reports of outbreaks in military personnel,[66] psychiatric care facility,[67] and ICU.[68]

Parainfluenza

- Most infections are caused by parainfluenza 1 and 3.[69] Parainfluenza 2 is less commonly identified, and parainfluenza 4 is a rare cause of respiratory infection.
- In adults, influenza-like symptoms are a common manifestation of parainfluenza infection.[70] In children, common presentations are croup and bronchiolitis.[69]
- In a population-based study of adults hospitalized for lower respiratory tract infection in 2 counties in Ohio, parainfluenza-1 and parainfluenza-3 were detected in 2.5% to 3.1% of tested patients. Parainfluenza-1 epidemic season spanned the summer–autumn. Parainfluenza-3 epidemic season spanned the spring–summer. Median age was 61.5 years for parainfluenza-1–infected patients and 77.5 years for parainfluenza-3–infected patients. Of those infected by parainfluenza-3, 59% had an infiltrate on chest radiograph, 23% required ICU stay, and none died.[71]

Metapneumovirus

- It has been identified in 4.5% of acute respiratory illnesses of adults prospectively followed as outpatient.[72]
- It has been identified in 4% of patients with community-acquired pneumonia.[73]
- Among outpatient adults, those of younger age tend to be more commonly infected by metapneumovirus, which has been presumably attributed to their closer contact with children. However, hospitalized patients with metapneumovirus infection are older.[72]

- Mean age in a series of community-acquired pneumonia and metapneumovirus infection: 62 years.[73]
- In the outpatient setting, cough and nasal congestion are the most common symptoms.[72]
- In patients with metapneumovirus infection and pneumonia, common symptoms are cough with sputum production, dyspnea, and fatigue.[73]

Human bocavirus

- Commonly identified in symptomatic and asymptomatic children but it seems to be a less common cause of respiratory symptoms in adults.[74]
- Human bocavirus infection is more common in the winter.[75]
- Common clinical presentations include upper respiratory tract symptoms, bronchiolitis, and pneumonia.[76] Cases of encephalitis have been reported.[77,78]
- It has been detected in acute respiratory illness of adults with immunosuppression and chronic lung disease.[79,80]
- A study showed that it can be often identified in the sinus tissue specimens of adult patients with chronic sinusitis.[81]

CLINICAL PRESENTATION
Clinical Manifestations

Patients with influenza infection in general (not just pneumonia) commonly present with cough, fever, fatigue, myalgia, runny nose, and sweating. Wheezing as a symptom can occur in close to half of the patients.[82] Patients with influenza pneumonia tend to have the same symptoms as patients with nonpneumonic influenza infection but an important distinction is that patients with pneumonia more often have dyspnea.[83] Perhaps, the greatest clinical clue for influenza in a patient with acute respiratory symptoms (or pneumonia) is whether the patient is presenting during an influenza epidemic. As an example, the absence of coughing and temperature greater than 37.8°C make influenza very unlikely in patients presenting with influenza-like illness outside an influenza epidemic but has a lesser impact on the likelihood of influenza if the same patient presented during an epidemic. However, the presence of these symptoms during an epidemic substantially increases the probability of influenza but has a lesser impact outside of an epidemic.[84]

Several studies have assessed the accuracy of clinical manifestations for the diagnosis of influenza in patients with acute respiratory symptoms. Some of the earlier studies were limited by retrospective design, leading to potential classification bias, or by the reliance on clinical manifestations for the final diagnosis of influenza, leading to incorporation bias.[85] More recent studies used a prospective design and viral polymerase chain reaction test as the reference standard. A prospective study enrolled 100 patients with influenza-like illness who presented to 3 different clinics. Viral polymerase chain reaction test was used for the diagnosis of influenza. The accuracy of several symptoms was tested. On multivariate analysis, only cough and temperature remained significant predictors of influenza.[86] In a prospective study of 258 patients who presented to the emergency department with acute respiratory symptoms, a symptom inventory and influenza polymerase chain reaction test was applied to the patients. Using polymerase chain reaction test as the reference standard, the accuracy of clinical judgment, decision rule, and rapid influenza test was provided. The presence of cough and fever had a positive likelihood ratio of 5.1 and a negative likelihood ratio of 0.7.[82] In a prospective study of 270 high-risk patients who presented to an emergency department with acute respiratory illness, clinicians were asked whether they thought patient had influenza. Viral polymerase chain reaction was the reference standard. A clinician diagnosis of influenza had a positive likelihood ratio of 1.63 and negative likelihood ratio of 0.82.[87] Likelihood ratios are an interesting way of providing the accuracy of symptoms or clinical diagnosis because they allow for the estimate of the probability of a disease after considering the pretest probability.[88] See **Fig. 3.** See **Table 3** for a summary of these studies.

Overall, the above studies indicate that the predictive value of symptoms, combination of symptoms, or clinical impression for the diagnosis of influenza is only modest for patients presenting with acute illness. Symptoms or clinical impression is not enough to rule in or rule out influenza. In fact, clinicians failed to clinically diagnose influenza in approximately two-thirds of influenza-confirmed patients in a prospective series.[87] Ultimately, clinicians need to pay close attention to surveillance data, and if there is evidence of influenza activity in the area where they practice, any acute febrile respiratory illness should place influenza because a high possibility in the differential diagnosis. This is line with recent guidelines that recommend different testing strategies according to whether there is circulation of seasonal influenza A and B.[89] In the United States, the Centers for Disease Control and Prevention provide weekly data on influenza activity according to regions in the country. This is available at https://www.cdc.gov/flu/weekly/index.htm. Other important aspects of clinical history include close contact with persons with acute febrile illness, and recent travel. Additionally, it is important to realize that in some tropical countries influenza circulates throughout the year.[90]

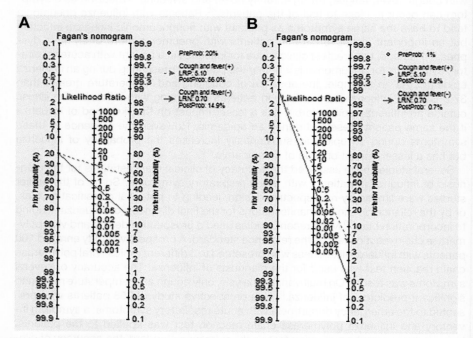

Fig. 3. Probability of influenza according to presence of combined cough and fever in patients presenting during influenza season (*A*) and outside the influenza season (*B*). (Data for likelihood ratios from Stein J, Louie J, Flanders S, et al. Performance characteristics of clinical diagnosis, a clinical decision rule, and a rapid influenza test in the detection of influenza infection in a community sample of adults. Ann Emerg Med. 2005;46(5):412-419.)

Table 3
Characteristics of studies that prospectively assessed the accuracy of symptoms for the diagnosis of influenza infection

Author, Year	Design	Setting	Sample	Inclusion Criteria	Reference	Results
Boivin et al,[86] 2000	Prospective cohort	Patients presenting to 3 outpatient clinics	100	Flu-like illness of <72h duration	PCR and culture from nasopharyngeal swab	*Cough and fever (>38°C):* Sens of 77.6% Spec of 55.0% PPV of 86.8% NPV of 39.3%
Stein et al,[82] 2005	Prospective cohort	Adult patients presenting to the emergency department	258	New illness within the past 3 wk associated with cough, fever, or upper respiratory tract symptoms		*Clinician judgment:* Sens of 29% (95% CI 18% to 43%) Spec of 92% (95% CI 87% to 95%) PLR of 3.8 (95% CI 1.9–7.5) NLR: of 0.8 (95% CI 0.6–0.9) *Decision rule* *(cough and fever):* Sens of 40% (95% CI 27% to 54%) Spec of 92% (95% CI 87% to 95%) PLR of 5.1 (95% CI 2.7–9.6) NLR of 0.7 (95% CI 0.5–0.8)

(continued on next page)

Table 3
(continued)

Author, Year	Design	Setting	Sample	Inclusion Criteria	Reference	Results
Dugas et al,[87] 2015	Prospective cohort	Adult patients presenting to the emergency department	270	Fever or any respiratory-related symptom	PCR from nasopharyngeal swab	*Clinical judgment:* Sens of 36% (95% CI 22%–52%) Spec of 78% (95% CI 72%–83%) PLR of 1.63 (95% CI 1.01–2.62) NLR of 0.82 (95% CI 0.65–1.04) *Influenza-like illness* *(fever ≥37.8°C with either* *cough or sore throat):* Sens of 31% (95% CI 18%–47%) Spec of 88% (95% CI 83%–92%) PLR of 2.61 (95% CI 1.47–4.64) NLR of 0.78 (95% CI 0.64–0.96)

Abbreviations: NLR, negative likelihood ratio; NPV, negative predictive value; PCR, polymerase chain reaction; PLR, positive likelihood ratio; PPV, positive predictive value; Sens, sensitivity; Spec, specificity.

The clinical manifestations and prognosis of COVID-19 vary according to the host immune status, the SARS-CoV-2 variant and subvariant, and age. In a community study, representative symptoms of COVID-19 in vaccinated persons during the Omicron variant period included runny nose (76.5%), headache (74.7%), sore throat (70.5%), sneezing (63%), persistent cough (49.8%), hoarse voice (42.6%), joint pain (41.2%), fever (29.3%), brain fog (24.9%), diarrhea (16.7%), loss of smell (16.6%), and dyspnea (4.9%). Symptoms such as loss of smell, fever, and brain fog were less common when compared with prior Delta variant period. Both the median duration of acute symptoms (6.87 days vs 8.89 days, $P<.01$) and the risk of hospitalization (1.9% vs 2.6%, $P = .03$) were lower in the Omicron period compared with the Delta period.[50]

A hallmark of respiratory syncytial virus infection is the presence of wheezing, which occurs in a higher frequency as compared with patients with influenza. Hospitalized patients with respiratory syncytial virus infection may present with clinical-radiological dissociation, in which patients may seem toxemic despite mild radiological abnormalities. In a cohort of 118 hospitalized patients with respiratory syncytial virus infection, the most common symptoms were cough (97%), dyspnea (95%), wheezing (73%), and nasal congestion (68%). On physical examination, wheezing was present in 82% of the patients. A temperature greater than 39°C was only present in 13% of the patients. It should be noted, however, that these percentages are for all hospitalized patients with respiratory syncytial virus infection. When assessing only those hospitalized patients with respiratory syncytial virus infection and pneumonia, wheezing and nasal congestion were less common.[91] In another study of 57 patients with respiratory syncytial virus infection and clinical diagnosis of pneumonia, the most common symptoms were cough (88%), dyspnea (82%), wheezing (79%), fever (61%), and runny nose (58%). On physical examination, the most common findings were wheezing (53%), rhonchi (46%), and crackles (40%).[92]

Just as in pneumonia caused by influenza or respiratory syncytial virus, there are no specific clinical manifestations of pneumonia caused by other respiratory viruses. In fact, symptoms and signs are not specific enough to differentiate viral from bacterial pneumonia.[93] The usual clinical manifestations of pneumonia, including fever greater than 37.8°C, heart rate greater than 100 beats per minute, crackles, and decreased breath sounds,[94] are to be expected in pneumonia caused by any of the respiratory viruses. In the end, the diagnosis of viral infection in patients with pneumonia relies on the recognition that respiratory viruses are a common cause of pneumonia and on the systematic performance of viral microbiology studies on these patients.

Radiological Manifestations

The chest radiograph of patients with viral pneumonia can show different patterns including ground-glass opacities, consolidation, and nodular opacities. In general, patients present with faint opacities, commonly described as a ground-glass pattern. The second most commonly reported pattern is consolidation. Nodular opacities are less common but can occur. The opacities are often patchy in distribution.[91,95–98] Bilateral involvement is fairly common, and some series in influenza pneumonia show that bilateral involvement is slightly more common than unilateral involvement.[95] However, other series in respiratory syncytial virus or coronavirus pneumonia show that unilateral involvement is more common.[91,96] Pleural effusions are not usual but have been reported.[98] On computed tomography of the chest, the most common pattern, ground-glass opacity, becomes even more noticeable, often in a patchy and bilateral distribution. Other patterns, such as consolidation, nodular opacities, and interlobular thickening, can also be present.[97] See **Figs. 4** and **5**.

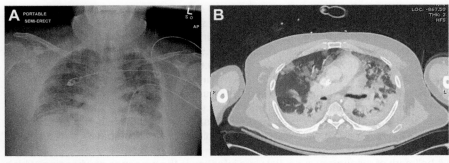

Fig. 4. Chest radiograph and computed tomography of the chest of a 42-year-old male patient admitted with pneumonia and 2009 H1N1 influenza infection leading to acute respiratory failure. Chest radiograph (A) reveals diffuse consolidation, and the computed tomography of the chest (B) reveals bilateral patchy ground-glass opacities and dense consolidation in the dorsal areas.

Similar to the clinical manifestations, the radiological findings are not specific and do not allow for the differentiation of viral from bacterial infection in patients with pneumonia let alone the identification of a specific virus. The radiological findings, however, can help corroborate the diagnosis of viral pneumonia. For instance, in a patient in which a viral pathogen has been identified by oropharyngeal swab, the demonstration of patchy ground-glass opacities in the lung is suggestive of a viral pneumonic infiltrate. Additionally, the radiological findings on chest CT have had a prominent role both in corroborating the diagnosis and the prognostication of patients with COVID-19. The typical radiological manifestations of COVID-19 include ground-glass opacities that are peripheral and predominate in the lower lobes.[99]

PATHOGEN-DIRECTED THERAPY
Influenza

The 3 main classes of antiviral drugs for the treatment of influenza include neuraminidase inhibitors, cap-dependent endonuclease inhibitors, and adamantanes.[7,100,101] Influenza viruses infect cells through the binding of its surface glycoprotein hemagglutinin to the

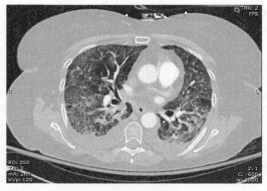

Fig. 5. Computed tomography of the chest revealing diffuse ground-glass opacities and small bilateral pleural effusion in a 62-year-old female patient with respiratory syncytial virus infection who developed pneumonia and acute respiratory distress syndrome.

sialic acid receptor. The attached virus is then released into the cells by another surface glycoprotein, neuraminidase, which is the target of neuraminidase inhibitors.[102] The cap-dependent endonuclease inhibitor baloxavir marboxil is hydrolyzed into an active form, baloxavir acid. The latter inhibits the endonuclease responsible for cleaving the mRNA bound to a cap-binding domain.[103] The cleavage of the bound mRNA is an important step in influenza virus transcription. The adamantanes, which include amantadine and rimantadine, block the M2 protein, a membrane protein with ion channel activity.[104] They exhibit activity against influenza A but not against influenza B. The antiviral drugs currently approved by the US Food and Drug Administration are the neuraminidase inhibitors oral oseltamivir, inhaled zanamivir and intravenous peramivir, and the cap-dependent endonuclease inhibitor baloxavir marboxil. The adamantanes are not recommended for the treatment of influenza because of high resistance of influenza A against these drugs.[105]

Several clinical trials assessed the effect of oseltamivir for influenza. A comprehensive systematic review summarized the effect of oseltamivir for prophylaxis and treatment in adults and children. For the assessment of time to alleviation of symptoms in adults with influenza, 8 studies were pooled, totaling 2208 patients in the oseltamivir group and 1746 in the placebo group. Oseltamivir led to earlier relief of symptoms (16.8 hours; 95% CI 8.4–25.1 hours; $P<.001$). For the assessment of pneumonia prevention in adults with influenza, 8 studies were pooled, which included 2694 patients in the oseltamivir group and 1758 in the placebo group. Oseltamivir led to a reduction in pneumonia (risk difference of 1% [0.22% to 1.49%]). For the assessment of hospitalization prevention in adults with influenza, 7 studies were pooled, which included 2663 patients in the oseltamivir group and 1731 in the placebo group. There was no difference in need for hospitalization (risk ratio: 0.92 [95% CI: 0.57–1.5]; $P = .73$). The pooling of 8 studies in adults, which included 2694 patients in the oseltamivir group and 1758 in the control group, showed that oseltamivir led to more nausea (risk ratio: 1.57 [95% CI: 1.14–2.15]; $P = .005$) and more vomiting (risk ratio: 2.43 [95% CI: 1.75–3.38]; $P<.001$).[106] In aggregate, these meta-analyses indicate that influenza-infected patients treated with oseltamivir have a modest benefit in relief of symptoms and prevention of pneumonia. This comes at the expense of more nausea and vomiting. It should be noted, however, that the patients included in these trials did not seem ill. For instance, studies that enrolled patients with immunosuppressive conditions such as HIV infection or malignancy were not included in the meta-analyses. The inclusion criterion for the pooled studies was the presence of influenza-like-illness rather than pneumonia. Additionally, only one death was reported among all trials that included the adult population.

An earlier systematic review included observational studies that evaluated antiviral therapy versus no therapy or other antiviral therapy in patients with laboratory-confirmed or a clinical diagnosis of influenza. This review of observational studies had important distinctions from the review of randomized clinical trials. First, here the authors pooled studies that included hospitalized patients, a high-risk population. The pooling of 3 studies (total of 681 patients) that adjusted for confounders showed that oseltamivir, as compared with no antiviral therapy, was associated with a reduction in mortality (odds ratio: 0.23 [CI: 0.13–0.43]).[107] The quality of the evidence generated by this review was generally low because it relied on observational studies, which are at risk of confounding despite adjustment in the analyses. However, these observational studies and their meta-analyses fill in important knowledge gaps, which were not and likely will not be addressed by clinical trials.

The efficacy of intravenous peramivir was evaluated in a trial that included 300 previously healthy adults aged 20 to 64 years with the onset of symptoms within the

48 hours before enrollment and a confirmed diagnosis of influenza. Patients were randomized to 300 mg of peramivir, 600 mg of peramivir, or placebo. The primary endpoint was time to alleviation of symptoms. The time to alleviation of symptoms was significantly lower on the groups that received peramivir compared with placebo: 59.1 hours (95% CI 0.9–72.4) in the group that received 300 mg of peramivir, 59.9 hours (95% CI 54.4–68.1) in the group that received 600 mg of peramivir, and 81.8 hours (95% CI 68.0–101.5) in the group that received placebo.[108]

The efficacy of inhaled zanamivir was evaluated in a trial that included 262 previously healthy patients with confirmed influenza. The primary endpoint was time to alleviation of major symptoms of influenza. The mean time to alleviation of symptoms was shorter in the inhaled zamamivir group compared with the placebo group (5.5 vs 6.3 days; $P = .05$).[109]

The efficacy of baloxavir was demonstrated in a phase 3 clinical trial that enrolled 1064 patients with acute uncomplicated influenza. The comparison was to placebo and oseltamivir. The primary endpoint was alleviation of symptoms. The median time to alleviation of symptoms with baloxavir was shorter when compared with placebo (65.4 hours vs 88.6 hours, $P < .001$) and similar when compared with oseltamivir (53.5 hours vs 53.8 hours).[101]

The Centers for Disease Control and Prevention recommends that treatment be initiated as soon as possible for those hospitalized; patients with severe, complicated, or progressive disease; and those at higher risk for influenza complications. For these patients, the first choice antiviral agent is oseltamivir given the relative paucity of data for inhaled zanamivir and intravenous peramivir.[105] We agree with the Centers for Disease Control and Prevention recommendations, and as such, we submit that all influenza-infected patients with pneumonia, a complication from influenza, should receive antiviral therapy. In the absence of a sensitive point-of-care polymerase chain reaction, clinicians have to decide whether to initiate empiric treatment of influenza pneumonia. Strong consideration should be given to surveillance data and risk factors for influenza. It is important to note that not only an influenza diagnosis is often missed but also clinicians often fail to prescribe antiviral influenza treatment when a clinical diagnosis of influenza is made and there is indication for treatment.[110,111] The benefit from treatment is greatest when it is started early but a survival benefit has been demonstrated with treatment up to 5 days after symptom initiation.[112] See **Fig. 6**.

Coronavirus Disease 2019

The treatment can be divided into outpatient and inpatient. In the outpatient setting, treatment should be selected for those at high risk of disease progression.[113] Factors and conditions leading to high risk of disease progression include older age (especially >50 years old), racial and ethnic minorities, residence in long-term care facility, underlying medical problems (eg, chronic lung and heart diseases), and immunocompromised status.[52] In the outpatient setting, the preferred treatment is ritonavir-boosted nirmatrelvir, which is an oral antiviral agent that inhibits the SARS-CoV-2-3CL protease. The inhibition of the cytochrome P450 3A4 by the ritonavir component leads to several interactions between ritonavir-boosted nirmatrelvir and other medications. Clinicians should review the patient's medication list, including prescribed and nonprescribed medications, before initiating treatment with ritonavir-boosted nirmatrelvir. If potential interactions are identified, strategies such as dose reduction or temporary discontinuation of a chronic medication while patient takes ritonavir-boosted nirmatrelvir, can be implemented. Second choice is remdesivir,[113,114] which is an intravenous antiviral drug that inhibits the RNA-dependent RNA polymerase of coronaviruses, thereby stopping the replication and transcription of the coronavirus genome.[115] The intravenous route

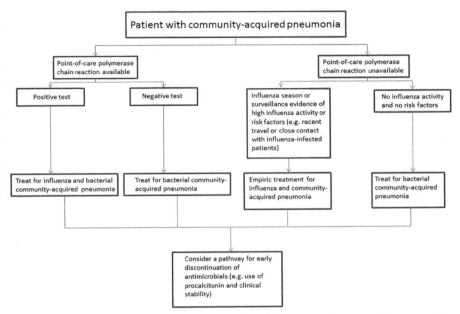

Fig. 6. Treatment approach in patients presenting with community-acquired pneumonia.

of administration can pose logistic barriers to the widespread use of this medication in the outpatient setting, particularly in times of surge of COVID-19 transmission. An alternative medication is molnupiravir, an oral antiviral agent that is converted from a ribonucleoside into N-hydroxycytidine. The latter form inhibits SARS-CoV-2 replication by biding to its genome. The modest efficacy of molnupiravir has led the National Institutes of Health to recommend molnupiravir only when the other options are not available or feasible to use.[113,114] Data from studies in animals show molnupiravir has the potential to cause fetal harm. The use of molnupiravir in pregnancy is not recommended. Concern for fetal harm with molnupiravir mandates pregnancy test in women of childbearing potential and contraception during treatment and for 4 days after treatment completion. Men should use contraception during treatment and for 3 months after treatment completion if they are sexually active and have a female partner of childbearing potential.[114,116]

In hospitalized patients, the treatment options of COVID-19 depend on the severity of the disease. In patients hospitalized for COVID-19 who have infiltrate on chest imaging or tachypnea or oxygen saturation less than 94%, the use of remdesivir led to a faster recovery. Remdesivir seems mainly beneficial early in the disease process and did not lead to better outcomes in patients on mechanical ventilation or extracorporeal membrane oxygenation.[117] The use of systemic corticosteroid leads to better outcomes in patients hospitalized for COVID-19. The largest trial assessing systemic corticosteroid in patients with COVID-19 enrolled 6425 patients. Dexamethasone led to a reduction in mortality in those requiring oxygen therapy or mechanical ventilation. The mortality benefit was more pronounced in those requiring mechanical ventilation.[118] Other immunosuppressive medications such as the interleukin-6 inhibitor tocilizumab and Janus kinase inhibitors (eg, Baricitinib) have improved outcomes in hospitalized patients with COVID-19[119,120] and are currently recommended for patients who deteriorate despite therapy with dexamethasone.[113]

Other Respiratory Viruses

For the treatment of pneumonia caused by respiratory viruses other than influenza and SARS-CoV-2, defining whether the patient is immunocompetent or immunosuppressed is important. In immunocompetent patients, current antiviral treatment options are limited, generally reserved for severely ill patients, and based on anecdotal data. For instance, case reports and series have reported the use of cidofovir for the treatment of severe pneumonia caused by adenovirus in nonimmunocompromised patients.[121,122] Even though patients had clinical improvement in these series, those studies were uncontrolled and thus do not allow a firm conclusion as to the efficacy of cidofovir. Antiviral treatment of pneumonia caused by viruses of the Herpesviridae family in immunocompetent hosts has been reported in severe cases.[123,124] In pregnant women with varicella-zoster-virus pneumonia, the mortality is high, and treatment with intravenous acyclovir is indicated.[125]

In immunosuppressed patients, aerosolized ribavirin, oral ribavirin, intravenous immunoglobulin, hyperimmunoglobulin, and palivizumab are treatment options that have been used in respiratory syncytial virus infection, particularly in patients with hematological malignancy or transplant recipients.[126] For cytomegalovirus pneumonia, treatment includes intravenous ganciclovir.[127] The addition of cytomegalovirus immunoglobulin to ganciclovir seems to lead to improved survival according to a case series.[128] An alternative treatment of cytomegalovirus pneumonia is intravenous foscarnet.[129] For the treatment of varicella pneumonia, the indicated treatment is intravenous acyclovir.[130] Similarly, herpes simplex virus pneumonia is treated with intravenous acyclovir.[131] The evidence for the use of these therapies is weak and comes in the form of observational studies. See **Fig. 7**.

DISCONTINUATION OF ANTIBIOTIC THERAPY

The identification of a viral pathogen in pneumonia does not always warrant deescalation or discontinuation of empirical antibiotics because dual bacterial-viral infection can occur. The clinical context and the identified viral pathogen should be factored in the decision to initiate and deescalate or discontinue empirical antibiotic. The prevalence of dual bacterial-viral infection varies according to the virus. For example, coinfection and superimposed infections are common with influenza. In a study that included 645 critically ill patients with 2009 influenza A (H1N1) virus infection, coinfection occurred in 17.5% of the patients. Of these, more than half were due to *Streptococcus pneumoniae*.[132] However, coinfection on presentation is not as common with SARS-CoV-2. A pooled analysis found that 7% of patients hospitalized with COVID-19 have bacterial coinfection.[133] Another pooled analysis found that on presentation bacterial coinfection was present in 5.9% (95%CI 3.8%–8.0%) in all hospitalized patients and 8.1% in critically ill patients (95%CI 2.3–13.8).[134] Bacterial coinfection is thus infrequent in SARS-CoV-2 infection, and for most patients diagnosed with COVID-19 pneumonia, empirical antibiotic therapy is not warranted on presentation.

The recognition that dual bacterial-viral may occur seems to be reflected in clinical practice. In an observational study before the COVID-19 pandemic, most patients with respiratory tract infection admitted to the hospital who turned out to have an identified viral pathogen did not have their antibiotics discontinued.[135] However, the use of a clinical pathway integrating the results of viral microbiology testing with clinical findings and procalcitonin testing could have a role in the safe discontinuation of antibiotics. It is now well established that the use of procalcitonin to guide initiation and discontinuation of antibiotic in patients with acute respiratory tract infection leads to less use of antibiotics without worsening the outcomes.[136]

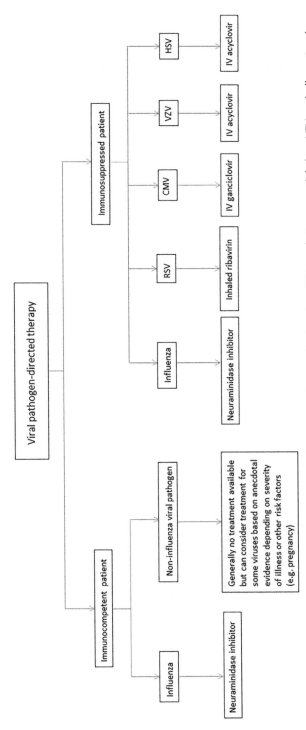

Fig. 7. Viral pathogen-directed therapy. CMV, cytomegalovirus; HSV, herpes simplex virus; RSV, respiratory syncytial virus; VZV, varicella-zoster virus.

In a randomized clinical trial of 300 hospitalized patients with lower respiratory tract infection, the use of combined procalcitonin and viral polymerase chain reaction tests was compared with standard care. Both groups had similar antibiotic exposure. However, a lower proportion of patients with a positive viral polymerase chain reaction test and low procalcitonin received antibiotic on discharge as compared with standard care.[137] This study suggests that the result of a viral polymerase chain reaction test has the impact to further influence decision-making even after procalcitonin and clinical evolution are factored in. It should be noted, however, that this was a feasibility study and patients with pneumonia were excluded. Additionally, viral polymerase chain reaction test result may not influence antibiotic decision in the absence of a protocol. This was shown in an observational, retrospective study in which only 10.5% of patients had antibiotic discontinued within 48 hours of a positive viral respiratory panel and a low procalcitonin result.[138]

Another randomized clinical trial assessed the effect of point-of-care respiratory viral panel in patients with acute respiratory illness or fever. The study enrolled 720 patients. There was no difference in the primary endpoint, which was the proportion of patients treated with antibiotics. However, the relevance of the primary outcome was impaired because many patients received antibiotics before the results of the point-of-care test. A significantly greater proportion of patients in the point-of-care group received only a single dose of antibiotics (10% vs 3%) or antibiotics for less than 48 hours (17% vs 9%).[139]

In summary, there is weak but mounting evidence that the use of nucleic acid amplification tests have the potential to aid in the decision to discontinue antibiotics in patients with respiratory infection (including pneumonia) but it is more likely to do so if integrated with clinical findings and procalcitonin. Additionally, continuing clinician education will be important to ensure implementation of strategies to minimize antibiotic exposure. Antibiotic stewardship programs can play an important role in minimizing inadequate antibiotic prescriptions for hospitalized patients through monitoring of emerging information and update of guidelines, revision of the relevant literature, and education of treating clinicians.[140]

CORTICOSTEROID THERAPY

An exuberant inflammatory response can play a major role in the morbidity and mortality of patients with pneumonia. Corticosteroid has been used as a way of mitigating the exacerbated inflammatory response in these patients. Recently, 2 large clinical trials that addressed systemic corticosteroid in severe CAP have been published. In one trial that included 795 patients, the use of dexamethasone for patients with CAP admitted to the ICU lead to a 28-day mortality benefit compared with placebo (6.2%; 95% CI, 3.9–8.6 in the vs 11.9%; 95% CI, 8.7–15.1; $P = .006$). This study excluded patients with influenza.[141] In another trial that included 584 patients with severe CAP, the use of methylprednisolone, as compared with placebo, did not lead to a significant improvement in 60-day mortality (16% in the methylprednisolone group vs 18% in the placebo group; $P = .61$) but the systemic corticosteroid was initiated later in this trial. This study did not exclude patients with influenza but only 4% of the patients tested positive for influenza.[142]

The 2009 H1N1 pandemic brought to light the use of systemic corticosteroid in influenza pneumonia. Some studies revealed that 40% to 50% of patients with severe influenza pneumonia received corticosteroid during the pandemic.[143,144] Unfortunately, although corticosteroid seems to be beneficial in patients with severe CAP, the same may not hold true for patients with influenza pneumonia, a condition in which corticosteroids might be detrimental as demonstrated in the systematic review. In this study, the authors pooled 10 observational studies (total of 1497 patients) and found that corticosteroid therapy was associated with higher odds of death (OR, 2.12; 95% CI, 1.36–3.29). Of note, the studies included in the meta-analysis were predominantly conducted during the 2009 H1N1 influenza pandemic and in the ICU setting.[145]

A clinical trial designed to evaluate the effect of systemic corticosteroid in ICU patients with the 2009 H1N1 influenza pneumonia was unable to enroll the planned number of patients, highlighting the difficulties in conducting a clinical trial during a pandemic.[144] A limitation of the observational studies assessing corticosteroid therapy in influenza pneumonia is the possibility of confounding by indication, that is, the possibility that sicker patients are more often prescribed systemic corticosteroid. This has the potential to cause the false impression that corticosteroid therapy leads to worse outcomes in influenza pneumonia. Some studies adjusted for confounding factors but residual confounding can still occur. In the absence of randomized clinical trials, and in view of the results of observational studies, it is our opinion that currently corticosteroid therapy should not be administered in influenza pneumonia.

As previously discussed, systemic corticosteroid leads to better outcomes in patients hospitalized for COVID-19.[118] The effect of corticosteroid in patients with non-influenza and non-SARS-CoV-2 viral pneumonia is unclear.

FUTURE RESEARCH

The advent of nucleic acid amplification tests improved our understanding of the epidemiology of viral infections in pneumonia and enabled an etiologic diagnosis of viral infection in a large proportion of patients with pneumonia. However, one of the downsides of nucleic acid amplifications tests was a relatively long turn around, limiting its clinical utility. This has been overcome by the development of "point-of-care" polymerase chain reaction tests that have a turnaround time of approximately 1 hour.[146] The assessment of these point-of-care tests in clinical pathways is a promising venue for clinical investigation. As these tests are being rapidly integrated into clinical practice, it is important to study their cost-effectiveness and whether they influence outcomes or decision-making. A potential downside of polymerase chain reaction test is that persistent viral shedding leading to positive result occurs in some patients despite symptom resolution and no evidence of contagiousness.[147]

Ongoing research on antiviral treatment is promising. Just as for bacterial infection, combination therapy has been studied in influenza infection with different goals such as preventing pathogen resistance,[148,149] mitigating the inflammatory response,[150] or achieving synergy.[151,152] There has been development of new compounds for the treatment of respiratory syncytial virus. These include a fusion inhibitor, which prevents the fusion of respiratory syncytial virus viral envelope with the host cell membrane, and a nucleoside analog, which prevents respiratory syncytial virus replication.[153,154]

SUMMARY

Viral respiratory infection is common in pneumonia and is present in approximately 25% of patients with community-acquired pneumonia. It is also common in immunosuppressed patients but the latter are susceptible not only to the usual community-acquired respiratory viruses but also to viruses of the Herpesviridae family. Recent data show that respiratory viruses are also identified in hospital-acquired infections. The clinical diagnosis of viral infection is challenging. Clinical prediction rules have been developed for the diagnosis of influenza infection but they showed only modest accuracy. Similarly, radiological studies are nonspecific. In the end, the diagnosis of viral infection relies on the recognition that respiratory viruses are commonly present in pneumonia, and on the systematic performance of viral microbiology studies, particularly nucleic acid amplifications tests. The treatment of influenza pneumonia is currently with a neuraminidase inhibitor. Treatment of COVID-19 is also available and differs according to the setting (inpatient vs outpatient). The treatment options for pneumonia caused by other viruses in immunocompetent patients with pneumonia are limited, and the data are largely anecdotal. In immunosuppressed patients with infection by respiratory syncytial virus or a virus of the Herpesviridae family, there are antiviral treatments available. There is ongoing research involved with the development and testing of new treatment strategies both for influenza and non-influenza viruses.

DISCLOSURE

R.Cavallazzi: Site investigator for a study that aims to assess the safety of a monoclonal antibody for community-acquired bacterial pneumonia.

REFERENCES

1. Iuliano AD, Roguski KM, Chang HH, et al. Estimates of global seasonal influenza-associated respiratory mortality: a modelling study. Lancet 2018; 391(10127):1285–300.
2. Jain S, Self WH, Wunderink RG, et al. Community-acquired pneumonia requiring hospitalization among U.S. adults. N Engl J Med 2015;373(5):415–27.
3. Horimoto T, Kawaoka Y. Influenza: lessons from past pandemics, warnings from current incidents. Nat Rev Microbiol 2005;3(8):591–600.
4. Zimmer SM, Burke DS. Historical perspective–Emergence of influenza A (H1N1) viruses. N Engl J Med 2009;361(3):279–85.
5. Centers for Disease Control and Prevention. Influenza activity in the United States during the 2022–23 season and composition of the 2023–24 influenza vaccine. https://www.cdc.gov/flu/spotlights/2023-2024/22-23-summary-technical-report.htm#print.
6. De Clercq E, Li G. Approved antiviral drugs over the past 50 years. Clin Microbiol Rev 2016;29(3):695–747.
7. Kamali A, Holodniy M. Influenza treatment and prophylaxis with neuraminidase inhibitors: a review. Infect Drug Resist 2013;6:187–98.
8. Bouvier NM, Palese P. The biology of influenza viruses. Vaccine 2008;26(Suppl 4):D49–53.
9. McLellan JS, Ray WC, Peeples ME. Structure and function of respiratory syncytial virus surface glycoproteins. Curr Top Microbiol Immunol 2013;372:83–104.
10. Jacobs SE, Lamson DM, St George K, et al. Human rhinoviruses. Clin Microbiol Rev 2013;26(1):135–62.
11. San Martín C. Latest insights on adenovirus structure and assembly. Viruses 2012;4(5):847–77.
12. Henrickson KJ. Parainfluenza viruses. Clin Microbiol Rev 2003;16(2):242–64.
13. de Haan CA, Kuo L, Masters PS, et al. Coronavirus particle assembly: primary structure requirements of the membrane protein. J Virol 1998;72(8):6838–50.
14. Wen X, Krause JC, Leser GP, et al. Structure of the human metapneumovirus fusion protein with neutralizing antibody identifies a pneumovirus antigenic site. Nat Struct Mol Biol 2012;19(4):461–3.
15. Gurda BL, Parent KN, Bladek H, et al. Human bocavirus capsid structure: insights into the structural repertoire of the parvoviridae. J Virol 2010;84(12):5880–9.

16. Melero JA, Mas V. The Pneumovirinae fusion (F) protein: a common target for vaccines and antivirals. Virus Res 2015;209:128–35.

17. Thibaut HJ, De Palma AM, Neyts J. Combating enterovirus replication: state-of-the-art on antiviral research. Biochem Pharmacol 2012;83(2):185–92.

18. Olson NH, Kolatkar PR, Oliveira MA, et al. Structure of a human rhinovirus complexed with its receptor molecule. Proc Natl Acad Sci U S A 1993;90(2):507–11.

19. Bosch BJ, van der Zee R, de Haan CA, et al. The coronavirus spike protein is a class I virus fusion protein: structural and functional characterization of the fusion core complex. J Virol 2003;77(16):8801–11.

20. Burk M, El-Kersh K, Saad M, et al. Viral infection in community-acquired pneumonia: a systematic review and meta-analysis. Eur Respir Rev 2016;25(140):178.

21. Yin YD, Zhao F, Ren LL, et al. Evaluation of the Japanese Respiratory Society guidelines for the identification of Mycoplasma pneumoniae pneumonia. Respirology 2012;17(7):1131–6.

22. Choi SH, Hong SB, Ko GB, et al. Viral infection in patients with severe pneumonia requiring intensive care unit admission. Am J Respir Crit Care Med 2012;186(4):325–32.

23. Karhu J, Ala-Kokko TI, Vuorinen T, et al. Lower respiratory tract virus findings in mechanically ventilated patients with severe community-acquired pneumonia. Clin Infect Dis 2014;59(1):62–70.

24. Ramirez JA, Wiemken TL, Peyrani P, et al. adults hospitalized with pneumonia in the united states: incidence, epidemiology, and mortality. Clin Infect Dis 2017; 65(11):1806–12.

25. Couch RB, Englund JA, Whimbey E. Respiratory viral infections in immunocompetent and immunocompromised persons. Am J Med 1997;102(3a):2–9, discussion 25-6.

26. Meyers JD, Flournoy N, Thomas ED. Nonbacterial pneumonia after allogeneic marrow transplantation: a review of ten years' experience. Rev Infect Dis 1982; 4(6):1119–32.

27. Kim DH, Messner H, Minden M, et al. Factors influencing varicella zoster virus infection after allogeneic peripheral blood stem cell transplantation: low-dose acyclovir prophylaxis and pre-transplant diagnosis of lymphoproliferative disorders. Transpl Infect Dis 2008;10(2):90–8.

28. Koc Y, Miller KB, Schenkein DP, et al. Varicella zoster virus infections following allogeneic bone marrow transplantation: frequency, risk factors, and clinical outcome. Biol Blood Marrow Transplant 2000;6(1):44–9.

29. Green ML. Viral pneumonia in patients with hematopoietic cell transplantation and hematologic malignancies. Clin Chest Med 2017;38(2):295–305.

30. Hong HL, Hong SB, Ko GB, et al. Viral infection is not uncommon in adult patients with severe hospital-acquired pneumonia. PLoS One 2014;9(4):e95865. https://doi.org/10.1371/journal.pone.0095865.

31. Dawood FS, Iuliano AD, Reed C, et al. Estimated global mortality associated with the first 12 months of 2009 pandemic influenza A H1N1 virus circulation: a modelling study. Lancet Infect Dis. Sep 2012;12(9):687–95.

32. Lee N, Hui D, Wu A, et al. A major outbreak of severe acute respiratory syndrome in Hong Kong. N Engl J Med 2003;348(20):1986–94.

33. Ksiazek TG, Erdman D, Goldsmith CS, et al. A novel coronavirus associated with severe acute respiratory syndrome. N Engl J Med 2003;348(20):1953–66.

34. Drosten C, Günther S, Preiser W, et al. Identification of a novel coronavirus in patients with severe acute respiratory syndrome. N Engl J Med 2003;348(20): 1967–76.

35. Zaki AM, van Boheemen S, Bestebroer TM, et al. Isolation of a novel coronavirus from a man with pneumonia in Saudi Arabia. N Engl J Med 2012;367(19):1814–20.

36. de Groot RJ, Baker SC, Baric RS, et al. Middle East respiratory syndrome coronavirus (MERS-CoV): announcement of the Coronavirus Study Group. J Virol 2013;87(14):7790–2.

37. Lim YX, Ng YL, Tam JP, et al. Human coronaviruses: a review of virus-host interactions. Diseases 2016;4(3). https://doi.org/10.3390/diseases4030026.

38. Guery B, Poissy J, el Mansouf L, et al. Clinical features and viral diagnosis of two cases of infection with Middle East Respiratory Syndrome coronavirus: a report of nosocomial transmission. Lancet 2013;381(9885):2265–72.

39. Assiri A, McGeer A, Perl TM, et al. Hospital outbreak of Middle East respiratory syndrome coronavirus. N Engl J Med 2013;369(5):407–16.

40. Bialek SR, Allen D, Alvarado-Ramy F, et al. First confirmed cases of Middle East respiratory syndrome coronavirus (MERS-CoV) infection in the United States, updated information on the epidemiology of MERS-CoV infection, and guidance for the public, clinicians, and public health authorities - May 2014. MMWR Morb Mortal Wkly Rep 2014;63(19):431–6.

41. World Health Organization. Middle East respiratory syndrome: global summary and assessment of risk - 16 November 2022. https://www.who.int/publications/i/item/WHO-MERS-RA-2022.1.

42. Centers for Disease Control and Prevention. Preliminary estimated influenza illnesses, medical visits, hospitalizations, and deaths in the United States – 2021-2022 influenza season. https://www.cdc.gov/flu/about/burden/2021-2022.htm#table01.

43. Casalino E, Antoniol S, Fidouh N, et al. Influenza virus infections among patients attending emergency department according to main reason to presenting to ED: A 3-year prospective observational study during seasonal epidemic periods. PLoS One 2017;12(8):e0182191.

44. Garg S, Jain S, Dawood FS, et al. Pneumonia among adults hospitalized with laboratory-confirmed seasonal influenza virus infection-United States, 2005-2008. BMC Infect Dis 2015;15:369.

45. Maruyama T, Fujisawa T, Suga S, et al. Outcomes and prognostic features of patients with influenza requiring hospitalization and receiving early antiviral therapy: a prospective multicenter cohort study. Chest. Feb 2016;149(2):526–34.

46. Blanton L, Mustaquim D, Alabi N, et al. Update: influenza activity - United States, October 2, 2016-February 4, 2017. MMWR Morb Mortal Wkly Rep 2017;66(6):159–66.

47. World Health Organization. WHO Coronavirus (COVID-19) Dashboard. https://covid19.who.int/.

48. Centers for Disease Control and Prevention. Covid Data Tracker. https://covid.cdc.gov/covid-data-tracker/#variant-proportions.

49. Hughes TD, Subramanian A, Chakraborty R, et al. The effect of SARS-CoV-2 variant on respiratory features and mortality. Sci Rep 2023;13(1):4503.

50. Menni C, Valdes AM, Polidori L, et al. Symptom prevalence, duration, and risk of hospital admission in individuals infected with SARS-CoV-2 during periods of omicron and delta variant dominance: a prospective observational study from the ZOE COVID Study. Lancet 2022;399(10335):1618–24.

51. Adjei S, Hong K, Molinari NM, et al. mortality risk among patients hospitalized primarily for COVID-19 during the omicron and delta variant pandemic periods - United States, April 2020-June 2022. MMWR Morb Mortal Wkly Rep 2022;71(37):1182–9.

52. Centers for Disease Control and Prevention. Underlying medical conditions associated with higher risk for severe covid-19: Information for healthcare professionals. https://www.cdc.gov/coronavirus/2019-ncov/hcp/clinical-care/under lyingconditions.html.
53. Tai DBG, Shah A, Doubeni CA, et al. The disproportionate impact of COVID-19 on racial and ethnic minorities in the United States. Clin Infect Dis 2021;72(4): 703–6.
54. Johnson AG, Linde L, Ali AR, et al. COVID-19 incidence and mortality among unvaccinated and vaccinated persons aged ≥12 years by receipt of bivalent booster doses and time since vaccination - 24 U.S. jurisdictions, October 3, 2021-December 24, 2022. MMWR Morb Mortal Wkly Rep 2023;72(6):145–52.
55. Falsey AR, Hennessey PA, Formica MA, et al. Respiratory syncytial virus infection in elderly and high-risk adults. N Engl J Med 2005;352(17):1749–59.
56. Zhou H, Thompson WW, Viboud CG, et al. Hospitalizations associated with influenza and respiratory syncytial virus in the United States, 1993-2008. Clin Infect Dis 2012;54(10):1427–36.
57. Gwaltney JM. Clinical significance and pathogenesis of viral respiratory infections. Am J Med 2002;112(Suppl 6A):13s–8s.
58. Monto AS. The seasonality of rhinovirus infections and its implications for clinical recognition. Clin Ther 2002;24(12):1987–97.
59. Gaunt ER, Hardie A, Claas EC, et al. Epidemiology and clinical presentations of the four human coronaviruses 229E, HKU1, NL63, and OC43 detected over 3 years using a novel multiplex real-time PCR method. J Clin Microbiol 2010; 48(8):2940–7.
60. Gerna G, Percivalle E, Sarasini A, et al. Human respiratory coronavirus HKU1 versus other coronavirus infections in Italian hospitalised patients. J Clin Virol 2007;38(3):244–50.
61. Ruuskanen O, Mertsola J, Meurman O. Adenovirus infection in families. Arch Dis Child 1988;63(10):1250–3.
62. Tan D, Zhu H, Fu Y, et al. Severe community-acquired pneumonia caused by human adenovirus in immunocompetent adults: a multicenter case series. PLoS One 2016;11(3):e0151199. https://doi.org/10.1371/journal.pone.0151199.
63. Cao B, Huang GH, Pu ZH, et al. Emergence of community-acquired adenovirus type 55 as a cause of community-onset pneumonia. Chest 2014;145(1):79–86.
64. Shields AF, Hackman RC, Fife KH, et al. Adenovirus infections in patients undergoing bone-marrow transplantation. N Engl J Med 1985;312(9):529–33.
65. Berciaud S, Rayne F, Kassab S, et al. Adenovirus infections in Bordeaux University Hospital 2008-2010: clinical and virological features. J Clin Virol 2012;54(4): 302–7.
66. Park JY, Kim BJ, Lee EJ, et al. Clinical features and courses of adenovirus pneumonia in healthy young adults during an outbreak among korean military personnel. PLoS One 2017;12(1):e0170592. https://doi.org/10.1371/journal.pone.0170592.
67. Klinger JR, Sanchez MP, Curtin LA, et al. Multiple cases of life-threatening adenovirus pneumonia in a mental health care center. Am J Respir Crit Care Med 1998;157(2):645–9.
68. Cassir N, Hraiech S, Nougairede A, et al. Outbreak of adenovirus type 1 severe pneumonia in a French intensive care unit, September-October 2012. Euro Surveill 2014;19(39). https://doi.org/10.2807/1560-7917.es2014.19.39.20914.
69. Weinberg GA, Hall CB, Iwane MK, et al. Parainfluenza virus infection of young children: estimates of the population-based burden of hospitalization. J Pediatr 2009;154(5):694–9.

70. Liu WK, Liu Q, Chen DH, et al. Epidemiology and clinical presentation of the four human parainfluenza virus types. BMC Infect Dis 2013;13:28.
71. Marx A, Gary HE Jr, Marston BJ, et al. Parainfluenza virus infection among adults hospitalized for lower respiratory tract infection. Clin Infect Dis 1999; 29(1):134–40.
72. Falsey AR, Erdman D, Anderson LJ, et al. Human metapneumovirus infections in young and elderly adults. J Infect Dis 2003;187(5):785–90.
73. Johnstone J, Majumdar SR, Fox JD, et al. Human metapneumovirus pneumonia in adults: results of a prospective study. Clin Infect Dis 2008;46(4):571–4.
74. Longtin J, Bastien M, Gilca R, et al. Human bocavirus infections in hospitalized children and adults. Emerg Infect Dis 2008;14(2):217–21.
75. Ghietto LM, Majul D, Ferreyra Soaje P, et al. Comorbidity and high viral load linked to clinical presentation of respiratory human bocavirus infection. Arch Virol 2015;160(1):117–27.
76. Jula A, Waris M, Kantola K, et al. Primary and secondary human bocavirus 1 infections in a family, Finland. Emerg Infect Dis 2013;19(8):1328–31.
77. Mori D, Ranawaka U, Yamada K, et al. Human bocavirus in patients with encephalitis, Sri Lanka, 2009-2010. Emerg Infect Dis 2013;19(11):1859–62.
78. Yu JM, Chen QQ, Hao YX, et al. Identification of human bocaviruses in the cerebrospinal fluid of children hospitalized with encephalitis in China. J Clin Virol 2013;57(4):374–7.
79. Windisch W, Schildgen V, Malecki M, et al. Detection of HBoV DNA in idiopathic lung fibrosis, Cologne, Germany. J Clin Virol 2013;58(1):325–7.
80. Krakau M, Brockmann M, Titius B, et al. Acute human bocavirus infection in MDS patient, Cologne, Germany. J Clin Virol 2015;69:44–7.
81. Falcone V, Ridder GJ, Panning M, et al. Human bocavirus DNA in paranasal sinus mucosa. Emerg Infect Dis 2011;17(8):1564–5.
82. Stein J, Louie J, Flanders S, et al. Performance characteristics of clinical diagnosis, a clinical decision rule, and a rapid influenza test in the detection of influenza infection in a community sample of adults. Ann Emerg Med 2005;46(5): 412–9.
83. Oliveira EC, Marik PE, Colice G. Influenza pneumonia: a descriptive study. Chest 2001;119(6):1717–23.
84. Michiels B, Thomas I, Van Royen P, et al. Clinical prediction rules combining signs, symptoms and epidemiological context to distinguish influenza from influenza-like illnesses in primary care: a cross sectional study. BMC Fam Pract 2011;12:4.
85. Ebell MH, Afonso A. A systematic review of clinical decision rules for the diagnosis of influenza. Ann Fam Med 2011;9(1):69–77.
86. Boivin G, Hardy I, Tellier G, et al. Predicting influenza infections during epidemics with use of a clinical case definition. Clin Infect Dis 2000;31(5):1166–9.
87. Dugas AF, Valsamakis A, Atreya MR, et al. Clinical diagnosis of influenza in the ED. Am J Emerg Med 2015;33(6):770–5.
88. McGee S. Simplifying likelihood ratios. J Gen Intern Med 2002;17(8):646–9.
89. Uyeki TM, Bernstein HH, Bradley JS, et al. Clinical practice guidelines by the infectious diseases society of america: 2018 update on diagnosis, treatment, chemoprophylaxis, and institutional outbreak management of seasonal influenzaa. Clin Infect Dis 2018;68(6):e1–47.
90. Saha S, Chadha M, Al Mamun A, et al. Influenza seasonality and vaccination timing in tropical and subtropical areas of southern and south-eastern Asia. Bull World Health Organ 2014;92(5):318–30.

91. Walsh EE, Peterson DR, Falsey AR. Is clinical recognition of respiratory syncytial virus infection in hospitalized elderly and high-risk adults possible? J Infect Dis 2007;195(7):1046–51.
92. Dowell SF, Anderson LJ, Gary HE Jr, et al. Respiratory syncytial virus is an important cause of community-acquired lower respiratory infection among hospitalized adults. J Infect Dis 1996;174(3):456–62.
93. Huijskens EGW, Koopmans M, Palmen FMH, et al. The value of signs and symptoms in differentiating between bacterial, viral and mixed aetiology in patients with community-acquired pneumonia. J Med Microbiol 2014;63(Pt 3):441–52.
94. Heckerling PS, Tape TG, Wigton RS, et al. Clinical prediction rule for pulmonary infiltrates. Ann Intern Med 1990;113(9):664–70.
95. Aviram G, Bar-Shai A, Sosna J, et al. H1N1 influenza: initial chest radiographic findings in helping predict patient outcome. Radiology 2010;255(1):252–9.
96. Woo PC, Lau SK, Tsoi HW, et al. Clinical and molecular epidemiological features of coronavirus HKU1-associated community-acquired pneumonia. J Infect Dis 2005;192(11):1898–907.
97. Chong S, Lee KS, Kim TS, et al. Adenovirus pneumonia in adults: radiographic and high-resolution CT findings in five patients. AJR Am J Roentgenol 2006; 186(5):1288–93.
98. Wang K, Xi W, Yang D, et al. Rhinovirus is associated with severe adult community-acquired pneumonia in China. J Thorac Dis 2017;9(11):4502–11.
99. Kanne JP, Bai H, Bernheim A, et al. COVID-19 imaging: what we know now and what remains unknown. Radiology 2021;299(3):E262–79.
100. Ikematsu H, Hayden FG, Kawaguchi K, et al. Baloxavir marboxil for prophylaxis against influenza in household contacts. N Engl J Med 2020;383(4):309–20.
101. Hayden FG, Sugaya N, Hirotsu N, et al. Baloxavir marboxil for uncomplicated influenza in adults and adolescents. N Engl J Med 2018;379(10):913–23.
102. Moscona A. Neuraminidase inhibitors for influenza. N Engl J Med 2005;353(13): 1363–73.
103. Todd B, Tchesnokov EP, Götte M. The active form of the influenza cap-snatching endonuclease inhibitor baloxavir marboxil is a tight binding inhibitor. J Biol Chem 2021;296:100486.
104. Wang C, Takeuchi K, Pinto LH, et al. Ion channel activity of influenza A virus M2 protein: characterization of the amantadine block. J Virol 1993;67(9):5585–94.
105. Centers for Disease Control and Prevention. Influenza antiviral medications: Summary for clinicians. https://www.cdc.gov/flu/professionals/antivirals/summary-clinicians.htm.
106. Jefferson T, Jones M, Doshi P, et al. Oseltamivir for influenza in adults and children: systematic review of clinical study reports and summary of regulatory comments. BMJ 2014;348:g2545.
107. Hsu J, Santesso N, Mustafa R, et al. Antivirals for treatment of influenza: a systematic review and meta-analysis of observational studies. Ann Intern Med 2012;156(7):512–24.
108. Kohno S, Kida H, Mizuguchi M, et al, S-021812 Clinical Study Group. Efficacy and safety of intravenous peramivir for treatment of seasonal influenza virus infection. Antimicrob Agents Chemother 2010;54(11):4568–74.
109. Hayden FG, Osterhaus AD, Treanor JJ, et al. Efficacy and safety of the neuraminidase inhibitor zanamivir in the treatment of influenzavirus infections. GG167 Influenza Study Group. N Engl J Med 1997;337(13):874–80.

110. Biggerstaff M, Jhung MA, Reed C, et al. Impact of medical and behavioural factors on influenza-like illness, healthcare-seeking, and antiviral treatment during the 2009 H1N1 pandemic: USA, 2009-2010. Epidemiol Infect 2014;142(1):114–25.

111. Lindegren ML, Schaffner W. Treatment with neuraminidase inhibitors for high-risk patients with influenza: why is adherence to antiviral treatment recommendations so low? J Infect Dis 2014;210(4):510–3.

112. Louie JK, Yang S, Acosta M, et al. Treatment with neuraminidase inhibitors for critically ill patients with influenza A (H1N1)pdm09. Clin Infect Dis 2012;55(9):1198–204.

113. National Institutes of Health. Coronavirus disease 2019 (covid-19) treatment guidelines. Clinical management of adults summary. https://www.covid19treatmentguidelines.nih.gov/management/clinical-management-of-adults/clinical-management-of-adults-summary/?utm_source=site&utm_medium=home&utm_campaign=highlights.

114. Cavallazzi R, Ramirez JA. How and when to manage respiratory infections out of hospital. Eur Respir Rev 2022;31(166). https://doi.org/10.1183/16000617.0092-2022.

115. Kokic G, Hillen HS, Tegunov D, et al. Mechanism of SARS-CoV-2 polymerase stalling by remdesivir. Nat Commun 2021;12(1):279.

116. The US Food and Drug Administration. Fact Sheet For Healthcare Providers: Emergency Use Authorization For Lagevrio™ (Molnupiravir) Capsules. 2022, March.

117. Beigel JH, Tomashek KM, Dodd LE, et al. Remdesivir for the treatment of covid-19 — final report. N Engl J Med 2020;383(19):1813–26.

118. Horby P, Lim WS, Emberson JR, et al. Dexamethasone in hospitalized patients with covid-19. N Engl J Med 2021;384(8):693–704.

119. Abani O, Abbas A, Abbas F, et al. Tocilizumab in patients admitted to hospital with COVID-19 (RECOVERY): a randomised, controlled, open-label, platform trial. Lancet 2021;397(10285):1637–45.

120. Kalil AC, Patterson TF, Mehta AK, et al. Baricitinib plus remdesivir for hospitalized adults with Covid-19. N Engl J Med 2020;384(9):795–807.

121. Kim SJ, Kim K, Park SB, et al. Outcomes of early administration of cidofovir in non-immunocompromised patients with severe adenovirus pneumonia. PLoS One 2015;10(4):e0122642.

122. Lee M, Kim S, Kwon OJ, et al. Treatment of adenoviral acute respiratory distress syndrome using cidofovir with extracorporeal membrane oxygenation. J Intensive Care Med 2017;32(3):231–8.

123. Grilli E, Galati V, Bordi L, et al. Cytomegalovirus pneumonia in immunocompetent host: case report and literature review. J Clin Virol 2012;55(4):356–9.

124. Hunt DP, Muse VV, Pitman MB. Case records of the Massachusetts General Hospital. Case 12-2013. An 18-year-old woman with pulmonary infiltrates and respiratory failure. N Engl J Med 2013;368(16):1537–45.

125. Broussard RC, Payne DK, George RB. Treatment with acyclovir of varicella pneumonia in pregnancy. Chest 1991;99(4):1045–7.

126. Khanna N, Widmer AF, Decker M, et al. Respiratory syncytial virus infection in patients with hematological diseases: single-center study and review of the literature. Clin Infect Dis 2008;46(3):402–12.

127. Tan BH. Cytomegalovirus Treatment. Curr Treat Options Infect Dis 2014;6(3):256–70.

128. Reed EC, Bowden RA, Dandliker PS, et al. Treatment of cytomegalovirus pneumonia with ganciclovir and intravenous cytomegalovirus immunoglobulin in patients with bone marrow transplants. Ann Intern Med 1988;109(10):783–8.

129. Farthing C, Anderson MG, Ellis ME, et al. Treatment of cytomegalovirus pneumonitis with foscarnet (trisodium phosphonoformate) in patients with AIDS. J Med Virol 1987;22(2):157–62.

130. Mohsen AH, McKendrick M. Varicella pneumonia in adults. Eur Respir J 2003; 21(5):886–91.

131. Ferrari A, Luppi M, Potenza L, et al. Herpes simplex virus pneumonia during standard induction chemotherapy for acute leukemia: case report and review of literature. Leukemia 2005;19(11):2019–21.

132. Martín-Loeches I, Sanchez-Corral A, Diaz E, et al. Community-acquired respiratory coinfection in critically ill patients with pandemic 2009 influenza A(H1N1) virus. Chest 2011;139(3):555–62.

133. Lansbury L, Lim B, Baskaran V, et al. Co-infections in people with COVID-19: a systematic review and meta-analysis. J Infect 2020;81(2):266–75.

134. Langford BJ, So M, Raybardhan S, et al. Bacterial co-infection and secondary infection in patients with COVID-19: a living rapid review and meta-analysis. Clin Microbiol Infect 2020;26(12):1622–9.

135. Yee C, Suarthana E, Dendukuri N, et al. Evaluating the impact of the multiplex respiratory virus panel polymerase chain reaction test on the clinical management of suspected respiratory viral infections in adult patients in a hospital setting. Am J Infect Control 2016;44(11):1396–8.

136. Schuetz P, Wirz Y, Sager R, et al. Procalcitonin to initiate or discontinue antibiotics in acute respiratory tract infections. Cochrane Database Syst Rev 2017; 10(10):Cd007498.

137. Branche AR, Walsh EE, Vargas R, et al. Serum procalcitonin measurement and viral testing to guide antibiotic use for respiratory infections in hospitalized adults: a randomized controlled trial. J Infect Dis 2015;212(11):1692–700.

138. Timbrook T, Maxam M, Bosso J. Antibiotic discontinuation rates associated with positive respiratory viral panel and low procalcitonin results in proven or suspected respiratory infections. Infect Dis Ther 2015;4(3):297–306.

139. Brendish NJ, Malachira AK, Armstrong L, et al. Routine molecular point-of-care testing for respiratory viruses in adults presenting to hospital with acute respiratory illness (ResPOC): a pragmatic, open-label, randomised controlled trial. Lancet Respir Med 2017;5(5):401–11.

140. Barlam TF, Al Mohajer M, Al-Tawfiq JA, et al. SHEA statement on antibiotic stewardship in hospitals during public health emergencies. Infect Control Hosp Epidemiol 2022;43(11):1541–52.

141. Dequin PF, Meziani F, Quenot JP, et al. Hydrocortisone in severe community-acquired pneumonia. N Engl J Med 2023;388(21):1931–41.

142. Meduri GU, Shih MC, Bridges L, et al. Low-dose methylprednisolone treatment in critically ill patients with severe community-acquired pneumonia. Intensive Care Med 2022;48(8):1009–23.

143. Brun-Buisson C, Richard JC, Mercat A, et al, REVA-SRLF A/H1N1v 2009 Registry Group. Early corticosteroids in severe influenza A/H1N1 pneumonia and acute respiratory distress syndrome. Am J Respir Crit Care Med 2011;183(9): 1200–6.

144. Annane D, Antona M, Lehmann B, et al, CORTIFLU Investigators, CRICs, AZUREA, REVA/SRLF networks. Designing and conducting a randomized trial

for pandemic critical illness: the 2009 H1N1 influenza pandemic. Intensive Care Med 2012;38(1):29–39.

145. Rodrigo C, Leonardi-Bee J, Nguyen-Van-Tam JS, et al. Effect of corticosteroid therapy on influenza-related mortality: a systematic review and meta-analysis. J Infect Dis 2015;212(2):183–94.

146. Somerville LK, Ratnamohan VM, Dwyer DE, et al. Molecular diagnosis of respiratory viruses. Pathology 2015;47(3):243–9.

147. Vibholm LK, Nielsen SSF, Pahus MH, et al. SARS-CoV-2 persistence is associated with antigen-specific CD8 T-cell responses. EBioMedicine 2021;64:103230.

148. Pires de Mello CP, Drusano GL, Adams JR, et al. Oseltamivir-zanamivir combination therapy suppresses drug-resistant H1N1 influenza A viruses in the hollow fiber infection model (HFIM) system. Eur J Pharm Sci 2018;111:443–9.

149. Duval X, van der Werf S, Blanchon T, et al. Efficacy of oseltamivir-zanamivir combination compared to each monotherapy for seasonal influenza: a randomized placebo-controlled trial. PLoS Med 2010;7(11):e1000362.

150. Hung IFN, To KKW, Chan JFW, et al. Efficacy of clarithromycin-naproxen-oseltamivir combination in the treatment of patients hospitalized for influenza A(H3N2) infection: an open-label randomized, controlled, phase IIb/III trial. Chest 2017;151(5):1069–80.

151. Nguyen JT, Hoopes JD, Le MH, et al. Triple combination of amantadine, ribavirin, and oseltamivir is highly active and synergistic against drug resistant influenza virus strains in vitro. PLoS One 2010;5(2):e9332.

152. Smee DF, Hurst BL, Wong MH, et al. Effects of double combinations of amantadine, oseltamivir, and ribavirin on influenza A (H5N1) virus infections in cell culture and in mice. Antimicrob Agents Chemother 2009;53(5):2120–8.

153. DeVincenzo JP, Whitley RJ, Mackman RL, et al. Oral GS-5806 activity in a respiratory syncytial virus challenge study. N Engl J Med 2014;371(8):711–22.

154. DeVincenzo JP, McClure MW, Symons JA, et al. Activity of oral ALS-008176 in a respiratory syncytial virus challenge study. N Engl J Med 2015;373(21):2048–58.

155. Self WH, Williams DJ, Zhu Y, et al. Respiratory viral detection in children and adults: comparing asymptomatic controls and patients with community-acquired pneumonia. J Infect Dis 2016;213(4):584–91.

156. Korteweg C, Gu J. Pathology, molecular biology, and pathogenesis of avian influenza A (H5N1) infection in humans. Am J Pathol 2008;172(5):1155–70.

157. van der Sluijs KF, van der Poll T, Lutter R, et al. Bench-to-bedside review: bacterial pneumonia with influenza - pathogenesis and clinical implications. Crit Care 2010;14(2):219.

158. Grabowska K, Högberg L, Penttinen P, et al. Occurrence of invasive pneumococcal disease and number of excess cases due to influenza. BMC Infect Dis 2006;6:58.

159. Jartti T, Lehtinen P, Vuorinen T, et al. Persistence of rhinovirus and enterovirus RNA after acute respiratory illness in children. J Med Virol 2004;72(4):695–9.

Coronavirus Disease-2019 in the Immunocompromised Host

Christopher D. Bertini Jr, MD[a], Fareed Khawaja, MD[b],
Ajay Sheshadri, MD, MS[c],*

KEYWORDS

- COVID-19 • SARS-CoV-2 • Immunocompromised host • Pneumonia
- Hematologic malignancy • Immunosuppression

KEY POINTS

- Immunocompromise refers to a host's inability to combat infections from a variety of partial or total immune defects and can occur in the setting of diseases such as hematologic malignancies, immunosuppression use, primary immunodeficiency syndromes, and human immunodeficiency virus infection.
- Hospitalization risk, intensive care unit admission, and mortality are substantially higher after severe acute respiratory syndrome coronavirus 2 pneumonia in immunocompromised hosts.
- Immunocompromised hosts are underrepresented in clinical trials of vaccines and other treatments, and therefore efficacy data are often inferred or based upon small studies.
- Vaccines and treatments are often effective in immunocompromised hosts, but persistent viral replication due to impaired immunity can hinder the efficacy of these interventions.

INTRODUCTION

Severe acute respiratory syndrome coronavirus 2 (SARS-CoV-2) is a respiratory virus that originated in Wuhan, China in 2019. Since that time, SARS-CoV-2 has been responsible for over 6 million deaths from coronavirus disease-2019 (COVID-19).[1] Respiratory viral infections, in general, place an outsized burden on

This article was previously published in Clinics in Chest Medicine 44:2 June 2023.
The authors have nothing to disclose.
[a] Department of Internal Medicine, UTHealth Houston McGovern Medical School, 6431 Fannin, MSB 1.150, Houston, TX 77030, USA; [b] Department of Infectious Diseases, Infection Control, and Employee Health, The University of Texas MD Anderson Cancer Center, 1515 Holcombe Boulevard, Unit 1469, Houston, TX 77030, USA; [c] Department of Pulmonary Medicine, The University of Texas MD Anderson Cancer Center, 1400 Pressler Street Unit 1462, Houston, TX 77030, USA
* Corresponding author.
E-mail address: asheshadri@mdanderson.org
Twitter: @ajaysheshadri (A.S.)

Infect Dis Clin N Am 38 (2024) 213–228
https://doi.org/10.1016/j.idc.2023.12.007
0891-5520/24/© 2023 Elsevier Inc. All rights reserved.

id.theclinics.com

immunocompromised hosts, and increase the mortality.[2] Therefore, there was significant concern from the outset of the pandemic that SARS-CoV-2 infection would similarly impact immunocompromised patients disproportionately. This review focuses on the specific impact of COVID-19 on immunocompromised patients.

The term "immunocompromise" describes patients who have an impaired or absent immune system, limiting a host's ability to combat pathogens. Immunodeficiencies are classified as either primary or secondary. Primary immunodeficiencies (PIDs) are intrinsic to the immune system. Examples include congenital conditions such as severe combined immunodeficiency (SCID), caused by various mutations which can impact many immune cell lineages, and common variable immune deficiency (CVID), which is caused by a diverse array of genetic conditions that result in varying degrees of hypogammaglobulinemia.[3] Secondary immunodeficiencies refer to those acquired through conditions that depress the immune system. These include hematological malignances, solid and hematopoietic transplantation, infection with the human immunodeficiency virus (HIV), chronic immunosuppressive medication use, and others. In these cases, the period of immunocompromise may be limited in duration; for example, a patient with leukemia may no longer be immunocompromised once their disease is in remission and leukocyte counts recover, or a patient receiving biologic immunosuppressive therapy may no longer be immunocompromised once therapy has completed and enough time has lapsed to allow for immune recovery. On the contrary, comorbidities that may impact immune function, such as diabetes, do not necessarily connote an immunocompromised state, but are worthy of consideration because they are often independently associated with poor outcomes after COVID-19.[4,5] **Table 1** shows examples of high-risk groups who we consider to be immunocompromised and their attendant immune deficits.

Immunocompromised hosts are at considerable risk for a variety of infections. For example, bacterial pneumonia has been estimated to account for 30% of intensive care unit (ICU) admissions in patients with cancer.[6] In another study of severe influenza pneumonia, 12.5% of patients admitted to the ICU were immunocompromised, indicative of a higher propensity toward critical illness after infection.[7] Indeed, mortality was over twofold higher among immunocompromised patients with influenza pneumonia. Other respiratory viruses also affect the immunocompromised; a recent retrospective cohort study of 1643 hematopoietic cell transplant (HCT) patients found increased mortality in allogeneic recipients infected with human rhinovirus (HRV) and adenovirus lower respiratory infections.[2] Finally, human herpesvirus-6 (HHV-6) and cytomegalovirus (CMV) have long been associated with increased mortality amongst HCT recipients.[8]

Considering that over 500 million cases of COVID-19 have been reported worldwide since the pandemic began, it is likely that several million immunocompromised hosts were infected, extrapolating from the estimate that 2.7% of the American adult population are immunocompromised.[9] Research within this specific vulnerable population has not been commensurate to the substantial body of literature for COVID-19 in general. This review will summarize the current scientific literature that discusses the impact of COVID-19 on immunocompromised hosts. We will discuss mechanisms for COVID-19's affinity for the immunocompromised, compare clinical data between immunocompromised and immunocompetent hosts, and examine the evidence supporting treatment strategies within immunocompromised hosts who develop COVID-19.

MECHANISMS OF IMMUNOCOMPROMISE

The innate immune response is driven by cells such as neutrophils, macrophages, and natural killer cells. The innate immune response is evolutionarily ancient and is often

Table 1
Examples of immunocompromised conditions and possible mechanisms of immunocompromise

Immunocompromised Condition	Mechanism of Immunocompromise	Immune Deficits
Hematologic malignancies	Marrow infiltration and cytotoxic chemotherapy	Lymphopenia Neutropenia Impaired cellular immunity Impaired humoral immunity
Hematopoietic cell transplantation	Corticosteroid use, immunosuppressive medications (eg, tacrolimus, sirolimus, and ibrutinib)	Lymphopenia Neutropenia Impaired cellular immunity Impaired humoral immunity
Solid organ transplant (kidney, lung, and heart)	Corticosteroid use, immunosuppressive medications (eg, tacrolimus, sirolimus, and cyclosporine)	Impaired cellular immunity Impaired humoral immunity
Human immunodeficiency virus (HIV)	Apoptosis of T cells	Lymphopenia Impaired cellular immunity Impaired humoral immunity
Autoimmune rheumatology diseases requiring immunosuppressive drug therapy	Use of immunosuppressive agents (eg, methotrexate, TNF-alpha inhibitors, and specific interleukin inhibitors)	Lymphopenia Impaired cellular immunity Impaired humoral immunity Impaired innate immunity
Primary immunodeficiency syndromes	Hereditary agammaglobulinemia, defective phagocytosis, and impaired leukopoiesis	Lymphopenia Neutropenia Impaired cellular immunity Impaired humoral immunity Impaired innate immunity

the first defense against many pathogens, including SARS-CoV-2. Impaired innate immunity may be correlated with COVID-19 severity. For example, in a study of 84 COVID-19 patients, of whom 44 were critically ill, the presence of immature neutrophils, defined by low CD13 expression and characterized by diminished antimicrobial and phagocytic activity, was associated with a critical illness.[10] Similar findings were seen in monocytes, and the diminished functional capacity of monocytes was correlated with increased risk for septic shock rate and mortality. Impaired type 1 interferon responses measured in the peripheral blood were also associated with severe illness in 50 patients with COVID-19 of variable severity.[11] On the contrary, more exuberant type 1 interferon responses that occur later in the course of infection have been associated with a worsening of lung injury, indicating that these innate immune responses may have salutary or harmful roles depending upon when they occur within the course of disease.[12] Of note, these studies were conducted in immunocompetent hosts and were performed during an acute infection, and although the findings indicate that innate immune impairments are associated with higher COVID-19 severity, these findings require validation in immunocompromised hosts who are evaluated before the onset of disease.

Cellular, or cell-mediated, immunity, typically refers to host response involving T cells, though notably many innate immune cells also have a direct cell-mediated anti-pathogen response. In many immunocompromised hosts, cellular immunity can be impaired and lead to worsened outcomes after COVID-19. In a study comparing over 1400 immunocompetent COVID-19 patients to 166 immunocompromised patients, lymphopenia was associated with threefold mortality increase in the latter.[13] The immunocompromised cohort consisted of patients with autoimmune rheumatologic diseases (ARD) (39.2%) as well as patients with hematologic malignancies (21.1%), solid malignances (19.3%), and solid organ transplant (SOT) recipients (18.1%). Specifically, CD8 cells may have an important role in determining outcomes after COVID-19. In a prospective cohort study of 106 patients with cancer, lower peripheral blood CD8 T-cell counts were correlated with a higher COVID-19 viral load and associated with higher mortality.[14] However, hematologic patients with cancer with preserved CD8 counts had low viral loads and decreased mortality, even among patients with impaired humoral immunity. Of note, 23% of patients with hematologic malignancy had no detectable anti-SARS-CoV-2 T-cell responses. In another cohort of 79 COVID-19 patients, 36 immunocompromised hosts had significantly fewer CD3+ T -cells and CD3+/CD4+ T cells compared with 20 patients above age 60 and 23 patients with diabetes.[15] T cells from immunocompromised patients produced less interferon-gamma compared with elderly patients, but there was no difference in interferon production between diabetic and immunocompromised patients. However, this study included patients with renal disease and cirrhosis as part of its definition of immunocompromised hosts. Further detailing the role CD8 cells play, a retrospective case-control study of 174 COVID-19 hospitalized patients in Spain showed that patients admitted to the ICU had lower CD8 counts compared with patients admitted to the general wards.[16] CD4 counts did not vary between ICU and non-ICU admitted patients. However, in general, the classification of immunocompromise should precede the infection, and in this study, most of the patients did not have a disease that would indicate immunocompromise.

In addition to impaired cellular immunity, immunocompromised hosts may have diminished humoral immunity, defined by an impaired ability to produce pathogen-specific antibodies against COVID-19 and other pathogens. For example, a study of 103 patients with cancer showed that delayed viral clearance was associated with loss of antibody production, despite adequate T cell response to infection.[17] Prolonged viremia was driven by B-cell depletion, potentially indicating that the resolution of infection depends upon adequate humoral immunity. In a study of lymphoma patients, B-cell-depleting therapies, such as rituximab, were associated with higher rates of hospital readmission and persistent SARS-CoV-2 positivity.[18] This diminished humoral response may increase the risk in for adverse outcomes; a study of 111 patients with lymphoma admitted to French hospitals for the treatment of COVID-19 found that anti-CD20 therapies increased the risk of mortality by over two-fold.[19] With regards to the development of humoral immunity after infection, Wunsch and colleagues[15] found in a cohort of 70 patients with SARS-CoV-2 infection IgG ELISA antibody responses measured after infection that 16 patients lacked antibodies. Of these 16 patients, 11 were immunocompromised. This lack of humoral immunity can in rare instances lead to immune escape by SARS-CoV-2 variants.

Long-term shedding of COVID-19 in immunocompromised patients has been well described in transplant recipients and patients with cancer with B cell depletion.[20–24] Many of these cases describe changes in viral spike protein despite repeated treatment with antivirals. For example, one renal transplant patient with COVID-19, over a 145-day course of infection, SARS-CoV-2 viral spike proteins showed increased resistance to neutralizing antibodies.[20] These mutations have been shown to mimic variants from Brazil and the United Kingdom, though no clear link between long-term shedding and the evolution of COVID-19 variants have been identified.[20] In addition to the potential for mutations in the spike protein, resistance to antiviral agents may also arise in patients with long-term shedding[24]; this was most recently described in a cancer patient with B cell depletion.[24] These examples cite the risk long-term shedding of COVID-19 poses in immunocompromised patients and the need for effective prevention and treatment methods.

Clinical Outcomes After Coronavirus Disease-2019 Infection in Immunocompromised Hosts

Immunocompromised patients generally develop more severe illness after SARS-CoV-2 infection than immunocompetent patients. However, the studies discussed here need to be interpreted in the context of which variants dominated during the time of study and the availability of vaccines and effective therapies. We will discuss COVID-19 disease severity in the immunocompromised and considerations amongst different types of immunocompromised patients.

Immunocompromised patients may have a higher ICU admission rate and longer hospital lengths of stay. A Turkish retrospective case-control study reported a 22% ICU admission rate among 156 immunocompromised patients compared with 9% ICU admission rate among 312 nonimmunocompromised patients between April 2020 and October 2020.[25] Length of stay was longer in the immunocompromised cohort as well. The immunocompromised cohort included people living with HIV (PLWH), cancer, rheumatologic disease, and those who were on immunosuppressive medications. Immunocompromised patients may also have higher mortality rates compared with those in the immunocompetent. For example, a separate Korean retrospective cohort study of 871 immunocompromised patients and 5564 nonimmunocompromised patients found that immunocompromised patients had a mortality of 9.6%, over four times higher than the 2.3% mortality rate observed in immunocompetent patients.[26] Immunocompromised patients included those with HIV/AIDs, malignancy, SOT, and immunosuppressive medication use. Smaller cohort studies have also shown a mortality rate three to four times higher in immunocompromised patients.[25]

Immunocompromised patients who are mechanically ventilated often present with more severe acute respiratory distress syndrome (ARDS). For example, a retrospective cohort of 1594 patients with COVID-19, of whom 166 were immunocompromised, found that the mean Sap02/Fi02 ratio was 251 in immunocompromised patients, compared with 276 in immunocompetent patients.[13] Mild ARDS (Sap02/FiO2 >235 mm Hg) occurred in 42.3% of the immunocompetent grouped, compared with 33.7% of the immunocompromised group, and moderate ARDS (Sap02/FiO2 >160 mm Hg) occurred in 25.6% of the immunocompetent group compared with 33.1% of the immunocompromised group. No significant difference was observed in the rate of severe ARDS (Sap02/FiO2 <100 mm Hg) between the two groups. Immunocompromised patients had higher mortality, and among immunocompromised patients, older age, the presence of ARDS, and severe lymphopenia were predictors of mortality. These studies show the shift to a higher disease severity among COVID-19 patients.

Hematologic malignancy

Patients with hematologic malignancy have been shown to have high rates of hospitalization for COVID-19. For example, a European multicenter analysis of 3801 patients with hematologic malignancies who developed COVID-19 reported a hospitalization rate of 74%.[27] Other studies have also reported high hospitalization rates; for example, Mato and colleagues[28] reported a 25% admission rate among

174 patients with chronic lymphocytic leukemia (CLL). ICU admission rate has high as 18% have been observed, with a median length of stays as long as 15 days.[27] Mortality is often high in hematologic patients with cancer. For example, in 174 patients with CLL, 33% of patients died during the analysis.[28] Similarly, a study of 3801 patients with hematologic malignancies showed a mortality rate of 31%, with the highest found in patients with AML or myelodysplastic syndrome (~40%).[27] Smaller cohort studies have confirmed a case fatality rate of about 40% among patients with hematologic malignancy. Lastly, patients with hematologic malignancies often require vasopressor support and renal replacement; in a cohort of patients with CLL, 27% required vasopressor support and 11% required hemodialysis.[28] Reassuringly, survival in patients with CLL may be improving with newer variants.[29]

Solid malignancy

Several studies have shown that solid malignancy COVID-19 patients have a high hospitalization rate. A French retrospective cohort study of 212 solid tumor patients with cancer, of whom about 75% were undergoing active treatment of cancer, found a similar 70% rate of hospitalization, but a lower rate of ICU admission (12%).[30] Half of this cohort had undergone chemotherapy in the first 3 months, and overall mortality was 30%.

Furthermore, Dai and colleagues[31] showed an ICU admission rate of 20% for 105 hospitalized patients with cancer, compared with 8% in 536 non-patients with cancer, and ICU survivors with cancer had a mean 27-day length of stay compared with 17 in ICU survivors without cancer. The cancer cohort in this study included patients with lung, breast, thyroid, blood, cervical and esophageal cancer. In addition, death occurred in 11% of the cancer cohort compared with 4% in the noncancer cohort. Of all the cancers, hematologic and lung cancers had the highest mortality rates at 33% and 18%, respectively. This suggests that though patients with lung cancer usually do not meet the definition of immunocompromise, their risk of death is substantially higher than in non-patients with cancer. Though it is not clear how lung cancer increases mortality in patients with COVID-19, it is possible that this is either due to the extent of preexisting lung disease or a direct effect from smoking.[32] Further work is necessary to understand the mechanisms driving increased in mortality in lung patients with cancer with COVID-19.

In general, patients with hematologic and lung cancers or metastatic cancers had more severe COVID-19 illness. To wit, Dai and colleagues[31] found that 10% of patients with cancer required mechanical ventilation, compared with less than 1% of non-patients with cancer. The authors also found that patients with cancer had higher rates of renal replacement therapy and extracorporeal membrane oxygenation compared with non-patients with cancer, in addition to symptoms such as fever or chest pain.

Risk factors that have been reported to correlate with disease severity in immunocompetent patients have been validated in patients with cancer.[33] For example, a Chinese comparative study showed that old age, d-dimer, elevated tumor necrosis factor (TNF) alpha and N terminal pro-brain natriuretic peptide (pro-BNP) may be correlated worsening hypoxemia in solid and hematological patients with cancer admitted with COVID 19.[34] Furthermore, in an analysis of 218 solid and hematologic patients with cancer, D-dimer levels were twice as high in patients with cancer who died; serum lactate and lactate dehydrogenase were also higher among decedents.[35] Furthermore, CRP and ferritin have been shown to be higher in immunocompromised patients compared with immunocompetent patients.[25] This suggests that serum biomarkers which correlate with disease severity in non-patients with cancer are also applicable to patients with cancer.

Hematopoietic cell transplantation
A study of 382 HCT recipients in Europe during the first few months of the pandemic showed a mortality of 22% in allogeneic transplant recipients and 28% in autologous transplant recipients; children had a mortality of 7%, lower than adults but exponentially higher than the mortality observed in children who were not HCT recipients.[36,37] Older age and more severe immunodeficiency were associated with a higher chance for death. Furthermore, an observational cohort study of 86 HCT recipients in Brazil showed that 70% required hospitalization and 14% required ICU admission.[38] Mortality in this cohort was 30%, with a 34% mortality rate among the 62 adult patients compared with 21% in the 24 pediatric patients. In general, large studies of HCT recipients who are infected with SARS-CoV-2 are lacking.

Solid organ transplant
SOT recipients also have poorer outcomes after COVID-19. In over 17,000 patients with SOT, of whom 1682 developed COVID-19, COVID-19 increased the rate of death by nearly ten-fold, and SOT recipients hospitalized with COVID-19 were about 2.5 times more likely to die than those hospitalized with non-SARS-CoV-2 pneumonia.[39] In-hospital mortality among those who developed COVID-19 was 17%, and 21% required ICU admission. SOT recipients with COVID-19 had an increased length of stay (LOS) compared with SOT patients with non-COVID-19 pneumonia (6 vs. 4 days). Similar to the general population, certain comorbidities increase hospitalization risk in SOT recipients. For example, a case-control series of 47 SOT recipients found that chronic kidney disease (CKD), type 2 diabetes mellitus (T2DM), and hypertension (HTN) were more prevalent in the hospitalized patients compared with the non-hospitalized control group.[40]

In 49 advanced heart failure (HF) patients admitted for COVID-19, heart transplant (HTx) patients had worse mortality compared with left ventricular assist device (LVAD) and HF patients.[41] Specifically, mortality for the HTx group was 18.9% compared with 12.5% for LVAD and 11.5% for HF, respectively. Similarly, HTx patients, who are often on immunosuppressive medications, have been shown to have higher ICU LOS compared with HF patients. Kidney transplant recipients (KTx) show similar vulnerability to COVID-19. An international registry of 9845 KTx recipients reported that 144 patients required hospitalization.[42] The mortality rate was 32%; 29% were intubated and 52% developed acute kidney injury. Lymphopenia, elevated lactate dehydrogenase and elevated procalcitonin were all correlated with increased mortality. Outcomes may be more severe among lung transplant (LTx) recipients, as a French cohort analysis of 35 LTx patients with COVID-19 reported a hospitalization rate of 88.6%.[43] 42% were admitted to the ICU, and 52% required mechanical ventilation. 14% of the 35 LTx patients died after COVID-19.

People living with human immunodeficiency virus
COVID-19 may more severely affect PLWH who have uncontrolled HIV as compared with their well-controlled counterparts. For example, in an Italian study of 69 PLWH, 38 hospitalized patients had an average nadir CD4 count of 167 compared 399 in those who were not hospitalized.[44] However, the hospitalization rate remains high even among PLWH on antiretroviral therapy (ART). In a large Spanish cohort of 77,590 PLWH on ART, 63% of the 236 PLWH diagnosed with COVID-19 required hospitalization.[45] Of those 151 hospitalized patients, the ICU admission rate was about 9% and the mortality rate was 11%. Of the 15 PLWH admitted to the ICU, the mortality rate was 33%. The median LOS for 116 patients who survived to hospital discharge was 7 days. Similar to the general population and other immunocompromised patients,

age and number of comorbidities were highly correlated with hospitalization, ICU admission, and death rates.

Autoimmune rheumatologic disease

Patients with rheumatologic illness are also at high risk for severe complications from COVID-19. For example, a cohort of 58,052 Danish patients with inflammatory rheumatologic diseases had a 50% higher probability of admission compared with the general Danish population of 4.5 million.[46] The risk was 30% higher for patients with rheumatoid arthritis and over 80% higher for patients with vasculitis. However, the use of immunosuppressive agents (TNF-alpha inhibitors and steroids) surprisingly did not impact admission rate. Hospitalized patients with rheumatoid arthritis, particularly those with lung or cardiovascular disease, may have the more severe infection than hospitalized patients without ARD. In a case-control study comparing 2,379 patients with ARD to those without, ARD increased the risk of hospitalization by 14%, ICU admission by 32%, acute kidney injury by 81%, and venous thromboembolism by 74%, but did not increase the risk for mechanical ventilation or death.[47] Severe outcomes were more common for patients on glucocorticoids, but not DMARDs (disease-modifying antirheumatic drugs). In a study of 52 patients with systemic ARD, of whom 75% were on immunosuppressive therapy and 31% on biologic therapies, the requirement for mechanical ventilation was threefold higher in patients with rheumatologic disease compared with matched controls. However, mortality was indistinguishable between the two groups. Similar to other patients, a greater number of comorbidities increases the likelihood of severe COVID-19 in patients with ARD. For example, in patients with inflammatory bowel disease with two or more comorbidities, such as heart disease, diabetes, and kidney disease, severe COVID-19 was more common than in patients with one or zero comorbidities.[48]

Primary immunodeficiency

Little data exist for patients who have non-HIV immunodeficiency. In an Italian case series of seven patients with PIDs, six were hospitalized, and three were admitted the ICU.[49] Of the hospitalized patients at time of publication, 1 patient died in hospital, three were discharged and two were still being treated. The length of stay ranged between 3 days to 25 days.

TREATMENT

In general, there is a paucity of randomized controlled trial data examining the efficacy of anti-SARS-CoV-2 treatments in immunocompromised hosts. For example, in a recent randomized controlled trial of high-risk individuals who developed COVID-19 and were randomized to nirmatrelivir/ritonavir or placebo, fewer than 30 patients met any criteria for immunocompromise as we outline above.[50] Most data comes from observational or case-control studies. In this section, we will discuss studies that show the efficacy of antiviral, monoclonal antibodies, and convalescent plasma to treat, preempt, or prevent COVID-19 in immunocompromised patients.

Little data exist regarding antiviral therapy and its efficacy specifically in the immunocompromised. One challenge with the use of antiviral therapy is that the kinetics of viral replication necessitate prompt therapy to ensure an adequate outcome[51]; there is no clear evidence that replication is more rapid in immunocompromised hosts, despite the possibility due to impaired innate and cellular immunity. In one series of 31 ARD patients treated with nirmatrelivir/ritonavir (29) and molnupiravir during the first 5 days of COVID-19 diagnosis, no patients were hospitalized, but most (94%) were fully vaccinated,[52] and no comparator arm was studied. Little efficacy data is available for remdesivir in immunocompromised hosts; a case study suggested that remdesivir can reduce viral load in immunocompromised patients with persistent infections.[53] A recent randomized, double-blind, placebo-controlled trial found that a 3-day course of remdesivir in non-hospitalized patients with COVID-19 with high-risk conditions reduced the risk for hospitalization or death by 87%; however, only 4% of patients were immunocompromised.[54] Given the possibility of prolonged viral replication, multiple courses or longer courses of remdesivir may be necessary in immunocompromised hosts, but prospective studies comparing these strategies to usual care are necessary. In general, the evidence for the efficacy of antiviral therapy in immunocompromised hosts is lacking, but antiviral therapies are reasonable to use given the high probability of adverse outcomes in immunocompromised hosts.

It is unclear as to whether anti-inflammatory drugs are as effective in immunocompromised COVID-19 patients as in the general population. For example, a multicenter cohort study of 80 KTx patients showed that the mortality rate among patients treated with the interleukin-6 inhibitor tocilizumab was around 33%,[55,56] whereas the overall mortality rate for KTx patients with COVID-19 has been estimated to be around 24%. However, it is likely there is a selection bias as sicker patients tend to be treated with monoclonal antibodies, and prospective studies with appropriate controls are lacking. Similarly, studies regarding the use of the interleukin-6 inhibitor sarilumab have also excluded patients on immunosuppressive medications. The Infectious Disease Society of America (IDSA) does not promote nor discourage the use of tocilizumab and sarilumab in immunocompromised due to lack of available evidence.[57] Janus Kinase Inhibitors such as baricitinib have not been well studied in the immunocompromised. Both the RECOVERY trial and COV-BARRIER trial showed that baricitinib reduced risk of death in COVID-19 patients; however, only RECOVERY included immunocompromised patients, whereas COV-BARRIER excluded them.[58,59] The IDSA points out that data supporting the use of Janus kinase inhibitors in immunocompromised hosts is lacking.

COVID-19 convalescent plasma (CCP) has been used in immunocompetent patients with variable evidence for efficacy. Although this may be useful in immunocompromised patients who cannot generate a humoral response, high-quality randomized, placebo-controlled trials have shown no benefit.[60] Lower quality studies have suggested efficacy under some circumstances. For example, in a propensity score-matched analysis of 112 patients with hematologic malignancies, most of whom received other nonplasma therapies, the use of convalescent plasma decreased mortality by 63% among patients who were exposed to anti-CD20 antibodies in the subgroup of patients with B-cell neoplasms.[61] Transfusion reactions were rare. A Swedish cohort of 28 immunocompromised COVID-19 patients showed that 46% had clinical improvement by at least one score one WHO scale on week after convalescent plasma administration.[62] No comparator arm was studied. The United States Food and Drug Administration Emergency Use Authorization authorizes CCP use in patients with immunosuppressive conditions, but data is limited and caution is necessary when extrapolating data from immunocompetent hosts.[57]

VACCINATION

Vaccinations are effective for reducing mortality in immunocompromised patients. For example, a retrospective British study examining vaccine efficacy in SOT patients including 39260 double vaccinated patients, 1141 single vaccinated patients and 3080 unvaccinated patients showed a 20% reduction in risk of death in vaccinated patients.[63] However, vaccination may not effectively decrease risk of positive SARS-

CoV-2 test, as the risk-adjusted infection incidence rate was 1.29. Moreover, although two doses of ChAdOx1-S vaccines reduced the risk of death, similar efficacy was not observed with BNT162b2.

However, vaccines may be less effective for the immunocompromised compared with the immunocompetent. For example, one comparison prospective study detailing humoral immune response between 54 immunocompetent patients and 57 immunocompromised patients showed that some immunocompromised patients, namely patients with PIDs and rheumatologic disease, show declining immunity to COVID-19 as time progresses after two administrations of BNT162b2 vaccine.[64] Among the immunocompetent patients, PLWH and CKD patients, all had detectable antibodies at 2 weeks and 3 months post vaccination. The mean CD4 count for the PLWH was 254. However, subgroup analysis showed that 50% of the rheumatologic patients and 94.5% of the (PID) group had antibodies at two weeks. An inferior response to SARS-CoV-2 vaccination in immunocompromised patients has been shown in other studies. For example, an Austrian prospective cohort studied antibody response to COVID-19 vaccination in 15 healthy controls compared this to 74 patients previously treated with rituximab.[65] All healthy patients developed antibodies, but only 39% of the rituximab group developed antibodies to spike proteins following vaccination.

Lastly, COVID-19 hospitalization following vaccination, commonly referred to as "breakthrough cases," are more frequent in the immunocompromised. For example, an American study of 45 vaccine breakthrough COVID-hospitalizations reported that 44% were immunocompromised, and an Israeli cohort of 152 hospitalized fully vaccinated patients reported that 40% were immunocompromised.[66,67] Of the 60 immunocompromised fully vaccinated patients in the Israeli cohort, 18 had a poor outcome, which was defined as either requiring mechanical ventilation or death. Knowing that the prevalence of immunocompromise in the United States is around 2%, it follows that breakthrough infection seems to occur much more frequently among immunocompromised patients. Two studies prove this point more definitively. In a study of 6,860 cases of breakthrough COVID-19 after vaccination, patients with hematologic malignancies had over a four-fold higher risk for breakthrough infection,[68] with the highest rates seen in patients with leukemia or myeloma. Proteasome inhibitors and other immunomodulators significantly increased the risk for breakthrough infection. Similarly, in a study of over 45,000 patients with cancer, primarily with solid tumors, the overall incidence of breakthrough COVID-19 was 13.6%.[69] Mortality rate may be higher after breakthrough infection in immunocompromised patients. A cohort study of 54 fully vaccinated hematologic and solid tumor patients with cancer who developed breakthrough COVID-19 reported a 65% hospitalization rate, 19% ICU admission rate and 13% mortality rate,[70] not markedly different from adverse event rates among unvaccinated patients with cancer.

Pre-Exposure Prophylaxis

A preexposure prophylaxis strategy may be effective to mitigate COVID-19 severity in the immunocompromised. The PROVENT trial is a 2:1 randomized double-blind placebo-controlled study of 5197 patients investigating the use of tixagevimab and cilgavimab, a cocktail of two monoclonal antibodies that bind to non-overlapping sites from the SARS-CoV-2 spike protein, in preventing symptomatic COVID-19 in the at-risk patients, such as those with chronic obstructive pulmonary disease, immunocompromise, or elderly. Results show that the medication has a 77% risk reduction compared with placebo and 83% reduction at 6 months analysis.[71] As a result, the Infectious Diseases Society of America guidelines and US Food and Drug Administration agree about its use for the immunocompromised to provide further protection.

However, only 7.4% of the cohort had any cancer, only 3.3% were receiving immuno-suppressive therapies, and only 0.5% had a PID; therefore, these results are not necessarily indicative of efficacy in all immunocompromised hosts. Nevertheless, the use of tixagevimab and cilgavimab is reasonable given the frequent lack of humoral response to vaccination in immunocompromised hosts.

Post-Acute Sequelae of Coronavirus Disease-2019

Post-acute Sequelae of COVID-19 (PASC) refer to a range of ongoing health problems that people experience usually in the weeks and months following SARS-CoV-2 pneumonia,.[72] PASC refers to symptoms that are not explained by an alternative diagnosis, including fatigue, shortness of breath, anosmia, chest pain, diarrhea, and fever.[73,74] In immunocompromised patients, persistent respiratory symptoms and fatigue may be the most common.[74] These symptoms can persist for an extended period of time and, in some cases, may persist indefinitely.

PASC presents unique challenges to immunocompromised patients. A study of 1557 COVID-19 survivors with cancer showed that 15% reported PASC symptoms at a median of 44 days after COVID-19 diagnosis, suggesting a higher incidence than in the general population.[74] The study also reported a higher hospitalization rate and mortality rate due to PASC, but this must be interpreted in the context of other factors related to cancer, such as the discontinuation of cancer treatment which was independently associated with mortality. Lastly, the analysis revealed a few characteristics that were more frequent in the 234 patients with PASC as compared with the 1323 patients without PASC. Compared with patients without COVID-19 sequalae, a larger portion of the PASC group was male (54.5% vs 47.2%), over the age 65 (55.1% vs 48.1%), and had two or more comorbidities (48.4% vs 36.4%).[74]

One possibility for why immunocompromised patients may experience PASC is the possibility of delayed viral clearance. Some reports have shown that immunocompromised patients may display persistent viral infection well after initial COVID-19 diagnosis. For example, in addition to prior examples, one follicular lymphoma patient showed an increase in SARS-CoV-2 viral load 54 days after symptoms onset, whereas another patient receiving showed persistent RT-PCR (reverse transcription polymerase chain reaction) positivity 238 days following SARS-Cov-2 diagnosis.[53,75] A recent report suggested that the presence of spike proteins could be associated with PASC; in a recent study of 37 PASC patients, 84% had evidence of circulating spike protein, as compared with 0 in 26 recovered COVID-19 patients.[76] Whether the circulating spike protein represents active SARS-CoV-2 replication or simply viral remnants is unclear. Further work is needed to understand PASC in patients with or without immunocompromise.

SUMMARY

COVID-19 often results in more severe infections in immunocompromised patients. Hospitalization rate, disease severity, and mortality rates are generally higher for the immunocompromised, especially those with hematologic malignancies, SOT recipients, and patients with ARD. Treatment strategies for these patients are similar to those in the immunocompetent, but high-quality data are lacking. Vaccinations are recommended but less effective in immunocompromised patients. As the pandemic continues, the vulnerability of immunocompromised patients should garner the attention of the medical and scientific communities. Studies focusing on immunocompromised patients will help illuminate the best strategies to mitigate harms in these high-risk patients.

CLINICS CARE POINTS

- Immunocompromised patients have often develop severe SARS-CoV-2 pneumonia, and the threshold to escalate the level of care should be low given the possibility for rapid deterioration.
- Despite the possibility of inferior rates of response to vaccination, vaccinatiion is recommended in most immunocompromsied patients.
- Though most antiviral and anti-inflammatory agents have not been specifically tested in immunocompromised hosts, these should be initiated early given the possibility for clinical worsening without prompt intervention.

REFERENCES

1. WHO. WHO Coronavirus disease (COVID-19) dashboard In:2022. Available at: https://covid19.who.int/.
2. Kim Y, Waghmare A, Xie H, et al. Respiratory viruses in hematopoietic cell transplant candidates: impact of preexisting lower tract disease on outcomes. Blood Adv 2022;6:5307-16.
3. Raje N, Dinakar C. Overview of immunodeficiency disorders. Immunol Allergy Clin N Am 2015;35(4):599-623.
4. Chinen J, Shearer WT. Secondary immunodeficiencies, including HIV infection. J Allergy Clin Immunol 2010;125(2):S195-203.
5. Mahamat-Saleh Y, Fiolet T, Rebeaud ME, et al. Diabetes, hypertension, body mass index, smoking and COVID-19-related mortality: a systematic review and meta-analysis of observational studies. BMJ Open 2021;11(10):e052777.
6. Azoulay E, Pickkers P, Soares M, et al. Acute hypoxemic respiratory failure in immunocompromised patients: the Efraim multinational prospective cohort study. Intensive Care Med 2017;43(12):1808-19.
7. Garnacho-Montero J, Leon-Moya C, Gutierrez-Pizarraya A, et al. Clinical characteristics, evolution, and treatment-related risk factors for mortality among immunosuppressed patients with influenza A (H1N1) virus admitted to the intensive care unit. J Crit Care 2018;48:172-7.
8. Seo S, Renaud C, Kuypers JM, et al. Idiopathic pneumonia syndrome after hematopoietic cell transplantation: evidence of occult infectious etiologies. Blood 2015;125(24):3789-97.
9. Harpaz R, Dahl RM, Dooling KL. Prevalence of immunosuppression among US adults, 2013. JAMA 2016;316(23):2547.
10. Peyneau M, Granger V, Wicky P-H, et al. Innate immune deficiencies are associated with severity and poor prognosis in patients with COVID-19. Scientific Rep 2022;12(1):638.
11. Hadjadj J, Yatim N, Barnabei L, et al. Impaired type I interferon activity and inflammatory responses in severe COVID-19 patients. Science 2020;369(6504):718-24.
12. Lee JS, Park S, Jeong HW, et al. Immunophenotyping of COVID-19 and influenza highlights the role of type I interferons in development of severe COVID-19. Sci Immunol 2020;5(49):eabd1554.
13. Martínez-Urbistondo M, Gutiérrez-Rojas A, Andrés A, et al. Severe lymphopenia as a predictor of COVID-19 mortality in immunosuppressed patients. J Clin Med 2021;10(16):3595.

14. Bange E, Han N, Wileyto EP, et al. CD8 T cells compensate for impaired humoral immunity in COVID-19 patients with hematologic cancer. In: Research Square; 2021.
15. Wünsch K, Anastasiou OE, Alt M, et al. COVID-19 in elderly, immunocompromised or diabetic patients—from immune monitoring to clinical management in the hospital. Viruses 2022;14(4):746.
16. Urra JM, Cabrera CM, Porras L, et al. Selective CD8 cell reduction by SARS-CoV-2 is associated with a worse prognosis and systemic inflammation in COVID-19 patients. Clin Immunol 2020;217(108486):108486.
17. Lyudovyk O, Kim JY, Qualls D, et al. Impaired humoral immunity is associated with prolonged COVID-19 despite robust CD8 T cell responses. Cancer Cell 2022;40(7):738–753 e735.
18. Lee CY, Shah MK, Hoyos D, et al. Prolonged SARS-CoV-2 infection in patients with lymphoid malignancies. Cancer Discov 2022;12(1):62–73.
19. Dulery R, Lamure S, Delord M, et al. Prolonged in-hospital stay and higher mortality after Covid-19 among patients with non-Hodgkin lymphoma treated with B-cell depleting immunotherapy. Am J Hematol 2021;96(8):934–44.
20. Weigang S, Fuchs J, Zimmer G, et al. Within-host evolution of SARS-CoV-2 in an immunosuppressed COVID-19 patient as a source of immune escape variants. Nat Commun 2021;12(1):6405.
21. Choi B, Choudhary MC, Regan J, et al. Persistence and evolution of SARS-CoV-2 in an immunocompromised host. N Engl J Med 2020;383(23):2291–3.
22. Han A, Rodriguez TE, Beck ET, et al. Persistent SARS-CoV-2 infectivity greater than 50 days in a case series of allogeneic peripheral blood stem cell transplant recipients. Curr Probl Cancer Case Rep 2021;3:100057.
23. Baang JH, Smith C, Mirabelli C, et al. Prolonged severe acute respiratory syndrome coronavirus 2 replication in an immunocompromised patient. J Infect Dis 2021;223(1):23–7.
24. Gandhi S, Klein J, Robertson AJ, et al. De novo emergence of a remdesivir resistance mutation during treatment of persistent SARS-CoV-2 infection in an immunocompromised patient: a case report. Nat Commun 2022;13(1):1547.
25. Oztürk S, Kant A, Comoglu S, et al. Investigation of the clinical course and severity of covid-19 infection in immunocompromised patients. Acta Med Mediterranea 2021;37:2593–7.
26. Baek MS, Lee M-T, Kim W-Y, et al. COVID-19-related outcomes in immunocompromised patients: a nationwide study in Korea. PLOS ONE 2021;16(10): e0257641.
27. Pagano L, Salmanton-García J, Marchesi F, et al. COVID-19 infection in adult patients with hematological malignancies: a European Hematology Association Survey (EPICOVIDEHA). J Hematol Oncol 2021;14(1):1–168.
28. Mato AR, Roeker LE, Lamanna N, et al. Outcomes of COVID-19 in patients with CLL: a multicenter international experience. Blood 2020;136(10):1134–43.
29. Roeker LE, Eyre TA, Thompson MC, et al. COVID-19 in patients with CLL: improved survival outcomes and update on management strategies. Blood 2021;138(18):1768–73.
30. Martin S, Kaeuffer C, Leyendecker P, et al. <scp>COVID</scp>-19 in patients with cancer: a retrospective study of 212 cases from a French <scp>SARS-CoV</scp>-2 cluster during the first wave of the <scp>COVID</scp>-19 pandemic. The Oncologist 2021;26(9):e1656–9.

31. Dai M, Liu D, Liu M, et al. Patients with cancer appear more vulnerable to SARS-CoV-2: a multicenter study during the COVID-19 outbreak. Cancer Discov 2020; 10(6):783–91.

32. Luo J, Rizvi H, Preeshagul IR, et al. COVID-19 in patients with lung cancer. Ann Oncol 2020;31(10):1386–96.

33. Yao Y, Cao J, Wang Q, et al. D-dimer as a biomarker for disease severity and mortality in COVID-19 patients: a case control study. J Intensive Care 2020;8(1).

34. Tian J, Yuan X, Xiao J, et al. Clinical characteristics and risk factors associated with COVID-19 disease severity in patients with cancer in Wuhan, China: a multicentre, retrospective, cohort study. Lancet Oncol 2020;21(7):893–903.

35. Mehta V, Goel S, Kabarriti R, et al. Case fatality rate of patients with cancer with COVID-19 in a New York hospital system. Cancer Discov 2020;10(7):935–41.

36. Ljungman P, De La Camara R, Mikulska M, et al. COVID-19 and stem cell transplantation; results from an EBMT and GETH multicenter prospective survey. Leukemia 2021;35(10):2885–94.

37. Smith C, Odd D, Harwood R, et al. Deaths in Children and Young People in England following SARS-CoV-2 infection during the first pandemic year: a national study using linked mandatory child death reporting data. Laurel Hollow, NY: Cold Spring Harbor Laboratory; 2021.

38. Karataş A, Malkan ÜY, Velet M, et al. The clinical course of COVID-19 in hematopoietic stem cell transplantation (HSCT) recipients. Turkish J Med Sci 2021;51(4): 1647–52.

39. Jering KS, McGrath MM, Mc Causland FR, et al. Excess mortality in solid organ transplant recipients hospitalized with COVID-19: a large-scale comparison of SOT recipients hospitalized with or without COVID-19. Clin Transplant 2022; 36(1):e14492.

40. Chaudhry ZS, Williams JD, Vahia A, et al. Clinical characteristics and outcomes of COVID-19 in solid organ transplant recipients: a cohort study. Am J Transplant 2020;20(11):3051–60.

41. Cunningham LC, George S, Nelson D, et al. Outcomes of COVID-19 in an advanced heart failure practice: a single center study. J Heart Lung Transplant 2022;41(4):S176.

42. Cravedi P, Mothi SS, Azzi Y, et al. COVID-19 and kidney transplantation: results from the TANGO international transplant consortium. Am J Transplant 2020; 20(11):3140–8.

43. Messika J, Eloy P, Roux A, et al. COVID-19 in lung transplant recipients. Transplantation 2021;105(1):177–86.

44. Di Biagio A, Ricci E, Calza L, et al. Factors associated with hospital admission for COVID-19 in HIV patients. AIDS 2020;34(13):1983–5.

45. Del Amo J, Polo R, Moreno S, et al. Incidence and severity of COVID-19 in HIV-positive persons receiving antiretroviral therapy : a cohort study. Ann Intern Med 2020;173(7):536–41.

46. Cordtz R, Lindhardsen J, Soussi BG, et al. Incidence and severeness of COVID-19 hospitalization in patients with inflammatory rheumatic disease: a nationwide cohort study from Denmark. Rheumatology 2021;60(SI):SI59–67.

47. D'Silva KM, Serling-Boyd N, Wallwork R, et al. Clinical characteristics and outcomes of patients with coronavirus disease 2019 (COVID-19) and rheumatic disease: a comparative cohort study from a US 'hot spot. Ann Rheum Dis 2020; 79(9):1156–62.

48. Brenner EJ, Ungaro RC, Gearry RB, et al. Corticosteroids, but not TNF antagonists, are associated with adverse COVID-19 outcomes in patients with

inflammatory bowel diseases: results from an international registry. Gastroenter-ology 2020;159(2):481–91.e483.

49. Quinti I, Lougaris V, Milito C, et al. A possible role for B cells in COVID-19? Lesson from patients with agammaglobulinemia. J Allergy Clin Immunol 2020;146(1): 211–3.e214.

50. Hammond J, Leister-Tebbe H, Gardner A, et al. Oral nirmatrelvir for high-risk, nonhospitalized adults with covid-19. N Engl J Med 2022;386(15):1397–408.

51. Neant N, Lingas G, Le Hingrat Q, et al. Modeling SARS-CoV-2 viral kinetics and association with mortality in hospitalized patients from the French COVID cohort. Proc Natl Acad Sci U S A 2021;118(8):1.

52. Fragoulis GE, Koutsianas C, Fragiadaki K, et al. Oral antiviral treatment in patients with systemic rheumatic disease at risk for development of severe COVID-19: a case series. Ann Rheum Dis 2022;81 (10):1477–9, annrheumdis-202.

53. Camprubí D, Gaya A, Marcos MA, et al. Persistent replication of SARS-CoV-2 in a severely immunocompromised patient treated with several courses of remdesivir. Int J Infect Dis 2021;104:379–81.

54. Gottlieb RL, Vaca CE, Paredes R, et al. Early remdesivir to prevent progression to severe covid-19 in outpatients. N Engl J Med 2022;386(4):305–15.

55. Pérez-Sáez MJ, Blasco M, Redondo-Pachón D, et al. Use of tocilizumab in kidney transplant recipients with COVID-19. Am J Transplant 2020;20(11):3182–90.

56. Hilbrands LB, Duivenvoorden R, Vart P, et al. COVID-19-related mortality in kid-ney transplant and dialysis patients: results of the ERACODA collaboration. Nephrol Dial Transplant 2020;35(11):1973–83.

57. Adarsh Bhimraj RLM, Amy Hirsch Shumaker, Valery Lavergne, LindseyBaden, Vincent Chi-Chung Cheng, Kathryn M. Edwards,Rajesh Gandhi,Jason Galla-gher,William J. Muller, John C. O'Horo, Shmuel Shoham, M. Hassan Murad, Reem A.Mustafa, Shahnaz Sultan, Yngve Falck-Ytter3. Infectious Diseases Soci-ety of America Guidelines on the Treatment and Management of Patients with COVID-19. 2022. Version 10.1.1 Available at: http://www.idsociety.org/ COVID19guidelines.

58. Kalil AC, Patterson TF, Mehta AK, et al. Baricitinib plus remdesivir for hospitalized adults with covid-19. N Engl J Med 2021;384(9):795–807.

59. Marconi VC, Ramanan AV, De Bono S, et al. Efficacy and safety of baricitinib in patients with COVID-19 infection: results from the randomised, double-blind, pla-cebo-controlled, parallel-group COV-BARRIER phase 3 trial. Laurel Hollow, NY: Cold Spring Harbor Laboratory; 2021.

60. Ortigoza MB, Yoon H, Goldfeld KS, et al. Efficacy and safety of COVID-19 conva-lescent plasma in hospitalized patients: a randomized clinical trial. JAMA Intern Med 2022;182(2):115–26.

61. Hueso T, Godron A-S, Lanoy E, et al. Convalescent plasma improves overall sur-vival in patients with B-cell lymphoid malignancy and COVID-19: a longitudinal cohort and propensity score analysis. Leukemia 2022;36(4):1025–34.

62. Ljungquist O, Lundgren M, Iliachenko E, et al. Convalescent plasma treatment in severely immunosuppressed patients hospitalized with COVID-19: an observa-tional study of 28 cases. Infect Dis 2022;54(4):283–91.

63. Callaghan CJ, Mumford L, Curtis RMK, et al. Real-world effectiveness of the pfizer-BioNTech BNT162b2 and oxford-AstraZeneca ChAdOx1-S vaccines against SARS-CoV-2 in solid organ and islet transplant recipients. Transplantation 2022;106(3):436–46.

64. Oyaert M, De Scheerder MA, Van Herrewege S, et al. Evaluation of humoral and cellular responses in SARS-CoV-2 mRNA vaccinated immunocompromised patients. Front Immunol 2022;13:858399.

65. Mrak D, Tobudic S, Koblischke M, et al. SARS-CoV-2 vaccination in rituximab-treated patients: B cells promote humoral immune responses in the presence of T-cell-mediated immunity. Ann Rheum Dis 2021;80(10):1345–50.

66. Tenforde MW, Patel MM, Ginde AA, et al. Effectiveness of SARS-CoV-2 mRNA vaccines for preventing covid-19 hospitalizations in the United States. Clin Infect Dis 2022;74(9):1515–24.

67. Brosh-Nissimov T, Orenbuch-Harroch E, Chowers M, et al. BNT162b2 vaccine breakthrough: clinical characteristics of 152 fully vaccinated hospitalized COVID-19 patients in Israel. Clin Microbiol Infect 2021;27(11):1652–7.

68. Song Q, Bates B, Shao YR, et al. Risk and outcome of breakthrough COVID-19 infections in vaccinated patients with cancer: real-world evidence from the national COVID cohort collaborative. J Clin Oncol 2022;40(13):1414–27.

69. Wang W, Kaelber DC, Xu R, et al. Breakthrough SARS-CoV-2 infections, hospitalizations, and mortality in vaccinated patients with cancer in the US between december 2020 and november 2021. JAMA Oncol 2022;8(7):1027–34.

70. Schmidt AL, Labaki C, Hsu CY, et al. COVID-19 vaccination and breakthrough infections in patients with cancer. Ann Oncol 2022;33(3):340–6.

71. Levin MJ, Ustianowski A, De Wit S, et al. LB5. PROVENT: phase 3 study of efficacy and safety of AZD7442 (Tixagevimab/Cilgavimab) for pre-exposure prophylaxis of COVID-19 in adults. Open Forum Infect Dis 2021;8(Supplement_1):S810.

72. Center for Disease Control and Prevention. Long COVID or Post-COVID Conditions. In:2022. Available at: https://www.cdc.gov/coronavirus/2019-ncov/long-term-effects/index.html.

73. Soriano JB, Murthy S, Marshall JC, et al. A clinical case definition of post-COVID-19 condition by a Delphi consensus. Lancet Infect Dis 2022;22(4):e102–7.

74. Pinato DJ, Tabernero J, Bower M, et al. Prevalence and impact of COVID-19 sequelae on treatment and survival of patients with cancer who recovered from SARS-CoV-2 infection: evidence from the OnCovid retrospective, multicentre registry study. Lancet Oncol 2021;22(12):1669–80.

75. Taramasso L, Sepulcri C, Mikulska M, et al. Duration of isolation and precautions in immunocompromised patients with COVID-19. J Hosp Infect 2021;111:202–4.

76. Swank Z, Senussi Y, Alter G, et al. Persistent circulating SARS-CoV-2 spike is associated with post-acute COVID-19 sequelae. Laurel Hollow, NY: Cold Spring Harbor Laboratory; 2022.

Moving?

Make sure your subscription moves with you!

To notify us of your new address, find your **Clinics Account Number** (located on your mailing label above your name), and contact customer service at:

Email: journalscustomerservice-usa@elsevier.com

800-654-2452 (subscribers in the U.S. & Canada)
314-447-8871 (subscribers outside of the U.S. & Canada)

Fax number: 314-447-8029

Elsevier Health Sciences Division
Subscription Customer Service
3251 Riverport Lane
Maryland Heights, MO 63043

*To ensure uninterrupted delivery of your subscription, please notify us at least 4 weeks in advance of move.

Printed and bound by CPI Group (UK) Ltd, Croydon, CR0 4YY

08/05/2025

01864751-0002